T0192368

Vegetarian Nutrition and Wellness

Vegetarian Nutrition and Wellness

Edited by
Winston J. Craig

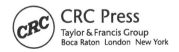

CRC Press
Taylor & Francis Group
Boca Raton London New York

CRC Press is an imprint of the
Taylor & Francis Group, an **informa** business

CRC Press
Taylor & Francis Group
6000 Broken Sound Parkway NW, Suite 300
Boca Raton, FL 33487-2742

First issued in paperback 2021

ISBN-13: 978-1-03-209528-8 (pbk)
ISBN-13: 978-1-138-03556-0 (hbk)

Library of Congress Cataloging-in-Publication Data

Names: Craig, Winston J., editor.
Title: Vegetarian nutrition and wellness / editor, Winston J. Craig.
Description: Boca Raton : Taylor & Francis, 2018. | Includes bibliographical references.
Identifiers: LCCN 2018005835 | ISBN 9781138035560 (hardback : alk. paper)
Subjects: | MESH: Diet, Vegetarian | Nutritional Physiological Phenomena | Conservation of Natural Resources
Classification: LCC RM236 | NLM QT 235 | DDC 613.2/62--dc23
LC record available at https://lccn.loc.gov/2018005835

**Visit the Taylor & Francis Web site at
http://www.taylorandfrancis.com**

**and the CRC Press Web site at
http://www.crcpress.com**

Contents

SECTION I   Environmental Issues

SECTION II   Prevention of Chronic Diseases

SECTION III   Plant Proteins

SECTION IV   Nutrient Profiles

SECTION V   Vegetarian Issues in Ethnic Groups

SECTION VI   Vegetarian Diets for Special Groups

Introduction

While millions of Americans, along with Europeans, Asian Indians, and others throughout the world, follow a vegetarian diet, many more are semivegetarian or consume at least one or two vegetarian meals each week. Consumers now have available to purchase a wide variety of plant protein foods (dried, canned, or frozen) based on gluten or a legume, such as soy. The current *Dietary Guidelines for Americans* endorses a healthy vegetarian diet as a healthy eating pattern that can be adapted based on cultural and personal preferences.

Section II of the book deals with how a vegetarian diet protects population groups from the major chronic diseases, such as cardiovascular diseases, obesity, and various cancers. Based on current scientific studies, both ecological and clinical studies, the various authors explain the health-promoting properties of plant-based diets, and compare and contrast the health outcomes obtained from consuming omnivorous diets with a vegetarian or vegan diet. Fruits and vegetables figure prominently in vegetarian diets and provide a substantial effect in the disease reduction and health-promoting properties of a plant-based diet.

A new interest in plant-based eating has developed recently from a desire to consume a more sustainable diet that is less destructive to the earth's natural resources. Chapters 2 and 3 address those concerns. Chapters 13 and 14 also deal with the issues surrounding the safety and effectiveness of consuming a vegetarian diet in athletic and sports performance. Furthermore, the adequacy of a vegetarian diet for pregnancy, lactation, infancy, and childhood is explained, along with recommendations for a healthy vegetarian diet.

A major component of the vegetarian diet is plant protein, which is typically supplied by legumes. Chapter 9 describes how beans and lentils are a treasure house of nutrients and provide many health-promoting properties. Chapter 8 focuses on the benefits of soy, a unique bean rich in isoflavones. Controversies surrounding soy are further explained in light of the current research.

Today, the greatest amount of research effort is expended to discover the health benefits of a plant-based diet; nevertheless, there continues to be concerns about the safety of some vegetarian diets, especially a vegan diet. A growing number of people are choosing the vegan or total vegetarian diet. Many areas of the world may have few, if any, fortified foods, and some consider supplements undesirable. Among such populations, concerns have been expressed about the long-term safety and appropriateness of a strict vegan diet. This book describes these issues and outlines how to prevent nutrient deficiencies (see Chapter 10).

Vegetarian Nutrition and Wellness was written for academic and clinical nutritionists, registered dietitians and other health professionals, graduate students in nutrition and public health, and upper-division dietetic and wellness students. Each chapter provides a comprehensive review of the scientific literature of a current topic. A concise summary is provided at the beginning of each chapter. It has been some time since a scholarly book on vegetarian nutrition entered the marketplace. The time is ripe for this new book to update the scientific community with a collage of well-documented topics on vegetarian nutrition.

Editor

Winston J. Craig is professor emeritus of nutrition at Andrews University in Berrien Springs, Michigan, and adjunct professor of nutrition, School of Public Health at Loma Linda University, California. Dr. Craig was chair of the Department of Nutrition and Wellness for 20 years and taught nutrition for 27 years at Andrews University and 5 years at Loma Linda University. He received his PhD degree from the University of Queensland in Brisbane, Australia, and a master of public health degree in nutrition from Loma Linda University. He currently holds membership in the American Society for Nutrition and held membership in the Academy of Nutrition and Dietetics for 30 years.

Dr. Craig has authored more than 300 articles for health publications, 7 chapters for various nutrition books, and 30 research articles for scholarly journals. Books he has written include *Nutrition and Wellness: A Vegetarian Way to Better Health*, *The Use and Safety of Common Herbs and Herbal Teas*, *Flavonoids, Food and Your Future*, *Herbs for Your Health: A Guide to the Therapeutic Use of 45 Commonly Used Herbs*, *Super Alimentos*, *Optimum Health*, *Maintaining a Healthy Lifestyle*, and *Eating for Good Health*. In 2009 and 2016, he coauthored the Academy of Nutrition and Dietetics position paper on vegetarian diets. His research interests include the health-promoting properties of phytochemicals, the role of a plant-based diet in preventing chronic diseases, and the disease-preventing properties of spices and herbs. His hobbies include hiking, camping, birding, and wildlife photography.

Contributors

Winston J. Craig
Department of Nutrition and Wellness
School of Health Professions
Andrews University
Berrien Springs, Michigan

Alison M. Duncan
Department of Human Health and
    Nutritional Sciences
University of Guelph
Guelph, Ontario, Canada

Kelly Virecoulon Giudici
School of Public Health
University of São Paulo
São Paulo, Brazil

Ella H. Haddad
Center for Nutrition, Lifestyle and
    Disease Prevention
School of Public Health
Loma Linda University
Loma Linda, California

Celine E. Heskey
Center for Nutrition, Lifestyle and
    Disease Prevention
School of Public Health
Loma Linda University
Loma Linda, California

Tony Jehi
Center for Nutrition, Lifestyle and
    Disease Prevention
School of Public Health
Loma Linda University
Loma Linda, California

D. Enette Larson-Meyer
Department of Family and Consumer
    Sciences
College of Agriculture and Natural
    Resources
University of Wyoming
Laramie, Wyoming

Reed Mangels
Department of Nutrition
School of Public Health and Health
    Sciences
University of Massachusetts
Amherst, Massachusetts

Dora Marinova
Curtin University
Perth, Australia

Michael J. Orlich
School of Public Health
and
School of Medicine
Loma Linda University
Loma Linda, California

Peter Pribis
Department of Individual, Family and
    Community Education
Nutrition Program
College of Education
University of New Mexico
Albuquerque, New Mexico

Sudha Raj
Department of Public Health, Food
    Studies and Nutrition
David B. Falk College of Sport and
    Human Dynamics
Syracuse University
Syracuse, New York

Talia Raphaely
Curtin University
Perth, Australia

Joan Sabaté
Center for Nutrition, Lifestyle and
    Disease Prevention
School of Public Health
Loma Linda University
Loma Linda, California

Angela V. Saunders
Corporate Nutrition
Sanitarium Health and Wellbeing
Berkeley Vale, New South Wales,
    Australia

Renae M. Thomas
School of Medicine
Loma Linda University
Loma Linda, California

Connie M. Weaver
Department of Nutrition Science
College of Health and Human Sciences
Purdue University
West Lafayette, Indiana

1 Vegetarian Diets
Trends in Acceptance and Perception. What Do the Dietary Guidelines Suggest?

Reed Mangels

CONTENTS

SUMMARY

The most recent edition of the *Dietary Guidelines for Americans* promotes the use of a vegetarian diet and identifies this diet as one of three healthy eating patterns that Americans can choose and adapt. There has been a significant shift in the perception of vegetarian diets by the scientific community and by the public. Vegetarian, vegan, and plant-based diets are increasingly being recommended as a part of the prevention and treatment of chronic diseases in the United States and globally. Research continues to accumulate, demonstrating the health-related and environmental benefits of these diets. The *2015–2020 Dietary Guidelines for Americans* endorses a "Healthy Vegetarian Eating Pattern" as one of three "healthy eating patterns that can be adapted based on cultural and personal preferences" (HHS and USDA, 2015). This support for a vegetarian diet as a desirable way to eat is indicative of the changes in the perception of vegetarian diets and of plant-based diets that have occurred over the past 10–20 years. These changes have occurred in many areas, including scientific research, the health professions, the general public, and government agencies in the United States, as well as in other countries.

1.1 BRIEF HISTORY OF VEGETARIAN DIETS

Early Greek and Roman philosophers and poets living more than two millennia ago promoted vegetarian diets for reasons related to ethics and health (Leitzmann, 2014). Their interest in vegetarianism may have been sparked by Indian vegetarian philosophers whose teachings were embraced by the ancient Greeks, including Pythagoras (Stuart, 2006). Medieval Jewish commentators, including Rashi and Maimondes, taught that the original diet that people were commanded to eat was a vegetarian diet (Schwartz, 1982). During the Renaissance era, Leonardo da Vinci condemned the eating of animals (Leitzmann, 2014), and in the eighteenth century, philosophers, including Wesley and Voltaire, promoted and adhered to vegetarian diets (Stuart, 2006; Leitzmann, 2014). Vegetarian societies were started in Europe and the United States in the 1800s, while vegan groups began to arise in the 1900s. The Seventh-day Adventist Church was founded in the mid-nineteenth century; church members were encouraged to adhere to a vegetarian diet (White, 1938).

In the 1950s and 1960s, Hardinge and Stare published a series of papers on vegetarians, which informed the scientific community about the adequacy of vegetarian diets and their effects on fiber and fat intake and cholesterol status (Hardinge et al., 1958, 1962). Register and others also showed the adequacy of vegetarian diets for humans in the 1960s and 1970s (Register and Sonnenberg, 1973).

Vegetarianism was embraced in the 1960s and 1970s by so-called "new vegetarians," who tended to be younger and have an alternative-lifestyle philosophy (Helman and Darnton-Hill, 1987). Reports of nutrition problems among these new vegetarians (Brown and Bergan, 1975; Helman and Darnton-Hill, 1987) led to concerns about the safety of vegetarian diets. This negative image has gradually changed as the result of scores of research papers showing the safety and adequacy of vegetarian diets. Today, vegetarian diets are recommended by a variety of groups, including the Academy of Nutrition and Dietetics (Melina et al., 2016) and the Canadian Diabetes Association (Rinaldi et al., 2016).

Worldwide, many cultures have used vegetarian or near-vegetarian diets for centuries. In some cases, this is due to the prohibitive cost of meat, making it an occasional part of the diet, at most. In other cases, religious teachings, including Hinduism, Buddhism, Judaism, Islam, Jainism, and Seventh-day Adventism, have promoted the use of vegetarian diets or have placed limitations on the types or timing of use of animal products.

1.2 CHANGES IN THE PERCEPTION OF VEGETARIAN DIETS

1.2.1 Scientific Community

Joan Sabaté of Loma Linda University has modeled shifts in the scientific community's perception of the nutrition and health status of vegetarians in affluent countries from the 1960s to the present (Sabaté, 2001, 2003; Leitzmann, 2014). In the 1960s and 1970s, vegetarian diets were believed to be of lower nutritional quality than meat-based diets and vegetarians were considered to be at a higher risk of nutrient deficiencies (Sabaté, 2003). There was limited examination of the health benefits of vegetarian diets. In the 1980s and 1990s, research began to be published on the benefits of vegetarian diets. The model shifted to suggest that vegetarians were at lower risk of an excess of unhealthy dietary components than were nonvegetarians but were at a higher risk of nutrient deficiency (Sabaté, 2003). There was still concern about the adequacy of vegetarian diets, but increasingly there was also concern about the risk of excessive intake of substances, including saturated fat, cholesterol, and protein, by nonvegetarians (Sabaté, 2003). In 2001, Sabaté proposed a new model for the future, one in which there is a more favorable risk-to-benefit ratio for the vegetarian diet than for a nonvegetarian diet (Sabaté, 2001). This model has been proposed to represent the situation today, near the beginning of the twenty-first century (Leitzmann, 2014). In this model, vegetarians are at lower risk for diseases of deficiency or excess than are meat eaters (Sabaté, 2003; Leitzmann, 2014).

Nutrition research has paralleled these shifts in perception of vegetarian health and nutrition. In the 1960s and 1970s, one-half of the articles published in biomedical literature on vegetarian nutrition dealt with nutrition adequacy (Sabaté et al., 1999). In the 1980s and 1990s, only about one-quarter of published articles on vegetarian nutrition focused on nutrition adequacy; many more examined the use of vegetarian diets in disease prevention and treatment (Sabaté et al., 1999). As Table 1.1 indicates, the growth in publications related to vegetarian and vegan nutrition is substantial.

Much of the early nutrition research tended to focus on the short-term effects of diets and on nutrient adequacy. Nutritional epidemiology developed as an area of research and allowed investigations that focused on the long-term effects of vegetarian diets on chronic disease (Sabaté, 2003). This ability to conduct and analyze long-term studies, along with the rising prevalence of type 2 diabetes, obesity, and other chronic diseases, led researchers to a greater focus on the role of food choice in long-term health. Large, long-term studies of vegetarians and nonvegetarians, such as the Adventist Health Study-1 (Fraser, 1999), the Adventist Health Study-2 (Orlich and Fraser, 2014), the Oxford Vegetarian Study (Appleby et al., 1999), the German Vegetarian Study (Chang-Claude et al., 1992), and EPIC-Oxford (Davey et al., 2003), have markedly increased knowledge related to vegetarian health and mortality and have changed the way that many health care professionals think about vegetarian diets.

TABLE 1.1

Number of Articles Indexed in PubMed Database Found with Search Term "Vegetarian Nutrition" or "Vegan Nutrition" and Published 1951–Present

Years	Vegetarian Nutrition	Vegan Nutrition
1951–1960	7	0
1961–1970	12	1
1971–1980	54	4
1981–1990	136	18
1991–2000	312	45
2001–2010	421	108
2011–2017[a]	371	137

[a] Includes material through March 12, 2017.

A recent estimate projected that global adoption of a more plant-based non-vegetarian diet could result in 5.1 million fewer deaths per year, use of a lacto-ovo vegetarian diet could reduce deaths by 7.3 million per year, and a vegan diet could result in 8.1 million fewer deaths per year (Springmann et al., 2016). Health care cost savings could be as much as $1 trillion per year with worldwide use of vegan diets, $973 billion with lacto-ovo vegetarian diets, and $735 billion with healthier nonvegetarian diets (Springmann et al., 2016). Reports such as this have stimulated interest in the health and economic benefits of vegetarian and near-vegetarian diets.

Another area of active research is that of the environmental impact of food choices. In 2006, the Food and Agriculture Organization (FAO) of the United Nations released an extensive report, titled *Livestock's Long Shadow: Environmental Issues and Opinions*, assessing livestock's impact on the environment (Steinfeld et al., 2006). This report showed that livestock production has a serious effect on land degradation, climate change, air pollution, water shortage and pollution, and the loss of biodiversity (Steinfeld et al., 2006). This report was followed by numerous studies using mathematical modeling to explore the effects of a transition toward more plant-based diets and away from animal products (Masset et al., 2014; Scarborough et al., 2014; Soret et al., 2014; Eshel et al., 2016; Springmann et al., 2016). As an example, researchers in the United Kingdom determined that worldwide use of a vegan diet would reduce food-related greenhouse gas emissions by 70% compared with what is projected for 2050 (Springmann et al., 2016). A lacto-ovo vegetarian diet would reduce these emissions by 63%, and a healthier nonvegetarian diet would reduce projected emissions by 29% (Springmann et al., 2016). Another study estimated that greenhouse gas emissions due to dietary choices were more than twice as high for meat eaters than for vegans (Scarborough et al., 2014).

There has been extensive research demonstrating the health, economic, and environmental benefits of vegetarian diets. This research has laid the foundation for changes in dietary recommendations.

1.2.2   PUBLIC PERCEPTION OF VEGETARIAN DIETS

Currently, about 3.3% of adults in the United States consistently follow a vegetarian diet, reporting that they never eat meat, fish, or poultry; about half of these vegetarians follow a vegan diet (The Vegetarian Resource Group, 2016). In 1994 and 1997, about 1% of U.S. adults were vegetarian; one-third to one-half of these vegetarians were vegans (Stahler, 1994; The Vegetarian Resource Group, 1997). Although these results are not directly comparable, they suggest that there has been an increase in the number of vegetarians and vegans in the United States over the past quarter century. There is also increased interest in vegetarianism, with more than one-third of U.S. adults always or sometimes eating vegetarian meals when they eat out (The Vegetarian Resource Group, 2016).

This more frequent use of vegetarian and vegan diets has been accompanied by a greater availability of specialty products for vegetarians and vegans in grocery stores and restaurants and by a proliferation of books, cookbooks, blogs, and websites devoted to all facets of vegetarian and vegan living. The public perception of vegetarian and vegan diets has shifted from a sense that vegetarian diets were used by a small minority of people for health or religious reasons to an increasingly more common acceptance of vegetarian and vegan diets as a popular healthy dietary choice.

Motivations of vegetarians and vegans vary. One survey of vegans in Germany reported that close to 90% of respondents listed animal welfare, animal rights, or animal agriculture as one of their main motives for being vegan. More than two-thirds said a motive for being vegan was personal health. Almost half mentioned environmental concerns as a motive. More than 80% of subjects had more than one main motive for being vegan, with 30% listing animals, personal health, and the environment as their primary motives (Janssen et al., 2016). A similar study of vegans in the United States found that about half of the study subjects reported personal health as their main reason for being vegan, while animal welfare concerns were the main motivation for 40% of the subjects (Dyett et al., 2013). This study only allowed respondents to choose a single motive for their veganism. A survey of vegetarians and vegans in the United States found that 56% reported avoiding meat for ethical reasons, 14% for health reasons, and 31% for a combination of ethics and health (Rothgerber, 2013).

For consumers with economic limitations, vegetarian and vegan diets can be a nutritious means of reducing food costs. In the U.S. Department of Agriculture's (USDA) low-cost eating plan, meats, poultry, and seafood account for more than 20% of the total cost (Flynn and Schiff, 2015). Replacing these foods with protein sources such as dried beans, nuts, seeds, and tofu can significantly reduce the cost of meals.

1.3   DIETARY GUIDELINES FOR AMERICANS

The changes in nutrition professionals' and the public's attitudes and knowledge about vegetarian nutrition are reflected in the *Dietary Guidelines for Americans*. The *Dietary Guidelines* are published every 5 years, starting in 1980, by the USDA and the U.S. Department of Health and Human Services (HHS) (Office of Disease Prevention and Health Promotion, 2015a). Each edition contains evidence-based dietary recommendations for Americans ages 2 and older. They are a statement of current federal policy on the role of dietary factors in health promotion and disease prevention. The overarching goals of the recommendations are to

- Promote health
- Prevent chronic disease
- Help people reach and maintain a healthy weight (Office of Disease Prevention and Health Promotion, 2015b)

The *Dietary Guidelines* form the basis of federal nutrition policy and affect local, state, and national activities to promote health and prevent disease. They also can affect product development and marketing by the food and beverage industry (Office of Disease Prevention and Health Promotion, 2015b).

Early editions of the *Dietary Guidelines* did not mention vegetarian diets. The Food Guide Pyramid was introduced along with the 1995 *Dietary Guidelines* and illustrated the concept of grains, vegetables, and fruits as the foundation of healthful diets (USDA and HHS, 1995).

Vegetarian diets were mentioned for the first time in 1995 when the text of the *Dietary Guidelines* said, "Vegetarian diets are consistent with the *Dietary Guidelines for Americans* and can meet Recommended Dietary Allowances for nutrients" (USDA and HHS, 1995). This statement was also included in the 2000 *Dietary Guidelines* (USDA and HHS, 2000). In the 1995 *Dietary Guidelines*, vegetarians were encouraged to pay special attention to sources of iron, zinc, and B vitamins; vegans were told to use vitamin B12 supplements and to ensure an adequate amount of vitamin D and calcium (USDA and HHS, 1995). The attitude toward vegetarian and vegan diets seemed supportive but cautious, with a focus on potential nutrient deficiency and an acknowledgment that "some Americans eat vegetarian diets for reasons of culture, belief, or health" (USDA and HHS, 1995). No attempt was made to promote vegetarian diets as a healthier choice.

The 2000 *Dietary Guidelines* continued to promote the use of plant foods as the foundation of meals (USDA and HHS, 2000). For the first time, calcium sources for those avoiding dairy products were mentioned. Sources included soy-based beverages with added calcium, tofu (if made with calcium sulfate), and dark green leafy vegetables, such as collards and turnip greens (USDA and HHS, 2000).

The 2005 *Dietary Guidelines* included a section on vegetarian diets that included explanations of different types of vegetarian diets, as well as how vegetarians could select nuts, seeds, and legumes (and eggs if desired) from what was called the "Meat and Beans Group." Nondairy sources of calcium were listed (USDA and HHS, 2005).

In 2010, the text of the *Dietary Guidelines* spoke positively about vegetarian diets, reporting that vegetarian eating patterns have been associated with lower rates of obesity, a reduction in blood pressure, and a reduced risk of cardiovascular disease (USDA and HHS, 2010). These benefits were attributed to vegetarians' lower intakes of saturated fat and energy; higher intakes of fiber, potassium, and vitamin C; and their generally lower body mass index (USDA and HHS, 2010). This edition of the *Dietary Guidelines* included lacto-ovo and vegan adaptations of the USDA Food Patterns. For 12 calorie levels, ranging from 1000 to 3200 kcal, the 2010 *Dietary Guidelines* provided recommended servings from each food group for lacto-ovo vegetarians and vegans (USDA and HHS, 2010).

The *2015–2020 Dietary Guidelines for Americans* endorses a Healthy Vegetarian Eating Pattern as one of three "healthy eating patterns that can be adapted based on cultural and personal preferences" (HHS and USDA, 2015). This Healthy Vegetarian Eating Pattern, along with two other recommended patterns, is suggested as a guide to planning and serving meals in schools, at worksites, and in other community settings (HHS and USDA, 2015). The Healthy Vegetarian Eating Pattern, as described by the *2015–2020 Dietary Guidelines*, includes vegetables, fruits, grains, dairy or fortified soymilk (or other plant-based dairy substitutes), and legumes, including soy products, nuts, and seeds. The eating pattern was developed based on foods and amounts of foods eaten by self-described vegetarians in the United States based on a large national study. The Healthy Vegetarian Eating Pattern is described as "similar in meeting nutrient standards to the Healthy U.S.-Style Pattern, but somewhat higher in calcium and fiber and lower in vitamin D due to differences in the foods included" (HHS and USDA, 2015).

The decision to include a vegetarian eating pattern as a recommended eating pattern was based on the Dietary Guidelines Committee's evidence-based assessment of the relationship between dietary patterns, such as a vegetarian pattern, and health outcomes (Dietary Guidelines Advisory Committee, 2015). Although the Dietary Guidelines Committee used an evidence-based approach to evaluate the foods and food components that improve the sustainability of dietary patterns (Dietary Guidelines Advisory Committee, 2015), information about sustainability and the environmental impact of food choices was not included in the final document.

1.4 DIETARY RECOMMENDATIONS FROM OTHER COUNTRIES

The United States is not the only country to promote plant-based diets. For example, the Dutch food-based dietary guidelines call for following a dietary pattern that includes more plant-based food and less animal-based food (Kromhout et al., 2016). They go on to recommend limiting the consumption of red meat, especially processed meat; eating legumes weekly and at least 15 g of nuts daily; and eating at least 200 g of fruit and 200 g of vegetables daily (Kromhout et al., 2016).

The United Kingdom's new Eatwell Guide tells users to "eat less red and processed meats" and "to eat more beans and pulses" (Public Health England, 2016). China's "Food Guide Pagoda" has cereals (in the form of rice, corn, bread, noodles, and crackers) and tubers as the base of the pagoda and, together with vegetables and fruits (on the second level), these are recommended to make up the majority of any meal (FAO, 2007a). The Swedish National Dietary Guidelines recommend eating lots of fruit, vegetables, and berries, and limiting red and processed meat to no more than 500 g per week, with only a small amount of this being processed meat (FAO, 2007b). The Dietary Guidelines for Costa Rica call for eating rice and beans, as they are the basis of the everyday diet, and eating at least five servings of fruits and vegetables of different colors every day (Intersectoral Commission on Dietary Guidelines, 2011).

1.5 CONCLUSIONS

There has been a shift in perception of vegetarian and vegan diets among scientific researchers, health care professionals, and the general public. These diets are increasingly being seen as mainstream alternatives and are used in the prevention and treatment of chronic diseases. They offer environmental advantages and can result in significant medical cost savings. The body of research on the benefits of vegetarian diets and their role in health promotion resulted in their being identified as one of the recommended eating patterns in the *2015–2020 Dietary Guidelines for Americans*.

REFERENCES

Appleby PN, Thorogood M, Mann J, Key TJ. 1999. The Oxford Vegetarian Study: An overview. *Am J Clin Nutr* 70(Suppl):525S–31S.

Brown PT, Bergan JG. 1975. The dietary status of "new" vegetarians. *J Am Diet Assoc* 67(5):455–9.

Chang-Claude J, Frentzel-Beyme R, Eilber U. 1992. Mortality pattern of German vegetarians after 11 years of follow-up. *Epidemiology* 3:395–401.

Davey GK, Spencer EA, Appleby PN, Allen NE, Knox KH, Key TJ. 2003. EPIC-Oxford lifestyle characteristics and nutrient intake in a cohort of 33,883 meat-eaters and 31,546 non meat-eaters in the UK. *Public Health Nutr* 6:259–68.

Dietary Guidelines Advisory Committee. 2015. Scientific report of the 2015 dietary guidelines advisory committee. Washington, DC: U.S. Government Printing Office.

Dyett PA, Sabaté J, Haddad E, Rajaram S, Shavlik D. 2013. Vegan lifestyle behaviors. An exploration of congruence with health-related beliefs and assessed health indices. *Appetite* 67:119–24.

Eshel G, Shepon A, Noor E, Milo R. 2016. Environmentally optimal, nutritionally aware beef replacement plant-based diets. *Environ Sci Technol* 50(15):8164–8.

FAO (Food and Agriculture Organization of the United Nations). 2007a. Food-based dietary guidelines—China. http://www.fao.org/nutrition/education/food-dietary-guidelines /regions/countries/China/en/ (accessed February 27, 2018).

FAO (Food and Agriculture Organization of the United Nations). 2007b. Food-based dietary guidelines—Sweden. http://www.fao.org/nutrition/education/food-dietary-guidelines /regions/countries/sweden/en/ (accessed February 27, 2018).

Flynn MM, Schiff AR. 2015. Economical healthy diets (2012): Including lean animal protein costs more than using extra virgin olive oil. *J Hunger Environ Nutr* 10:467–82.

Fraser GE. 1999. Associations between diet and cancer, ischemic heart disease, and all-cause mortality in non-Hispanic white California Seventh-day Adventists. *Am J Clin Nutr* 70(Suppl):532S–8S.

Hardinge MG, Chambers AC, Crooks H, Stare FJ. 1958. Nutritional studies of vegetarians. III. Dietary levels of fiber. *Am J Clin Nutr* 6(5):523–5.

Hardinge MG, Crooks H, Stare FJ. 1962. Nutritional studies of vegetarians. IV. Dietary fatty acids and serum cholesterol levels. *Am J Clin Nutr* 10:516–24.

Helman AD, Darnton-Hill I. 1987. Vitamin and iron status in new vegetarians. *Am J Clin Nutr* 45:785–9.

HHS (U.S. Department of Health and Human Services) and USDA (U.S. Department of Agriculture). 2015. *2015–2020 Dietary Guidelines for Americans*. 8th ed. Washington, DC: U.S. Government Printing Office.

Intersectoral Commission on Dietary Guidelines. 2011. Guías alimentarias para Costa Rica. https://www.ministeriodesalud.go.cr/gestores_en_salud/guiasalimentarias/guia _alimentarias_2011_completo.pdf (accessed March 14, 2017).

Janssen M, Busch C, Rödiger M, Hamm U. 2016. Motives of consumers following a vegan diet and their attitudes towards animal agriculture. *Appetite* 105:643–51.

Kromhout D, Spaaij CJ, de Goede J, Weggemans RM. 2016. The 2015 Dutch food-based dietary guidelines. *Eur J Clin Nutr* 70(8):869–78.

Leitzmann C. 2014. Vegetarian nutrition: Past, present, future. *Am J Clin Nutr* 100(Suppl):496S–502S.

Masset G, Vieux F, Verger EO, Sole, LG, Touazi D, Darmon N. 2014. Reducing energy intake and energy density for a sustainable diet: A study based on self-selected diets in French adults. *Am J Clin Nutr* 99(6):1460–9.

Melina V, Craig W, Levin S. 2016. Position of the Academy of Nutrition and Dietetics: Vegetarian diets. *J Acad Nutr Diet* 116:1970–80.

Office of Disease Prevention and Health Promotion. 2015a. About the dietary guidelines. Evolution. https://health.gov/dietaryguidelines/evolution.asp (accessed March 13, 2017).

Office of Disease Prevention and Health Promotion. 2015b. About the dietary guidelines. Purpose. https://health.gov/dietaryguidelines/purpose.asp (accessed March 13, 2017).

Orlich MJ, Fraser GE. 2014. Vegetarian diets in the Adventist Health Study 2: A review of initial published findings. *Am J Clin Nutr* 100(Suppl):353S–8S.

Public Health England. 2016. Eatwell guide. https://www.gov.uk/government/uploads/system/uploads/attachment_data/file/528193/Eatwell_guide_colour.pdf (accessed March 14, 2017).

Register UD, Sonnenberg LM. 1973. The vegetarian diet. Scientific and practical considerations. *J Am Diet Assoc* 62(3):253–61.

Rinaldi S, Campbell EE, Fournier J, O'Connor C, Madill J. 2016. A comprehensive review of the literature supporting recommendations from the Canadian Diabetes Association for the use of a plant-based diet for management of type 2 diabetes. *Can J Diabetes* 40:471–7.

Rothgerber H. 2013. A meaty matter. Pet diet and the vegetarian's dilemma. *Appetite* 68:76–82.

Sabaté J. 2001. The public health risk-to-benefit ratio of vegetarian diets: Changing paradigms. In *Vegetarian Nutrition*, ed. Sabaté J, 19–30. Boca Raton, FL: CRC Press.

Sabaté J. 2003. The contribution of vegetarian diets to health and disease: A paradigm shift? *Am J Clin Nutr* 78(Suppl):502S–7S.

Sabaté J, Duk A, Lee CL. 1999. Publication trends of vegetarian nutrition articles in biomedical literature, 1966–1995. *Am J Clin Nutr* 70(Suppl):601S–7S.

Scarborough P, Appleby PN, Mizdrak A, Briggs AD, Travis RC, Bradbury KE, Key TJ. 2014. Dietary greenhouse gas emissions of meat-eaters, fish-eaters, vegetarians and vegans in the UK. *Climatic Change* 125:179–92.

Schwartz RH. 1982. *Jewish Vegetarians.* Smithtown, NY: Exposition Press.

Soret S, Mejia A, Batech M, Jaceldo-Siegl K, Harwatt H, Sabate J. 2014. Climate change mitigation and health effects of varied dietary patterns in real-life settings throughout North America. *Am J Clin Nutr* 100(Suppl):490S–5S.

Springmann M, Godfray HC, Rayner M, Scarborough P. 2016. Analysis and valuation of the health and climate change cobenefits of dietary change. *Proc Natl Acad Sci USA* 113:4146–51.

Stahler C. 1994. How many vegetarians are there? http://www.vrg.org/nutshell/poll.htm (accessed March 13, 2017).

Steinfeld H, Gerber P, Wassenaar T, Castel V, Rosales M, de Haan C. 2006. *Livestock's Long Shadow: Environmental Issues and Opinions.* Rome: Food and Agriculture Organization.

Stuart T. 2006. *The Bloodless Revolution. A Cultural History of Vegetarianism from 1600 to Modern Times.* New York: W.W. Norton & Company.

USDA (U.S. Department of Agriculture) and HHS (U.S. Department of Health and Human Services). 1995. *Nutrition and Your Health: Dietary Guidelines for Americans.* 4th ed., Home and Garden Bulletin No. 232. Washington, DC: U.S. Department of Agriculture, Department of Health and Human Services.

USDA (U.S. Department of Agriculture) and HHS (U.S. Department of Health and Human Services). 2000. *Nutrition and Your Health: Dietary Guidelines for Americans.* 5th ed., Home and Garden Bulletin No. 232. Washington, DC: U.S. Department of Agriculture, Department of Health and Human Services.

USDA (U.S. Department of Agriculture) and HHS (U.S. Department of Health and Human Services). 2005. *Dietary Guidelines for Americans, 2005.* 6th ed. Washington, DC: U.S. Government Printing Office.

USDA (U.S. Department of Agriculture) and HHS (U.S. Department of Health and Human Services). 2010. *Dietary Guidelines for Americans, 2010.* 7th ed. Washington, DC: U.S. Government Printing Office.

The Vegetarian Resource Group. 1997. How many vegetarians are there? http://www.vrg.org/journal/vj97sep/979poll.htm (accessed March 13, 2017).

The Vegetarian Resource Group. 2016. How many adults in the U.S. are vegetarian and vegan? http://www.vrg.org/nutshell/Polls/2016_adults_veg.htm (accessed March 13, 2017).

White EG. 1938. *Counsels on Diets and Foods: A Compilation from the Writings of Ellen G. White.* Hagerstown, MD: Review and Herald.

Section I

Environmental Issues

2 Impact of Vegetarian Diets on the Environment

Dora Marinova and Talia Raphaely

CONTENTS

SUMMARY

This chapter explores the environmental impacts of different diets, providing an overview of implications related to climate change and greenhouse gas (GHG) emissions, land and water use, and biodiversity loss. Original estimates are included for the global warming potential of GHGs associated with two selected foods (beef and wheat) on a 20-year horizon, consistent with methane's life span in the earth's atmosphere, as well as the population that the planet can support on a plant-based diet. Irrespective of the type of environmental impact considered, the consumption of animal-based products, and meat in particular, is associated with a heavier ecological footprint that exceeds the capacity of the planet and its ability to feed the global population. A switch to vegetarian options can significantly ameliorate the ability of the earth's biosphere and atmosphere to provide habitat for all living species.

2.1 INTRODUCTION

All living species draw resources from the planet and its atmosphere—in the form of nutrients, water, and sunlight—for their development and survival. Food is essential to provide energy and sustain life (Merriam-Webster, 2017). Animals, including invertebrates (e.g., insects, mollusks, corals, crustaceans, arachnids, and worms) and vertebrates (amphibians, reptiles, fish, birds, and mammals), eat directly or indirectly other living species to maintain their life (Rastogi, 2004) and, by so doing, consume resources from the planet. Humans, a mammal animal species, have evolved to consume foods based on plant and animal matter and are generally described as omnivorous (as distinct from herbivorous animals, which eat only plants, and carnivorous, which eat other animals). Omnivores can also include fungi and algae in their diets (Bradford, 2016). A major feature of their biology is that they can adapt to the variety of foods available, which gives them a greater chance of survival and the ability to adjust to natural and social conditions (National Geographic, 2017).

Omnivores can also be described as opportunistic feeders whose anatomical and physiological characteristics, such as teeth, glands, and intestines, allow them to consume any food that is available, be it of plant or animal origin (McArdle, 2000). Hence, humans' choice of food is determined by factors such as availability, taste preferences, health concerns, and social factors, as well as environmental and ethical considerations. In societies where there is an abundance of food options, such as in the West, individual taste preferences seem to be a leading factor in decisions about what to eat, although eating history and health-related knowledge also play a role (Nestle et al., 1998).

In this day and age, however, we have witnessed an enormous expansion of the human race, reaching 7.5 billion in 2017 (Worldometers, 2017), and of the animals raised for food, estimated at 71 billion in 2014, 70 billion of which are slaughtered annually for consumption (FAO, 2017). Our eating choices, and particularly the consumption of meat, have serious implications not only for individual health but also for the ecological environment (Raphaely and Marinova, 2016). Many people make the conscious decision to exclude meat from their diet, that is, to be vegetarian, and even to abstain from all animal-based products, that is, to be vegan. While herbivores can only survive on plants, vegetarians explicitly make the choice not to eat meat. Although there are many health benefits from such a choice (e.g., Marsh et al., 2016), the aim of this chapter is to investigate the implications of a vegetarian diet for the natural environment. We do this by analyzing and comparing the impacts of human diet on climate change, land use, water, and biodiversity.

2.2   CLIMATE CHANGE

Climate change is the biggest threat to human well-being (Watts et al., 2015), and its anthropogenic roots are related to greenhouse gas (GHG) emissions, which, captured in the earth's atmosphere, prevent infrared radiation from being released and cause temperature increases (Lallanila, 2016). While there is widespread awareness about the contribution of carbon dioxide (CO_2) to global warming, there is much less attention given to the other GHGs. Other major GHGs, and much more powerful than CO_2, are methane (CH_4) and nitrous oxides (N_xO).

Although natural sources (e.g., wetlands, termites, and oceans) create methane, human activities are responsible for 64% of the total emissions of this GHG (Bousquet et al., 2006). More than a quarter (i.e., 27%) of all human-created methane emissions are the result of enteric fermentation in livestock animals, such as cows, goats, and sheep (Bousquet et al., 2006). In the process of plant digestion, the microorganisms in the stomach of these animals produce methane, which is released in the atmosphere through either exhalation or flatus (What's Your Impact, 2017). Nitrous oxide (N_2O) is similarly naturally present in the atmosphere; however, human activities, including agriculture, emit additional quantities of this GHG, estimated to be around 265 times more powerful than CO_2 (IPCC, 2014). A major source of nitrous oxide emissions is nitrogen-based fertilizers used for the production of food and animal feed (Grace and Barton, 2014). Estimates show that in Australia, for every tonnes of nitrogen applied as fertilizer, 25 kg is lost to the atmosphere, where it combines with oxygen and forms nitrous oxide (Grace and Barton, 2014). With animal products representing a longer and inefficient calorie conversion chain (Eshel et al., 2014) of plants to livestock and then to humans—in contrast to the shorter and more efficient conversion from plants to humans (Schmidinger et al., 2018)—growing more plants for animal feed generates an additional need for nitrogen use.

Hence, the livestock raised for human consumption are a major contributor to climate change. Consequently, people who eat meat contribute disproportionately more to global GHG emissions. These emissions are generated throughout the entire food cycle, including preproduction (e.g., fertilizers, pesticides, herbicides, and energy used for animal feed, buildings, and machinery), production (e.g., land clearing, enteric fermentation, manure management, and biomass burning), and postproduction (e.g., processing, packaging, transport, refrigeration, preparation, and waste) (Green et al., 2016).

There are numerous studies based on individual countries or geographic regions that estimate the GHG emissions of vegetarianism compared with nonvegetarian diets and foods. Examples include

- North America—Soret et al. (2014) showed that a vegetarian diet reduces GHG emissions by 29%, compared with a nonvegetarian diet.
- United Kingdom—According to Scarborough et al. (2014), the dietary GHG emissions of meat eaters are approximately 50% higher than those of vegetarians, and 100% higher than those of vegans.
- Continental Europe—Vieux et al. (2012) found that meat was the strongest contributor to diet-related GHG emissions; however, when substituted with fruit and vegetables to the same caloric content (which is an unlikely scenario), there were only small variations in emissions.
- Nordic European countries—For Sweden in particular, Hallström et al. (2014) link the 25% recommended dietary cut to reducing intake of saturated fat, which approximately halves the diet-related GHG emissions.
- Australia—Hendrie et al. (2014) estimated that red meat alone contributes 55% of the diet-related personal GHG emissions.
- New Zealand—The modeling conducted by Wilson et al. (2013) shows significant differences in GHG emissions between vegetarian and vegan diets built to satisfy key nutrient content requirements and diets comprising more familiar foods for New Zealanders, where the main meal is mince, sausage, or fish. The vegetarian and vegan diets were generating, respectively, 3 and 2.6 times less GHG emissions than the diets with more familiar foods.
- India—The life cycle analysis conducted by Pathak et al. (2010) shows that a nonvegetarian meal with mutton has 80% higher GHG emissions than a vegetarian meal.

Furthermore, Clark and Tilman (2017) conducted a meta-analysis of life cycle assessments of 742 agricultural systems—86% from highly industrialized Europe,

North America, Australia, and New Zealand and 14% from Asia, South America, and Africa—and 90 unique products for "cradle-to-farm gate" activities, excluding post–farm emissions. They concluded that ruminant meats have GHG emission impacts that are 20 to 100 times higher than those of plant-based foods.

According to Joyce et al. (2008) and Green et al. (2016), given that reducing the intake of animal products, and beef in particular, has the potential to lower GHG emissions, consumers need to be educated. Educational interventions combined with social marketing (Bogueva et al., 2017, 2018) are urgently needed, as even organizations and people who claim to be environmentalist and concerned about climate change continue to ignore the GHG contributions of diets (Andersen and Kuhn, 2014).

The study by Springmann et al. (2017) further argues that in order to combat the emissions associated with different animal-based foods and mitigate their contribution to climate change, price surcharges in the form of environmental taxes are needed. Beef, milk, lamb, and poultry would require surcharges of 40%, 20%, 14%, and 8%, respectively (Springmann et al., 2017).

There are two methodological problems with all current studies of the GHG contribution of different diets and food options that underrepresent the contribution of meat and animal products to climate change. The first relates to the methodology used to substitute animal products, for example, meat, when estimating what kind of transition toward more sustainable eating is required. Some models take a very narrow or unrealistic approach with unlikely and often nutritionally unjustified assumptions. For example, Vieux et al. (2012) substituted a 20% reduction in meat consumption for continental Europe by only fruits and vegetables, rather than broader vegetarian foods using the same high-calorie intake above the required level for energy needs. Similarly, Tom et al. (2016) substituted reduction in meat consumption in the United States with greater intake of fruits, vegetables, dairy, and fish or seafood (rather than all vegetarian options, including legumes, grains, nuts, and roots) on a caloric basis. When cross-checked with servings recommended by the U.S. dietary guidelines, the analysis by Hamm (2016) shows that the replacement of pork (a meat with a much lower GHG footprint than beef) produces significantly less GHG emissions even for the vegetables (cucumbers, eggplant, celery, and lettuces) claimed to be significantly more GHG-intensive than meat on a per calorie basis. When the analysis is properly conducted and compared with an omnivorous eating behavior, the diet with the lowest GHG emissions is vegetarian (Tilman and Clark, 2014).

The second methodological issue relates to how the impact of methane is estimated in the calculations of the GHGs associated with various diets and foods. Once emitted, all GHGs remain in the atmosphere long enough to form a mix that is more or less similar all over the world, irrespective of the source of air pollution (USEPA, 2017a). Climate scientists estimate the impact of the GHG mix through the global warming potential of the individual gases, referred to as CO_2 equivalence (CO_2e). All studies so far, with the exception of Goodland and Anhang (2009), who estimated livestock's contribution to global GHGs at 51%, use a CO_2e approach based on 100 years. In other words, the impact of methane is spread over 100 years to produce a global warming potential coefficient that compares it with CO_2. This coefficient is estimated at around 25 (IPCC, 2007; revised to 28 in IPCC, 2014). However, while CO_2 and nitrous oxides (e.g., N_2O) remain in the earth's atmosphere for hundreds of years, methane has a much shorter perturbation life span of around 12 years, after which it gradually decomposes (IPCC, 2014). While in the atmosphere, methane is also a precursor of ozone and enhances water vapor, which are in themselves GHGs (USEPA, 2017b). Therefore, it is more appropriate to estimate the impact of methane on a shorter time horizon consistent with its presence in the atmosphere, namely, 20 years. By using a 100-year instead of a 20-year equivalency—as has been the case with all estimates of diet contributions to climate change—the impact of methane is drastically diminished and, consequently, livestock's impact on climate change is significantly underestimated. The global warming coefficient for methane on a 20-year horizon is 84 (IPCC, 2014), compared with the 25 used in all existing assessments of the dietary contributions to GHG emissions.

With global demand for meat and animal products increasing as a result of improved living standards, higher incomes, and urbanization (Steinfeld et al., 2006), it is worth estimating the global warming potential of a vegetarian option, such as wheat, against beef, which has the highest GHG footprint (Eshel et al., 2014; Doran-Browne et al., 2015). Table 2.1 presents this comparison in the case of Australia. It is important to note that the comparison between beef and wheat is made on the basis of essential nutrients represented by the recommended daily intake of protein; fiber; vitamins A, C, and E; calcium; iron; magnesium; and potassium, as well as only protein, in response to the common myth about animal products being the only source of proteins (Bogueva and Phau, 2016; Bogueva et al., 2017) and energy (calorie or joules). Over a 20-year time horizon, beef generates 113 times more GHG emissions than wheat for the same amounts of nutrients and is 326 times more GHG-intensive than wheat as an energy source.

All existing evidence, including the Australian example (Table 2.1), shows that vegetarian dietary options are more appropriate for the Anthropocene—the geological period highly dominated by human activities (Castree, 2015)—in order to address global concerns about climate change. All efforts to keep temperature increases within a reasonable level, such as below 2°C and the desired 1.5°C under the Paris Agreement (UNFCC, 2017), would require food to be included in the policy agenda, with vegetarian food choices strongly encouraged.

TABLE 2.1

CO$_2$ Equivalence Comparisons between Wheat and Beef for Australia

	Wheat	Beef over 100 Years	Beef over 20 Years
CO$_2$e per nutrient (protein; fiber; vitamins A, C, and E; calcium; iron; magnesium; potassium)	1	79	113
CO$_2$e per protein	1	56	78
CO$_2$e per unit of energy (J or calorie)	1	227	326

Source: Doran-Browne NA et al., *Climatic Change* 129 (1–2): 73–87, 2015; Australian National Greenhouse Gas Inventory, National Greenhouse Gas Inventory—Kyoto Protocol classifications, Database, 2014, http://ageis.climatechange.gov.au (accessed June 13, 2017).

2.3 LAND USE

Clearing of native vegetation and conversion of vast areas into pastures, arable land, and food-growing lots is a continuing process with increasing population numbers. The scale of these land changes is often invisible for the urban dwellers, where the majority of the global population now lives. For example, in recent years in Australia 86% of clearing is for pastures, 10% for crops, and 4% for forest, mining, infrastructure, and settlements (Hamblin, 2001). This fact alone indicates the vast differences in land use between livestock and plant-based farming. In fact, the livestock sector is the single largest anthropogenic user of land. Furthermore, "twenty-six percent of the planet's ice-free land is used for livestock grazing and 33 percent of croplands are used for livestock feed production" (FAO, 2012, n.p.).

A comparison between the land requirements for different diets shows that the standard American (or Western) diet requires 3 acres per person and uses 18 times more land than a vegan or plant-only diet requiring 1/6 acre, or 6 times more land than a vegetarian diet, which includes dairy and eggs and requires a 1/2 acre (Andersen and Kuhn, 2014). The many calls and explicit preferences for organic methods of farming that require more land (Clark and Tilman, 2017) cannot be fulfilled for the world's 7.5 billion people on an omnivorous diet. In fact, with 7.68 billion acres of arable land available on the planet (One Simple Idea, 2017), the current global population cannot be fed on an American diet; on a vegan diet, however, the earth can feed 12.8 billion—an additional 5 billion people. The choice is simple. We face world hunger by either inefficiently allocating and using resources on an American type of a diet or feeding the entire global population for the foreseeable future—demographers project the world population to reach 10.9 billion by 2100 (Thomas, 2014) and stabilize with the increase of quality of life (Colleran, 2016).

2.4 WATER USE

All agricultural production, including plant- and animal-based foods and feed, requires freshwater. Although desalination is increasingly being used as a water supply option for growers (e.g., Sundrop Farms tomatoes in South Australia supplying mainstream supermarket chains; described by Matthews [2014]) and livestock farms (Department of Food and Agriculture, 2016), unless powered entirely by renewable energy, it contributes to GHG emissions and climate change. Furthermore, the discharge of the brine from desalination plants poses significant environmental concerns and can potentially damage the land, waterways, and water bodies, affecting other species (Department of Food and Agriculture, 2016). Hence, the demand for freshwater remains a major consideration when analyzing the environmental impacts of various diets.

With almost every country around the world experiencing water shortages or declines in availability, this very precious resource should be used wisely (Pimentel et al., 1997). The amount of water required to produce 1 kg of food varies between countries and depending on the agricultural methods used. What is, however, clear is that animal-based foods use much more water resources than any crops (Chapagain and Hoekstra, 2004). The methods used to estimate the water footprint of foods also vary.

At the lower end of the spectrum are the estimates by Chapagain and Hoekstra (2004), which show beef's water content at 13,193 L/kg in the United States, 17,122 L/kg in Australia, and 15,497 L/kg for the world average, compared with maize at 489, 744, and 909 L/kg, respectively. According to Pimentel and Pimentel (2003), the production of 1 kg of animal protein in the United States requires directly on average about 100 times more water than 1 kg of grain protein—an estimate at the top end of the spectrum. Per unit of calorie, beef in the American diet requires, respectively, 4, 8, and 40 times more irrigated water than rice, potato, and wheat (Eshel et al., 2014).

Our understanding of the water types, cycles, and use in growing and producing food is likely to improve in the future, leading to better consistency in estimates. Notwithstanding this, the environmental message is clear—a vegetarian diet, including avoiding beef in particular, requires significantly less water. The Australian Less Meat Less Heat website (2017) also argues for a climatarian diet that helps combat climate change and saves precious water resources.

2.5 BIODIVERSITY

With climate change being a top global priority for human survival, biodiversity loss is often forgotten or seen as an area relevant only to those interested in nature conservation. The reality, however, is that biodiversity loss has become one of the main limiting factors of life on earth as we know it. Biodiversity is negatively impacted both by changes in the climate—which cause shifts in species' habitat, distribution, and abundance—and by conversion of land for agricultural purposes, which causes habitat loss (Machovina et al., 2015). Within the planetary boundaries considered essential for the safe operation of human society, the rate of species' extinction—or biodiversity loss—is alarming and already significantly exceeds the acceptable levels (Rockström et al., 2009). The issue is even more serious given the fact that we still do not know "how much can be lost before ecosystems collapse, nor which species are the key players in a given ecosystem" (Pearce, 2010, n.p.). Rockström et al. (2009) estimate biodiversity loss in the Anthropocene as 100 extinctions per million species per year, against a previous rate of only 0.3. As a result, "up to 30 per cent of all mammal, bird and amphibian species will be threatened with extinction this century" (Pearce, 2010, n.p.), while another study warns that 15%–37% of species will be committed to extinction as early as 2050 (Thomas et al., 2004).

While scientists are trying to understand the importance of various species and how life comes together within the boundaries of our small planet, one industry has gone strongly on a destruction path, demolishing rain forests and woodland savannahs in Brazil (Brügger et al., 2016), clearing native vegetation in Australia, and threatening the habitat of all species in biodiversity hotspots in the tropical areas of the Americas, Africa, and Asia (Machovina et al., 2015). With the projected rates of increase in meat consumption in the developing world, some countries may require doubling of the land currently used for livestock (Machovina et al., 2015).

The sheer number of farmed and slaughtered animals overcrowds and pollutes the natural ecosystems, which cannot cope with the ecological burden imposed by the human desire for meat. There is ample evidence that diets rich in meat and animal products are contributing to species' extinction (World Preservation Foundation, 2013), while vegetarian diets are better suited for protecting biodiversity and the natural environment, reducing climate change, and minimizing air, soil, land, and water pollution (Leitzmann, 2003). In fact, "human carnivory … [is] the single biggest threat to much of the world's flora and fauna" (Morell, 2015, n.p.).

In response to the increasing awareness about the direct link between meat, human health, and the environment (Raphaely and Marinova, 2016), beef consumption, in particular, seems to have peaked around the world and is now on the decline (Marinova and Raphaely, 2018). Traditionally, high red meat–eating countries, such as Germany, the United States, and Australia, are witnessing decreases and replacement with poultry options, which have less impact on climate change (Rousseau, 2016). The high risks associated with the use of antibiotics in intensive farming (Review on Antimicrobial Resistance, 2015) is also likely to soon curb the trend in poultry consumption. People around the world are changing their eating habits and switching to vegetarian and vegan options, encouraged by leaders from the fields of science, arts, ethics, music, and sports (Leitzmann, 2014).

2.6 CONCLUSION

Plant-based diets appear to be environmentally more sustainable because they use fewer resources and have a smaller ecological footprint (Sabaté and Soret, 2014). A shift toward adopting vegetarian and vegan diets will improve both human well-being and the health of the planet. It will significantly decrease food-related GHG emissions, reduce demand for freshwater and land, and slow down biodiversity losses. Whether such a transition would happen suddenly or gradually will depend on a wide range of factors, such as education, information dissemination, social marketing, nutritional policies, and leadership, as well as barriers linked to vested interests, inertia, and gluttony. The battle for a positive outlook for the human race and all other living species in the biosphere we all share has started and is "perhaps one of the most rational and moral paths for a sustainable future" on planet Earth (Sabaté and Soret, 2014).

REFERENCES

Andersen K, Kuhn K. 2014. *Cowspiracy: The Sustainability Secret*, directed by Kip Andersen and Keegan Kuhn. Santa Rosa, CA: AUM Films and First Spark Media.

Australian National Greenhouse Gas Inventory. 2014. National Greenhouse Gas Inventory— Kyoto Protocol classifications. Database. http://ageis.climatechange.gov.au (accessed June 13, 2017).

Bogueva D, Marinova D, Raphaely T. 2017. Reducing meat consumption: The case for social marketing. *Asia Pacific Journal of Marketing and Logistics* 29 (3): 477–500.

Bogueva D, Marinova D, Raphaely T, eds. 2018. *Handbook of Research on Social Marketing and Its Influence on Animal Origin Food Product Consumption*. Hershey, PA: IGI Global.

Bogueva D, Phau I. 2016. Meat myths and marketing. In *Impact of Meat Consumption on Health and Environmental Sustainability*, ed. T Raphaely, D Marinova, 264–276. Hershey, PA: IGI Global.

Bousquet P, Ciais P, Miller JB, Dlugokencky EJ, Hauglustaine DA, Prigent C, van der Werf GR et al. 2006. Contribution of anthropogenic and natural sources to atmospheric methane variability. *Nature* 443: 439–443. doi: 10.1038/nature05132.

Bradford A. 2016. Omnivores: Facts about flexible eaters. *Live Science*. https://www
.livescience.com/53483-omnivores.html.

Brügger P, Marinova D, Raphaely T. 2016. Meat production and consumption: An ethical
educational approach. In *Impact of Meat Consumption on Health and Environmental
Sustainability*, ed. T Raphaely, D Marinova, 295–312. Hershey, PA: IGI Global.

Castree N. 2015. Anthropocene: A primer for geographers. *Geography* 100: 66–75.

Chapagain AK, Hoekstra AY. 2004. *Water Footprints of Nations*, Vol. 1, *Main Report*. Delft,
The Netherlands: UNESCO-IHE, Institute for Water Education. http://waterfootprint
.org/media/downloads/Report16Vol1.pdf (accessed June 13, 2017).

Clark M, Tilman D. 2017. Comparative analysis of environmental impacts of agricultural
production systems, agricultural input efficiency, and food choice. *Environmental
Research Letters* 12: 064016. http://iopscience.iop.org/article/10.1088/1748-9326
/aa6cd5/pdf (accessed August 23, 2017).

Colleran H. 2016. The cultural evolution of fertility decline. *Philosophical Transactions of
the Royal Society B* 371 (1692): 1–12.

Department of Food and Agriculture. 2016. Groundwater desalination and regulation for
farm water supply in Western Australia. Government of Western Australia. https://
www.agric.wa.gov.au/soil-salinity/groundwater-desalination-and-regulation-farm
-water-supply-western-australia (accessed June 13, 2017).

Doran-Browne NA, Eckard R, Behrendt R, Kingwell RS. 2015. Nutrient density as a metric
for comparing greenhouse gas emissions from food production. *Climatic Change* 129
(1–2): 73–87.

Eshel G, Shepon A, Makov T, Milo R. 2014. Land, irrigation water, greenhouse gas, and
reactive nitrogen burdens of meat, eggs, and dairy production in the United States.
Proceedings of the National Academy of Sciences of the United States of America 111
(33): 11996–12001.

FAO (Food and Agriculture Organization of the United Nations). 2012. Livestock and landscapes. Sustainability pathways. http://www.fao.org/docrep/018/ar591e/ar591e.pdf
(accessed June 14, 2017).

FAO (Food and Agriculture Organization of the United Nations). 2017. FAOSTAT: Livestock
primary. Dataset. http://www.fao.org/faostat/en/#data/QL (accessed June 10, 2017).

Goodland R, Anhang J. 2009. Livestock and climate change: What if the key actors in climate change are ... cows, pigs, and chickens? *World Watch*, November/December.
http://www.worldwatch.org/files/pdf/Livestock%20and%20Climate%20Change.pdf
(accessed July 13, 2017).

Grace P, Barton L. 2014. Meet N_2O, the greenhouse gas 300 times worse than CO_2. *The
Conversation*, December 9. http://theconversation.com/meet-n2o-the-greenhouse-gas
-300-times-worse-than-co2-35204 (accessed June 12, 2017).

Green C, Hallett J, Joyce J, Hannelly T, Carey G. 2016. The greenhouse gas emissions of
various dietary practices and intervention possibilities to reduce this impact. In *Impact
of Meat Consumption on Health and Environmental Sustainability*, ed. T Raphaely,
D Marinova, 1–26. Hershey, PA: IGI Global.

Hallström E, Röös E, Börjesson P. 2014. Sustainable meat consumption: A quantitative analysis of nutritional intake, greenhouse gas emissions and land use from a Swedish perspective. *Food Policy* 47: 81–90.

Hamblin A. 2001. Land theme report. Australia State of the Environment Report 2001.
Canberra, ACT: Department for the Environment. https://soe.environment.gov.au/sites/g
/files/net806/f/soe2011-report-land.pdf?v=1488162024 (accessed March 21. 2018).

Hamm M. 2016. Commentary: Energy use, GHG and blue water impacts if US diet aligns
with new USDA dietary recommend. East Lansing: Michigan State University, Centre
for Food Systems. http://foodsystems.msu.edu/news/commentary_energy_use_ghg
_and_blue_water_impacts (accessed January 25, 2017).

Hendrie GA, Ridoutt BG, Wiedmann TO, Noakes M. 2014. Greenhouse gas emissions and the Australian diet—Comparing dietary recommendations with average intakes. *Nutrients* 6 (1): 289–303.

IPCC (Intergovernmental Panel on Climate Change). 2007. Climate change 2007: Working Group I: The physical science basis. Fourth Assessment Report. Geneva: IPCC. https://www.ipcc .ch/publications_and_data/ar4/wg1/en/ch2s2-10-2.html (accessed June 12, 2017).

IPCC (Intergovernmental Panel on Climate Change). 2014. Climate change 2014: Synthesis report. Contribution of Working Groups I, II and III to the Fifth Assessment Report of the Intergovernmental Panel on Climate Change. Geneva: IPCC. https://www.ipcc.ch/pdf /assessment-report/ar5/syr/SYR_AR5_FINAL_full_wcover.pdf

Joyce AW, Dixon S, Comfort J, Hallett J. 2008. The cow in the room: Public knowledge of the links between dietary choices and health and environmental impacts. *Environmental Health Insights* 1: 31–34.

Lallanila M. 2016. What is the greenhouse gas effect? *Live Science*. https://www.livescience .com/37743-greenhouse-effect.html (accessed June 10, 2017).

Leitzmann C. 2003. Nutrition ecology: The contribution of vegetarian diets. *American Journal of Clinical Nutrition* 78 (3): 657S–659S.

Leitzmann C. 2014. Vegetarian nutrition: Past, present, future. *American Journal of Clinical Nutrition* 100 (Suppl. 1): 496S–502S.

Less Meat Less Heat. 2017. Facts. http://www.lessmeatlessheat.org/facts/ (accessed June 14, 2017).

Machovina B, Feeley KJ, Ripple WJ. 2015. Biodiversity conservation: The key is reducing meat consumption. *Science of the Total Environment* 536: 419–431.

Marinova D, Raphaely T. 2018. Taxing meat and animal food products. In *Handbook of Research on Social Marketing and Its Influence on Animal Origin Food Product Consumption*, ed. D Bogueva, D Marinova, T Raphaely, 121–134. Hershey, PA: IGI Global.

Marsh K, Saunders A, Zeuschner C. 2016. Red meat and health: Evidence regarding red meat, health, and chronic disease risk. In *Impact of Meat Consumption on Health and Environmental Sustainability*, ed. T Raphaely, D Marinova, 131–177. Hershey, PA: IGI Global.

Matthews J. 2014. Tomatoes watered by the sea: Sprouting a new way of farming. *The Conversation*, February 17. http://theconversation.com/tomatoes-watered-by-the-sea -sprouting-a-new-way-of-farming-23119 (accessed June 13, 2017).

McArdle J. 2000. Humans are omnivores. The Vegetarian Resource Group. http://www.vrg .org/nutshell/omni.htm.

Merriam-Webster. 2017. Food. https://www.merriam-webster.com/dictionary/food (accessed June 10, 2017).

Morell V. 2015. Meat-eaters may speed worldwide species extinction, study warns. *Science*, August 11. http://www.sciencemag.org/news/2015/08/meat-eaters-may-speed-worldwide -species-extinction-study-warns (accessed June 11, 2015).

National Geographic. 2017. Omnivore: Secondary consumer. National Geographic Society. https://www.nationalgeographic.org/encyclopedia/omnivore/ (accessed June 10, 2017).

Nestle M, Wing R, Birch L, DiSogra L, Mateo S, Drewnowski A, Middleton S, Sigman-Grant M, Sobal J, Winston M, Economos C. 1998. Behavioural and social influences on food choice. *Nutrition Review* 56 (5): S50–S74.

One Simple Idea. 2017. Environment. http://one-simple-idea.com/Environment1.htm (accessed June 14, 2017).

Pathak H, Jain N, Bhatia A, Patel J, Aggarwal PK. 2010. Carbon footprints of Indian food items. *Agriculture, Ecosystems & Environment* 139 (1–2): 66–73.

Pearce F. 2010. Earth's nine life-support systems: Biodiversity. *New Science* 2749, February 24. https://www.newscientist.com/article/dn18574-earths-nine-life-support -systems-biodiversity/ (accessed June 13, 2017).

Pimentel D, Houser J, Preiss E, White O, Fang H, Mesnick L, Barsky T, Tariche S, Schreck J, Alpert S. 1997. Water resources: Agriculture, the environment, and society. *BioScience* 47 (2): 97–106.

Pimentel D, Pimentel M. 2003. Sustainability of meat-based and plant-based diets and the environment. *American Journal of Clinical Nutrition* 78 (3): 660S–663S.

Raphaely T, Marinova D, eds. 2016. *Impact of Meat Consumption on Health and Environmental Sustainability*. Hershey, PA: IGI Global.

Rastogi VB. 2004. *Modern Biology*. 7th ed. New Delhi: Pitambar Publishing.

Review on Antimicrobial Resistance. 2015. Antimicrobials in agriculture and the environment: Reducing unnecessary use and waste. https://amr-review.org/sites/default /files/Antimicrobials%20in%20agriculture%20and%20the%20environment%20-%20 Reducing%20unnecessary%20use%20and%20waste.pdf (accessed April 17, 2017).

Rockström J, Steffen W, Noone K, Persson A, Chapin FS III, Lambin EF, Lenton TM et al. 2009. A safe operating space for humanity. *Nature* 461: 472–475. doi: 10.1038/461472a.

Rousseau O. 2016. Food trends: Meat consumption up, beef declines. *Global Meat News*, April 13. http://www.globalmeatnews.com/Analysis/Food-trends-meat-consumption-up -beef-declines (accessed June 13, 2017).

Sabaté J, Soret S. 2014. Sustainability of plant-based diets: Back to the future. *American Journal of Clinical Nutrition* 100 (Suppl. 1): 476S–482S.

Scarborough P, Appleby PN, Mizdrak A, Briggs ADM, Travis RC, Bradbury KE, Key TJ. 2014. Dietary greenhouse gas emissions of meat-eaters, fish-eaters, vegetarians and vegans in the UK. *Clim Change* 125 (2): 179–192.

Schmidinger K, Bogueva D, Marinova D. 2018. Future food—Meat without livestock. In *Handbook of Research on Social Marketing and Its Influence on Animal Origin Food Product Consumption*, ed. D Bogueva, D Marinova, T Raphaely, 344–361. Hershey, PA: IGI Global.

Soret S, Mejia A, Batech M, Jaceldo-Siegel K, Harwatt H, Sabaté J. 2014. Climate change mitigation and health effects of varied dietary patterns in real-life settings throughout North America. *American Journal of Clinical Nutrition* 100 (Suppl. 1): 490S–495S.

Springmann M, Mason-D'Croz D, Robinson S, Weibe K, Godfray HCJ, Rayner M, Scarborough P. 2017. Mitigation potential and global health impacts from emissions pricing of food commodities. *Nature Climate Change* 7 (1): 69–76.

Steinfeld H, Gerber P, Wassenaar T, Castel V, Rosales M, de Hann C. 2006. *Livestock's Long Shadow: Environmental Issues and Options*. Rome: Food and Agriculture Organization of the United Nations (FAO).

Thomas B. 2014. World population won't stabilise this century after all. *Discover: Science for the Curious*. http://blogs.discovermagazine.com/d-brief/2014/09/18/world-population -wont-stabilize-this-century/ (accessed June 14, 2017).

Thomas CD, Cameron A, Green RE, Bakkenes M, Beaumont LJ, Collingham YC, Erasmus BFN et al. 2004. Extinction risk from climate change. *Nature* 427 (6970): 145–148.

Tilman D, Clark M. 2014. Global diets link environmental sustainability and human health. *Nature* 515 (7528): 518–522. doi: 10.1038/nature13959.

Tom M, Fischbeck PS, Hendrickson CT. 2016. Energy use, blue water footprint, and greenhouse gas emissions for current food consumption patterns and dietary recommendations in the US. *Environment Systems & Decisions* 36 (1): 92–103.

UNFCC (United Nations Framework Convention on Climate Change). 2017. The Paris Agreement. http://unfccc.int/paris_agreement/items/9485.php (accessed June 13, 2017).

USEPA (U.S. Environmental Protection Agency). 2017a. Greenhouse gas emissions: Overview of greenhouse gases. https://www.epa.gov/ghgemissions/overview-green house-gases (accessed June 12, 2017).

USEPA (U.S. Environmental Protection Agency). 2017b. Greenhouse gas emissions: Understanding global warming potential. https://www.epa.gov/ghgemissions/under standing-global-warming-potentials (accessed June 12, 2017).

Vieux F, Darmon N, Touazi D, Soler LG. 2012. Greenhouse gas emissions of self-selected individual diets in France: Changing the diet structure or consuming less? *Ecological Economics* 75: 91–101.

Watts N, Adger WN, Agnolucci P, Blackstock J, Byass P, Cai W, Chaytor S et al. 2015. Health and climate change: Policy responses to protect public health. *Lancet* 386 (10006): 1861–1914.

What's Your Impact? 2017. Mean sources of methane emissions. http://whatsyourimpact.org /greenhouse-gases/methane-emissions#footnote1_bfom592 (accessed June 10, 2017).

Wilson N, Nghiem N, Mhurchu CN, Eyles H, Baker MG, Blakely T. 2013. Foods and dietary patterns that are healthy, low-cost and environmentally sustainable: A case study of optimization modelling for New Zealand. *PLoS One* 8 (3): 1–10.

Worldometers. 2017. Current world population. http://www.worldometers.info/world -population/ (accessed June 10, 2017).

World Preservation Foundation. 2013. Biodiversity in planetary ecosystems: Life on earth as we know it. https://news.godsdirectcontact.net/why-a-vegan-diet-is-the-best-solution -for-halting-biodiversitly-loss/ (accessed June 13, 2017).

3 The Sustainability of Vegetarian Diets

Joan Sabaté and Tony Jehi

CONTENTS

SUMMARY

This chapter defines sustainable diets and compares the production of animal and plant foods in terms of efficiency and environmental impacts. From a review of the literature, it is concluded that the production of meat protein is less energy efficient than that of plant protein, as it requires much more fossil fuel, water, and land. The chapter also discusses the environmental impacts of food on pollution, biodiversity, and climate change. Relative to plant protein production, animal protein production has a greater detrimental effect on the environment. Research suggests that switching from an animal-based diet to a plant-based diet could significantly attenuate the environment costs and greenhouse gas (GHG) emissions.

3.1 INTRODUCTION

People believed that our planet had inexhaustible physical resources and was able to endlessly satisfy the growing needs of the human population. However, this assumption has been shown to be false, as humans rely on nonrenewable energy sources to perform daily activities and to fuel the transportation, food, and pharmaceutical industries. Almost every human task relies on fossil fuels and disrupts the ecological balance. This increased adoption of nonrenewable resources comes with a price. The impacts are causing irreversible outcomes and contributing to environmental change.

By the year 2050, the world population is anticipated to reach 9 billion (U.S. Census Bureau, 2017), requiring more food to feed the additional 2 billion people. However, there are major problems in the current food system as the energy required to produce food exceeds that acquired from it. This signifies that our current diets are not sustainable and that there is a pressing need to find an alternative dietary lifestyle.

This chapter describes the current food system production patterns to understand whether they are sustainable. It also compares the production of animal and plant foods in terms of efficiency and environmental impacts. Finally, it evaluates the environmental impacts of vegetarian diets in comparison with meat-based diets.

3.1.1 WHAT ARE SUSTAINABLE DIETS?

The World Commission on Environment and Development defined sustainability as the efficiency to satisfy the needs of the present without causing deleterious repercussions that would sabotage the future; thus, it is the ability to foster a prosperous present while conquering three global concerns (poverty, global environmental deterioration, and rapid population growth) that would impact the future (Langhelle, 2000). However, the meaning of sustainability could be interpreted disparately based on the different economic, ecologic, or societal sectors; for instance, consumers define it differently than farmers or food manufacturers (Sabaté and Soret, 2014).

In 2010, the Food and Agriculture Organization (FAO) defined sustainable diets as "those diets with low environmental impacts which contribute to food and nutrition security and to healthy life for present and future generations. Sustainable diets are protective and respectful of biodiversity and ecosystems, culturally acceptable, accessible, economically fair and affordable; nutritionally adequate, safe and healthy; while optimizing natural and human resources page 7" (Burlingame and Dernini, 2012).

This chapter focuses on environmental sustainability and its two dimensions: efficiency and environmental protection. Efficiency is assessed by the ratio of outputs to inputs. In the production of foods, the inputs represent the natural resources utilized, and the outputs comprise the foods. As for the environmental protection dimension, it represents the perpetuation of ecological systems that allow life on the biosphere and is assessed by measuring the different environmental indicators, such as global warming potential, biodiversity, and eutrophication. When assessing the environmental sustainability of any diet, we will measure these dimensions not only in the production of the foods that compose the diets, but also in the processing, packaging, transportation, preparation, and disposing of these foods.

3.1.2 ARE CURRENT FOOD PRODUCTION PATTERNS SUSTAINABLE?

For thousands of years, traditional agriculture was based on a variety of crops and animals on the same farm. The efficiency of these farms was high since foods were produced with low inputs comprised solely of solar energy, rainwater, and animal wastes used as fertilizers (Altieri, 2004). Thus, agriculture during that era fell under the definition of sustainability (Sabaté and Soret, 2014). However, the last century witnessed a drastic change in agricultural and husbandry practices, with industrialism altering the form of farms as they became a monoculture enterprise that physically separated crops and animals. Nowadays, single farms are built to produce single food items (Horrigan et al., 2002). These specialized farms are much larger in size. The input provision stages, along with production and processing, are closely organized and controlled through shared ownership of assets and formal contracts. The main stimulator for these structural alterations in agriculture was the financial benefits and the augmented demand for meat. These changes contributed to drastic increases in productivity level but not in efficiency (MacDonald and McBride, 2009). Industrialized farms are relying on nonrenewable fuel to power the tractors and other agricultural machinery and electricity to power animal farms. Thus, from the energy perspective, the current food production system is highly inefficient.

Traditional agriculture was much more energy efficient, as more energy was obtained from food than used to produce it. One farmer was able to feed his entire family by relying on his labor and the energy provided by nature. Currently, the reliance of industrial agriculture on fossil fuel energy contributes to a decreased ratio of energy outputs from the food to nonrenewable energy inputs (Steinhart and Steinhart, 1974). This imbalance of energy ratio is magnified when taking into consideration other components of the food system. On-farm production amounts to 20% of the total food system energy usage (40% of it is the energy that goes into making chemical fertilizers and pesticides). Large amounts of energy go into food processing (16%), transportation (14%), packaging (7%), retail and restaurants (10%), and household storage and preparation (32%), of the total food system energy usage. For every 10.3 quads of the total energy used to produce food, only 1.4 quads of food energy is created, yielding an overall energy efficiency ratio of <1:7 (Center for Sustainable Systems, 2016).

Thus, the current food system uses much more energy than it gives back in food energy. From the energy perspective, the industrial food system is very inefficient (Horrigan et al., 2002).

3.2 ENVIRONMENTAL INDICATORS: COMPARING ANIMAL VERSUS PLANT FOODS

Diets or food patterns are composed of foods in different forms and proportions. This section focuses on the assessment of animal and plant foods in order to understand their efficiency and environmental impacts of their production.

3.2.1 EFFICIENCY

Raising animals for human food is intrinsically an inefficient process. As we move up in the trophic chain, there is a progressive loss of energy. Moreover, modern husbandry (animal farms) is based on intensive feeding of grain crops to animals. These grains could be a source of food for humans instead. The same standards apply to the production of other animal products, such as dairy.

The following sections assess the efficiency of producing animal foods (meats and animal products) versus plant foods for human consumption in relation to fossil fuel requirement, water use, and land use.

3.2.1.1   Fossil Fuel Use

In order to raise livestock, much fossil energy is utilized. As depicted in Table 3.1, the animal foods vary regarding energy requirements, with broiler chicken production being the most efficient; the latter requires an input of 4 kcal of fossil energy to yield 1 kcal of protein. However, when it comes to beef and lamb production, the ratio is much higher. This is due to the reliance on grains for feeding animals. The mean of fossil energy for all animal protein production systems required to yield 1 kcal of protein is 25 kcal; this is 11 times greater than that for plant protein, which utilizes only 2.2 kcal of fossil energy to generate 1 kcal of protein (Pimentel and Pimentel, 2003). Table 3.1 also displays the amounts of grains fed to animals relative to the meat yield: 13 kg of grain is required to produce just 1 kg of beef.

We previously conducted a study for the purpose of assessing the resource efficiency and environmental repercussions of generating 1 kg of edible protein from two plant (beans and almonds) and three animal (eggs, chicken, and beef) protein sources. We collected primary data and applied them to commodity production statistics (Sabaté et al., 2015). Table 3.2 and Figure 3.1 display the results of the study. Producing 1 kg of bean protein requires 0.3 L of fuel; 1 kg of almond, egg, or chicken protein uses double this amount of fuel, while 1 kg of beef requires 2.7 L of fuel. Thus, relative to beans, the production of beef protein utilizes around nine times more fuel.

3.2.1.2   Water Use

In the United States, agriculture uses freshwater in levels exceeding any other activity (Pimentel et al., 1997). Only 1.3% of that water is directly utilized by livestock to satisfy their cooling, drinking, and cleaning requirements (Hoekstra, 2009). When adding the water required to grow foods for the feeding of the livestock animals, the number is augmented drastically.

The animals consume foods such as hay and different types of grains. Around 1000 and 1350 L of water are needed for the production of 1 kg of hay and grain,

---

TABLE 3.1
Ratio of Different Inputs to Animal Outputs in U.S. Husbandry Practices

	Fossil Fuel Energy: Protein Energy	Grain Fed: Meat Produced
Beef	40:1	13:1
Eggs	39:1	11:1
Pork	14:1	5.9:1
Milk	14:1	–
Turkeys	10:1	3.8:1
Chickens	4:1	2.3:1

Source: Pimentel D and Pimentel M, *Am J Clin Nutr* 78 (3):660S–63S, 2003.

TABLE 3.2
Inputs and Animal Waste Generated to Produce 1 kg of Protein from Each Commodity

	Kidney Beans	Almonds	Eggs	Chicken	Beef
Food Yields					
Raw weight from farms (kg)	4.12	4.75	8.00	9.72	13.15
Raw weight from retailers (kg)	4.12	4.75	8.00	6.42	5.40
Cooked weight (kg)	10.95	4.75	8.00	4.17	3.40
Protein (kg)	1	1	1	1	1
Environmental Factors					
Land (m²)	15.5	21.2	37.6[a]	32.2[a]	282.6[a]
Water (m³)	10.4	23.3	11.1[b]	13.5[b]	109.0[b]
Fuel[c] (L)	0.3	0.6	0.6	0.7	2.7
Fertilizer[d] (g)	160.5	426.0	263.6	320.3	1945.1
Pesticide (g)	8.9	103.6	12.7	15.5	93.0
Animal waste (kg)	–	–	17.1	21.8	105.1

Source: Sabaté J et al., *Public Health Nutr* 18 (11):2067–73, 2015. With permission.
[a] Land used for raising animals and growing animal feed.
[b] Water used for raising animals and growing animal feed.
[c] Total fuel includes gasoline and diesel used on the farm for agricultural and livestock production.
[d] Total fertilizer includes nitrogen, phosphorous, and potassium.

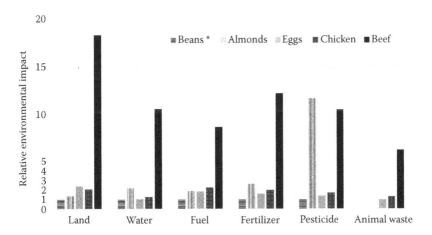

FIGURE 3.1 Relative environmental impacts to produce protein from plants and animals. Beans* has the reference value 1. (Elaborated from data in Sabaté J et al., *Public Health Nutr* 18 (11):2067–73, 2015. With permission.)

respectively (Thomas, 1987). Producing 1 kg of fresh beef requires 13 kg of grain and 30 kg of hay (Pimentel, 1980). Thus, compared with grain protein, the production of animal protein requires much more water (Pimentel and Pimentel, 1996).

Our study shows that producing 1 kg of protein from beef requires 109 m^3 of water, while 1 kg of protein from almonds and kidney beans requires 23 and 10 m^3 of water, respectively. Thus, beef protein requires more than 10 times the amount of water than bean protein (Figure 3.1). As for chicken and eggs, they require less water (14 and 11 m^3, respectively) than beef to produce 1 kg of protein (Table 3.2) (Sabaté et al., 2015).

3.2.1.3 Land Use

On a global basis, the livestock sector utilizes approximately 3900 million ha of land, which represents more than three-quarters of all agricultural land. Most of this land is used as grazing-based ruminant systems, which provide modest quantities of food and edible energy for humankind (Herrero et al., 2015). This abuse of land has not come without repercussions. In the United States, it is estimated that 60% of pastureland suffers from accelerated erosion and overgrazing. As discussed in a later section, livestock production is a chief contributor to soil erosion and land degradation (Pimentel and Kounang, 1998).

In our study, we compared the land requirement in square meters needed to produce 1 kg of protein between different commodities. Producing 1 kg of protein from beef requires 283 m^2 of land utilized to raise animals and grow animal feed. To produce 1 kg of protein from almonds and kidney beans, 21 and 16 m^2 of land are required, respectively (Table 3.2) (Sabaté et al., 2015). Thus, generating 1 kg of beef protein needs more than 18 times the area of land than does generating 1 kg of bean protein. As for producing 1 kg of protein from eggs and chicken, more than twice the area of land is required than for kidney beans (Figure 3.2).

3.2.2 Environmental Protection

This section compares the differential protection and degradation impacts of producing plant foods and meats on the environment. We consider the effects of the foods' impact on pollution (waste generation, chemical fertilizer use, and pesticide use), biodiversity, and climate change.

3.2.2.1 Pollution

3.2.2.1.1 Waste Generation

Producing meat is a major contributor to waste generation, which impacts the environment. In the United States, 7 billion livestock produce 130 times more waste than that generated by 300 million human beings (U.S. General Accounting Office, 1999). The majority of this waste remains untreated (Steinfeld et al., 2006), leading to damaging effects on the environment and polluting the water, soil, and air (Delgado et al., 2001). The World Health Organization (WHO) and the U.S. Department of Agriculture described the seriousness of this issue by stating that the augmented levels of phosphorus, potassium, and nitrogen, along with minute

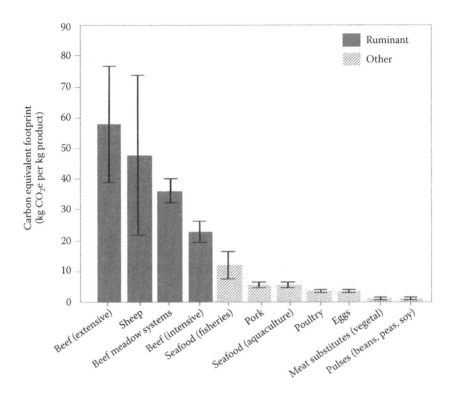

FIGURE 3.2 GHG emissions from protein-rich foods. (From Ripple WJ et al., *Nat Clim Change* 4 (1):2–5, 2014. With permission.)

concentrations of antibiotics and metals, represent a critical public health concern (Pimentel, 1999; U.S. General Accounting Office, 1999; Delgado et al., 2001; Steinfeld et al., 2006).

Livestock wastes generate gases that have local and global impacts. Locally, nuisance odors are produced due to ammonia (Delgado et al., 2001). The conversion of substantial food amounts into reactive nitrogen products, like ammonia from manure, is a chief contributor to aquatic and terrestrial pollution. Sutton and Dibb (2013) concluded that livestock production is accountable for about one-third of global biodiversity loss; 50% of UK food greenhouse gas (GHG) emissions are attributed to meat consumption, and it costs £1.28 billion to the National Health Service in early deaths associated with high meat intake.

Moreover, gases such as methane, carbon, and nitrous oxide have global impacts and have been associated with the global change phenomenon (Delgado et al., 2001; Horrigan et al., 2002; Eshel and Martin, 2006; Steinfeld et al., 2006).

When quantifying the level of waste production among different meat products, we found that producing 1 kg of protein from beef generates 105 kg of animal wastes, while producing 1 kg of protein from chicken and eggs yields 22 and 17 kg of animal wastes, respectively (Table 3.2). Thus, beef protein generates more than six times the amount of wastes than egg protein (Figure 3.1).

3.2.2.1.2 Chemical Fertilizer Use

In order to satisfy the feeding needs of the livestock sector, and because of the reduced natural fertility of the soil in the United States, chemical fertilizers have been excessively applied over the past six decades (Pimentel and Pimentel, 1983). This excessive use and reliance on fertilizers (nitrogen, potassium, and phosphate) that are synthesized from nonrenewable resources (Viglizzo et al., 2003) has produced serious outcomes, like air pollution (Cowling et al., 2001), groundwater contamination (Baroni et al., 2007), and an attenuation in biodiversity (Mineau and McLaughlin, 1996). For instance, the impacts of nitrogen accumulation in water include "red tides" in estuaries and "alga blooms" in lakes (Zhu and Chen, 2002).

Animal protein production requires large amounts of fertilizer. The production of 1 kg of protein from beef requires 1945 g of fertilizer, while producing 1 kg of protein from kidney beans requires 161 g of fertilizer (Table 3.2) (Sabaté et al., 2015), or 9.3% the amount of fertilizer required for beef production (Figure 3.1). Producing chicken protein requires lower amounts of fertilizers relative to beef. One kilogram of protein from chicken requires 320 g of fertilizers (Table 3.2), which is double the amount required for bean protein (Figure 3.1).

Copper is used in fertilizer and is utilized as a feed additive. Producing meat protein causes the emission of this trace element at a rate that is 100 times greater than that from plant protein production (Reijnders, 2001). This produces soil pollution, along with damaging effects on animals and certain plants (Lepp, 1981). Moreover, the use of phosphate rock through feed additives and synthetic fertilizers has had a damaging impact on the environment's biodiversity (Tilman et al., 2001). Producing meat protein requires seven times more phosphate rock than that utilized for soy-based vegetable protein (Reijnders, 2001).

3.2.2.1.3 Pesticide Use

Pesticide is defined by the Environmental Protection Agency (EPA) as a substance or a group of substances utilized for the purpose of pest prevention, annihilation, repellence, or mitigation (U.S. Environmental Protection Agency, 2017a). Fungicides, herbicides, and insecticides are all examples of pesticides (U.S. Environmental Protection Agency, 2017b).

The end of the twentieth century witnessed a drastic increase in the application of pesticides, with almost 2.5 million tons annually applied to crops (Paoletti and Pimentel, 2000). Their utilization has increased by 33-fold in the past 70 years (Pimentel et al., 1992).

The repercussions of this intensive application are not easily assessed and include augmented pest resistance (Pimentel et al., 1993; Foster et al., 1998), ground and surface water contamination (Levitan et al., 1995), bioamplification (Foster et al., 1998), and worker safety issues (Kishi and Ladou, 2001).

Producing animal foods requires much higher amounts of pesticides relative to plant foods. For instance, meat protein requires much more biocides (six times higher) than soybean protein (Reijnders, 2001). Biocides are utilized as disinfectants and pesticides on crops and are also applied in the animal husbandry sector; these pesticides pose a detrimental threat on the environment (Reijnders, 2001; Tilman et al., 2001).

Our study showed that producing 1 kg of protein from beef requires 93 g of pesticides, while producing 1 kg of protein from beans needs only 9 g of pesticides (Table 3.2) (Sabaté et al., 2015). Hence, generating 1 kg of beef protein requires more than 10 times the amount of pesticides than does generating 1 kg of bean protein (Figure 3.1).

3.2.2.2 Biodiversity

The change in land use presents the greatest immediate threat to biodiversity. This change is occurring due to the expansion of the livestock industry, which is considered to be a chief factor behind land degradation. Thus, the progressive expansion and growth of livestock production is associated with devastating concomitants (Steinfeld et al., 1998). A report by the FAO of the United Nations considered the livestock industry to be the principal anthropogenic utilizer of agricultural land (70%) and the land surface (30%) on the biosphere (Steinfeld et al., 2006).

Feeding animals requires grazing, which by itself is a threat to nature's ecosystems (Meehan and Platts, 1978). It contributes to large amounts of fine sediments that alter the aquatic communities' structure and attenuate biotic activity (Saunders and Smith, 1962) by contributing to a decreased productivity and water permeability of channel material utilized by fish to deposit eggs (McNeil and Ahnell, 1964; Cooper, 1965).

Other environmental impacts include the serious alterations in the ecosystems, desertification, deforestation, the dominance of woody plants over herbaceous plants, soil erosion or compaction, and the sedimentation of wetlands, coastal areas, and waterways (Uri and Lewis, 1998; Asner et al., 2004; Steinfeld et al., 2006), along with the expansion and propagation of invasive plants and animals (Gilchrist, 2005).

Another noteworthy effect of the livestock industry is increased deforestation. This has been progressively occurring mostly in wet tropic areas, resulting from the growth of pasture in forests and woodlands and the felling of trees to expand areas dedicated for livestock production (Reid et al., 2013). Currently, the main reason behind deforestation is planting crops (like soybeans) for the purpose of providing feed for cattle and sheep (Hecht, 2005). The places where this has been frequently occurring include Latin America (Amazon and other areas, like Cerrado Savanna woodlands and Pantanal), Asia, and Africa (Seidl et al., 2001).

The repercussions of destroying tropical rain forest are not inconsequential. Half of the world's species inhabit these areas that form just 7% of the planet's surface (Myers, 1988a, 1988b). Thus, even a minor land deforestation could destroy a vast number of species due to the high number or unit area. It is even estimated that thousands are demolished annually in these areas due to deforestation (Henderson-Sellers et al., 1988).

In order to perpetuate forest openings, farmers progressively create fires; the problems associated with such an action include the drought of the adjacent forests and their augmented susceptibility to develop second fires that usually have higher intensity (Cochrane et al., 1999). These fire storms are another chief factor for the destruction of species and for the expansion of exotic weeds (Cochrane and Schulze, 1998).

Nevertheless, there are other impacts of livestock and deforestation on biodiversity that are indirect and relatively less clear than those mentioned above.

These comprise the effects on genes, species, and populations (Reid et al., 2013). For instance, deforestation alters the habitats of many species, making them vulnerable to extinction due to their inability to adjust to the new environment (Vesk and Westoby, 2001). Another indirect impact is exerted through climate change; deforestation is a contributor to the latter, which in return highly affects biodiversity (Shukla et al., 1990; Gorte and Sheikh, 2010).

3.2.2.3   Climate Change

The global food system is considered a chief cause of climate change (Eshel and Martin, 2009; Garnett, 2011). Agriculture contributes to 20% of total anthropogenic GHG emissions, and the other constituents of the food system add 9% more, reaching a total global aggregate of the food sector of 29% of these emissions (Vermeulen et al., 2012). Climate change impacts the ability to progressively attain sufficient quantities of nutritious foods, thus affecting food security (Schmidhuber and Tubiello, 2007).

GHG emissions are strongly associated with the dietary choices adopted (Steinfeld et al., 2006). What it takes to produce a kilogram of meat or grains, including land use (Pimentel and Kounang, 1998), water use (Pimentel and Pimentel, 1996), deforestation (Reid et al., 2013), waste production (U.S. General Accounting Office, 1999), and packaging, is related to these emissions. Two distinct food items could have similar health impacts yet a wide variation in environmental and climate change effects due to the differences in the processes required to produce, manufacture, and even deliver them to the public.

Figure 3.2 compares GHG emissions from different protein-rich foods. It shows that ruminant meats have the highest emission levels, with extensive beef (based on grazing) contributing to the most elevated emissions. On the other hand, protein foods like meat substitutes and pulses led to the least GHG emissions.

The industrialization of agriculture led to negative repercussions on the environment and contributed to climate change. The main factor behind this is the livestock industry, which is considered, in the United States, to be the chief contributor of GHG emissions such as carbon dioxide, nitrous oxide, methane, and ammonia (Steinfeld et al., 2006). The gasoline and diesel used to fuel farm equipment (tractors, irrigating pumps, etc.) cause high emissions of carbon dioxide.

Moreover, microbes in the livestock's digestive system ferment feed. The methane produced is emitted by the exhaling and belching of the animal (Steinfeld et al., 2006). Methane is also produced when the manure that is stored as liquid in lagoons and ponds is anaerobically decomposed. This major GHG represents one-tenth of all U.S. GHG emissions. Methane possesses 23 times the potency of carbon dioxide even though it has a smaller residence time (Armor, 1995). It is estimated that animal agriculture is accountable for the production of 100 million tons of methane annually. With the progressive increase in demand and consumption rate of meat (fivefold augmentation in worldwide meat intake the past five decades), methane emissions are expected to further increase (Mohr, 2005; Yusuf et al., 2012).

As for nitrous oxide, it is produced mainly through microbial processes of nitrification and denitrification; the main source of this gas is nitrogen-based fertilizers used to grow animal feed (Defra, 2011). Nitrous oxide has 286 times the global warming potential of carbon dioxide and stays in the atmosphere for around

114 years. Ammonia, another GHG, is released to the environment through the urine of livestock. Other than contributing to climate change, this gas is also a precursor of fine particulate matter (PM2.5) that impacts human health (Schlesinger, 2007).

The reduction the level of GHGs is imperative in order to combat the global warming phenomenon. For instance, attenuating methane levels might be one of the most potent factors for preventing further climate change from happening. Reducing the intake of meat would yield an effective decline in methane emissions. Thus, by switching to meatless diets, one of the main sources of global warming could be highly attenuated, leading in return to a reduction in climate change (Mohr, 2005).

3.3   SUSTAINABILITY OF VEGETARIAN DIETS

Vegetarian diets exclude meats and sometimes other animal products, such as dairy and eggs. Since the production of plant foods compared with animal foods uses less resources and has less negative environmental impacts, it could be inferred that vegetarian diets are more sustainable than meat-based diets. However, not all vegetarians consume foods in the same proportions. For instance, the adoption of a diet rich in dairy products, such as some lacto-vegetarian diets, might be less sustainable than diets that include low amounts of meat. This section focuses on the differential environmental impacts of vegetarian versus animal-based diets as consumed by free-living individuals. It considers the effects of whole diets rather than specific food items. Most of the research in the area has been related to GHG emissions, with less attention to the use of resources.

One study measured the environmental impacts of different dietary patterns among California Adventists' participants in the Adventist Health Study cohort. Using California state agricultural data and state commodity production statistics, comparisons were made on the environmental effects to produce the different foods of a vegetarian diet versus nonvegetarian diet (Marlow et al., 2009). Results showed that for the combined differential production of 11 food items for which consumption differs among vegetarians and nonvegetarians, the nonvegetarian diet required 2.9 times more water, 2.5 times more primary energy, 13 times more fertilizer, and 1.4 times more pesticides than did the vegetarian diet (Marlow et al., 2009). In a subsequent publication, the researchers showed that the average diet containing animal products required on a weekly basis an additional 10,252 L of water, 9,910 kJ of energy, 186 g of fertilizer, and 6 g of pesticides in comparison with the vegetarian diet. The greatest contribution to the difference between these two diets came from the consumption of animal products, particularly beef. The researchers concluded that a nonvegetarian diet exerts a higher cost on the environment than a vegetarian diet (Marlow et al., 2014).

A UK study with subjects of the EPIC-Oxford cohort evaluated and compared the dietary GHG emissions embodied in the production of different types of diets. The mean of GHG emissions was highest for meat eaters and lowest for vegans. Specifically, the GHG emissions in kilograms of carbon dioxide equivalents per day (kg CO_2e/day) for the different dietary patterns were 7.19 for high meat eaters, 5.63 for medium meat eaters, 4.67 for low meat eaters, 3.91 for fish eaters, 3.81 for vegetarians, and 2.89 for vegans. Thus, the GHG emissions for the total diets of high meat consumers were double those for vegans. The authors concluded that switching to vegan diets can contribute to an attenuation of these emissions (Scarborough et al., 2014).

Moreover, using data from 73,308 participants of the Adventist Health Study-2, researchers compared the differential impacts of several dietary patterns on GHG emissions (Soret et al., 2014). The investigators strived to characterize the differential global warming effects of three dietary patterns (vegetarian, semivegetarian, and nonvegetarian) that varied in the quantity of animal and plant foods. In order to accomplish that, the GHG emissions of 210 foods, from the food frequency questionnaire, were calculated through life cycle assessments and using published data. For the nonvegetarian diets, the energy contribution from meats and plant foods was 6.5% and 77%, respectively. As for the semivegetarian diet and the vegetarian diet, they contributed 1% and 88%, and 0% and 91% of energy, respectively. The mean annual GHG emissions were 1113 kg CO_2e for nonvegetarians, 872 kg CO_2e for semivegetarians, and 788 kg CO_2e for vegetarians. Compared with the nonvegetarian diet, the semivegetarian diet had a 21.6% reduction and the vegetarian diet a 29.2% reduction in total GHG emissions. The relative food group contribution to GHG emissions for the three dietary patterns is shown in Figure 3.3. As expected, the overall pattern of food emissions reflected the underlying differential consumption of meats and plant foods. The proportional contribution to GHG emissions from dairy and eggs and other foods was similar among the three diets (Soret et al., 2014).

Other investigations have also reported differential GHG emissions of plant-based diets compared with meat-based diets. A number of reports have estimated the GHG

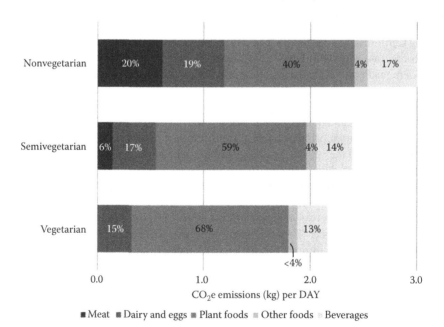

FIGURE 3.3 GHG emission (kg CO_2e/day) comparison between different food groups and dietary patterns, adjusted to 2000 kcal. CO_2e, carbon dioxide equivalent emissions. (From Soret S et al., *Am J Clin Nutr* 100 (Suppl. 1):490S–95S, 2014. With permission.)

emission reductions at the global level by the adoption of different types of plant-based diets in comparison with meat-based diets. Hedenus et al. (2014) portrayed an attenuation in food-associated GHG emissions of 3.4–5.2 $GtCO_2$-eq (CO_2 warming equivalents expressed in grams [g] or gigatonnes [Gt] of CO_2 carbon equivalents) by the year 2050 when switching to a diet that is composed of less meat and more cereals and pulses. Moreover, others estimated an attenuation of 4.2–8.4 $GtCO_2$-eq in the year 2050 if Mediterranean, pescetarian, or vegetarian diets were followed, with the latter having the most potent impact on the reductions (Tilman and Clark, 2014). An attenuation of 5.8–6.4 $GtCO_2$-eq in the year 2050 could be anticipated if the dietary alterations are followed on a global scale (Bajželj et al., 2014). Springmann et al. (2016) projected that switching to diets lower in meat would reduce the emissions by 3.3–8.0 $GtCO_2$-eq (compared with emissions in 2005–2007). This estimation is likely to underestimate the actual change, as the beneficial impact of a decreased deforestation rate is not taken into account.

3.4 CONCLUSION

Plant-based diets are more sustainable than meat-based diets, as they are more energy efficient, require less natural resources, and have less impact on the environment. The anticipated increase in the world's population and the expected increase in the demand for meat represent a major concern that could impact food sustainability and security. A dietary transition to a plant-based diet could diminish this possibility. Adopting a healthy vegetarian diet that is environmentally friendly and energy efficient would be a desirable goal.

Agricultural and nutritional policies that pave the way for a worldwide transition toward meatless diets, besides the environmental benefits, will also improve the health, food supply, and social justice outcomes for the global population. The implementation of such policies is not an easy process; it is rife with political obstacles but is probably the most rational, safe, science-based, and moral track for reaching a sustainable future for the human race.

REFERENCES

Altieri MA. 2004. Linking ecologists and traditional farmers in the search for sustainable agriculture. *Front Ecol Environ* 2 (1):35–42.

Armor JN. 1995. Emissions of greenhouse gases in the United States. *Appl Catal B* 6 (1):N2.

Asner GP, Elmore AJ, Olander LP, Martin RE, Harris AT. 2004. Grazing systems, ecosystem responses, and global change. *Annu Rev Environ Resour* 29:261–99.

Bajželj B, Richards KS, Allwood JM, Smith P, Dennis JS, Curmi E, Gilligan CA. 2014. Importance of food-demand management for climate mitigation. *Nat Clim Change* 4 (10):924–29.

Baroni L, Cenci L, Tettamanti M, Berati M. 2007. Evaluating the environmental impact of various dietary patterns combined with different food production systems. *Eur J Clin Nutr* 61 (2):279–86.

Burlingame B, Dernini S. 2012. Sustainable diets and biodiversity: Directions and solutions for policy, research and action. In *Proceedings of the International Scientific Symposium: Biodiversity and Sustainable Diets United against Hunger*, p7, Rome, November 3–5, 2010. Rome: Food and Agriculture Organization.

Center for Sustainable Systems, University of Michigan. 2016. U.S. food system factsheet. Publication no. CSS01-06. http://css.umich.edu/sites/default/files/css_doc/CSS01-06 .pdf.

Cochrane MA, Alencar A, Schulze MD, Souza CM, Nepstad DC, Lefebvre P, Davidson EA. 1999. Positive feedbacks in the fire dynamic of closed canopy tropical forests. *Science* 284 (5421):1832–35.

Cochrane MA, Schulze MD. 1998. Forest fires in the Brazilian Amazon. *Conserv Biol* 12 (5):948–50.

Cooper AC. 1965. The effect of transported stream sediments on the survival of sockeye and pink salmon eggs and alevin. New Westminster, BC: International Pacific Salmon Fisheries Commission.

Cowling E, Galloway J, Furiness C, Barber M, Bresser T, Cassman K, Erisman JW et al. 2001. Optimizing nitrogen management in food and energy production and environmental protection: Summary statement from the Second International Nitrogen Conference. *Scientific World Journal* 1:1–9.

Defra (Department for Environment, Food and Rural Affairs). 2011. *Agricultural Statistics and Climate Change.* 1st ed. London: Defra. http://www.defra.gov.uk/statistics /foodfarm/enviro/climate/.

Delgado C, Rosegrant M, Steinfeld H, Ehui S, Courbois C. 2001. Livestock to 2020: The next food revolution. *Outlook Agric* 30 (1):27–29.

Eshel G, Martin PA. 2006. Diet, energy, and global warming. *Earth Interact* 10 (9):1–17.

Eshel G, Martin PA. 2009. Geophysics and nutritional science: Toward a novel, unified paradigm. *Am J Clin Nutr* 89 (5):1710S–16S.

Foster V, Mourato S, Tinch R, Ozdemiroglu E, Pearce D. 1998. Incorporating external impacts in pest management choices. In *Bugs in the System: Redesigning the Pesticide Industry for Sustainable Agriculture*, 94. eds. W Vorley and D Keeney. Abingdon, UK: Routledge.

Garnett T. 2011. Where are the best opportunities for reducing greenhouse gas emissions in the food system (including the food chain)? *Food Policy* 36:S23–32.

Gilchrist P. 2005. Involvement of free-flying wild birds in the spread of the viruses of avian influenza, Newcastle disease and infectious bursal disease from poultry products to commercial poultry. *Worlds Poult Sci J* 61 (02):198–214.

Gorte RW, Sheikh PA. 2010. Deforestation and climate change. Washington, DC: Congressional Research Service.

Hecht SB. 2005. Soybeans, development and conservation on the Amazon frontier. *Dev Change* 36 (2):375–404.

Hedenus F, Wirsenius S, Johansson DJA. 2014. The importance of reduced meat and dairy consumption for meeting stringent climate change targets. *Clim Change* 124 (1–2):79–91.

Henderson-Sellers A, Dickinson RE, Wilson MF. 1988. Tropical deforestation: Important processes for climate models. *Clim Change* 13 (1):43–67.

Herrero M, Wirsenius S, Henderson B, Rigolot C, Thornton P, Havlík P, De Boer I, Gerber PJ. 2015. Livestock and the environment: What have we learned in the past decade? *Annu Rev Environ* 40:177–202.

Hoekstra AY. 2009. Human appropriation of natural capital: A comparison of ecological footprint and water footprint analysis. *Ecol Econ* 68 (7):1963–74.

Horrigan L, Lawrence RS, Walker P. 2002. How sustainable agriculture can address the environmental and human health harms of industrial agriculture. *Environ Health Perspect* 110 (5):445.

Kishi M, Ladou J. 2001. International pesticide use. Introduction. *Int J Occup Environ* 7 (4):259.

Langhelle O. 2000. Sustainable development and social justice: Expanding the Rawlsian framework of global justice. *Environ Values* 9 (3):295–323.

Lepp NW. 1981. Copper. In *Effect of Heavy Metal Pollution on Plants*, 111–43. Berlin: Springer.

Levitan L, Merwin I, Kovach J. 1995. Assessing the relative environmental impacts of agricultural pesticides: The quest for a holistic method. *Agric Ecosyst Environ* 55 (3):153–68.

MacDonald JM, McBride WD. 2009. The transformation of US livestock agriculture scale, efficiency, and risks. *Econ Inf Bull* (43).

Marlow HJ, Harwatt H, Soret S, Sabaté J. 2014. Comparing the water, energy, pesticide and fertilizer usage for the production of foods consumed by different dietary types in California. *Public Health Nutr* 18 (13):2425–32.

Marlow HJ, Hayes WK, Soret S, Carter RL, Schwab ER, Sabaté J. 2009. Diet and the environment: Does what you eat matter? *Am J Clin Nutr* 89 (5):1699S–703S.

McNeil WJ, Ahnell WH. 1964. Success of pink salmon spawning relative to size of spawning bed materials. Washington, DC: U.S. Department of Interior, Fish and Wildlife Service.

Meehan WR, Platts WS. 1978. Livestock grazing and the aquatic environment. *J Soil Water Conserv* 33 (6):274–78.

Mineau P, McLaughlin A. 1996. Conservation of biodiversity within Canadian agricultural landscapes: Integrating habitat for wildlife. *J Agric Environ Ethics* 9 (2):93–113.

Mohr N. 2005. A new global warming strategy. EarthSave International Report. Chatsworth, CA: EarthSave International.

Myers N. 1988a. Tropical deforestation and climatic change. *Environ Conserv* 15 (04):293–98.

Myers N. 1988b. Tropical deforestation and remote sensing. *For Ecol Manage* 23 (2–3):215–25.

Paoletti MG, Pimentel D. 2000. Environmental risks of pesticides versus genetic engineering for agricultural pest control. *J Agric Environ Ethics* 12 (3):279–303.

Pimentel D. 1999. Environmental and economic benefits of sustainable agriculture. In *Sustainability in Question: The Search for a Conceptual Framework*, 153. Eds Kohn J, Gowdy J, Hinterberger F, and Van der Straaten J Edward Elgar; Cheltenham, UK.

Pimentel, D 1980. *Handbook of Energy Utilization in Agriculture*. Boca Raton, FL: CRC Press.

Pimentel D, Acquay H, Biltonen M, Rice P, Silva M, Nelson J, Lipner S, Giordano A, D'Amore M. 1992. Environmental and economic costs of pesticide use. *Bioscience* 42 (10):750–60.

Pimentel D, Houser J, Preiss E, White O, Fang H, Mesnick L, Barsky T, Tariche S, Schreck J, Alpert S. 1997. Water resources: Agriculture, the environment, and society. *Bioscience* 47:97–106.

Pimentel D, Kounang N. 1998. Ecology of soil erosion in ecosystems. *Ecosystems* 1 (5):416–26.

Pimentel D, McLaughlin L, Zepp A, Lakitan B, Kraus T, Kleinman P, Vancini F, Roach WJ, Graap E, Keeton WS, Selig G. 1993. Environmental and economic effects of reducing pesticide use in agriculture. *Agric Ecosyst Environ* 46 (1):273–88.

Pimentel D, Pimentel M. 1983. The future of American agriculture. In *Sustainable Food Systems*, ed. D Knorr, 3–27. Westport, CT: Avi Publishers.

Pimentel D, Pimentel M. 1996. *Food, Energy and Society*. Niwot: Colorado University Press.

Pimentel D, Pimentel M. 2003. Sustainability of meat-based and plant-based diets and the environment. *Am J Clin Nutr* 78 (3):660S–63S.

Reid SR, Bedelian C, Said MY, Kruska RL, Mauricio RM, Castel V, Olson J, Thornton PK. 2013. Global livestock impacts of biodiversity. In *Livestock in a Changing Landscape*: *Drivers, Consequences, and Responses*, 115. eds. H Steinfeld, HA Mooney, F Schneider, and LE Neville. Washington, DC: Island Press.

Reijnders L. 2001. Vegetarian nutrition. In *Environmental Impacts of Meat Production and Vegetarianism*, ed. J Sabate, 441–62. Amsterdam: CRC Press.

Sabaté J, Soret S. 2014. Sustainability of plant-based diets: Back to the future. *Am J Clin Nutr* 100 (Suppl. 1):476S–82S.

Sabaté J, Sranacharoenpong K, Harwatt H, Wien M, Soret S. 2015. The environmental cost of protein food choices. *Public Health Nutr* 18 (11):2067–73.

Saunders JW, Smith MW. 1962. Physical alteration of stream habitat to improve brook trout production. *Trans Am Fish Soc* 91 (2):185–88.

Scarborough P, Appleby PN, Mizdrak A, Briggs ADM, Travis RC, Bradbury KE, Key TJ. 2014. Dietary greenhouse gas emissions of meat-eaters, fish-eaters, vegetarians and vegans in the UK. *Clim Change* 125 (2):179–92.

Schlesinger RB. 2007. The health impact of common inorganic components of fine particulate matter (PM2.5) in ambient air: A critical review. *Inhal Toxicol* 19 (10):811–32.

Schmidhuber J, Tubiello FN. 2007. Global food security under climate change. *Proc Natl Acad Sci U S A* 104 (50):19703–8.

Seidl AF, de Silva JSV, Moraes AS. 2001. Cattle ranching and deforestation in the Brazilian Pantanal. *Ecol Econ* 36 (3):413–25.

Shukla J, Nobre C, Sellers P. 1990. Amazon deforestation and climate change. *Science* 247 (4948):1322–25.

Soret S, Mejia A, Batech M, Jaceldo-Siegl K, Harwatt H, Sabaté J. 2014. Climate change mitigation and health effects of varied dietary patterns in real-life settings throughout North America. *Am J Clin Nutr* 100 (Suppl. 1):490S–95S.

Springmann M, Godfray HCJ, Rayner M, Scarborough P. 2016. Analysis and valuation of the health and climate change cobenefits of dietary change. *Proc Natl Acad Sci U S A* 113 (15):4146–51.

Steinfeld H, de Haan C, Blackburn H. 1998. Livestock and the environment, issues and options. In *Perspectives on Sustainable Development*, 283–301. ed. E Lutz. Washington, DC: European Commission Directorate-General for Development.

Steinfeld H, Gerber P, Wassenaar T, Castel V, Rosales M, De Haan C. 2006. *Livestock's Long Shadow: Environmental Issues and Options.* Rome: Food and Agriculture Organization.

Steinhart CE, Steinhart JS. 1974. *Energy: Sources, Use, and Role in Human Affairs.* North Scituate, MA: Duxbury Press.

Sutton C, Dibb S. 2013. Prime cuts: Valuing the meat we eat. England, UK: WWF-UK and Food Ethics Council.

Thomas GW. 1987. Water: Critical and evasive resource on semi-arid lands. In *Water and Water Policy in World Food Supplies*, ed. WR Jordan, 83–90. College Station: Texas A&M University Press.

Tilman D, Clark M. 2014. Global diets link environmental sustainability and human health. *Nature* 515 (7528):518–22.

Tilman D, Fargione J, Wolff B, D'Antonio C, Dobson A, Howarth R, Schindler D, Schlesinger WH, Simberloff D, Swackhamer D. 2001. Forecasting agriculturally driven global environmental change. *Science* 292 (5515):281–84.

Uri ND, Lewis JA. 1998. The dynamics of soil erosion in US agriculture. *Sci Total Environ* 218 (1):45–58.

U.S. Census Bureau. 2017. Total midyear population for the world: 1950–2050. International database. http://www.census.gov/population/international/data/idb/worldpoptotal.php (revised July 25, 2017).

U.S. Environmental Protection Agency 2017a. What is a Pesticide. Retrieved March, 2018 from https://www.epa.gov/minimum-risk-pesticides/what-pesticide.

U.S. Environmental Protection Agency 2017b. Types of Pesticide Ingredients. Retrieved March, 2018 from https://www.epa.gov/ingredients-used-pesticide-products/types-pesticide -ingredients.

U.S. General Accounting Office. 1999. Animal Agriculture Waste Management Practices. Pl. Washington, DC. Retrieved March, 2018 from https://www.gao.gov/archive/1999/rc99205.pdf.

Vermeulen SJ, Campbell BM, Ingram JSI. 2012. Climate change and food systems. *Annu Rev Environ* 37 (1):195.

Vesk PA, Westoby M. 2001. Predicting plant species' responses to grazing. *J Appl Ecol* 38 (5):897–909.

Viglizzo EF, Pordomingo AJ, Castro MG, Lértora FA. 2003. Environmental assessment of agriculture at a regional scale in the Pampas of Argentina. *Environ Monit Assess* 87 (2):169–95.

Yusuf R, Noor Z, Abba AH, Abu Hassan MA, Mohd Din MF. 2012. Greenhouse gas emissions: Quantifying methane emissions from livestock. *Am J Eng Appl Sci* 5 (1):1–8.

Zhu ZL, Chen DL. 2002. Nitrogen fertilizer use in China—Contributions to food production, impacts on the environment and best management strategies. *Nutr Cycl Agroecosyst* 63 (2–3):117–27.

Section II

Prevention of Chronic Diseases

4 Vegetarian Diet and Risk of Cardiovascular Disease

Ella H. Haddad

CONTENTS

SUMMARY

Evidence for the protective effect of vegetarian dietary patterns in the prevention and management of cardiovascular conditions is derived from multiple lines of research, including observational studies, prospective cohorts, and clinical trials. These benefits do not simply stem from foods avoided by vegetarians but more importantly from foods consumed by vegetarians. A heart-healthy vegetarian diet must include a variety of whole-grain cereals, legumes, vegetables, fruits, nuts, and seeds; limit refined products and added sugars; and avoid solid fats. This review addresses the potential benefits of plant foods on cardiovascular risk factors.

4.1   INTRODUCTION

Ever since the early 1950s, when Hardinge and Stare (1954) reported low blood cholesterol concentrations in individuals adhering to vegetarian diets, research on the cardiovascular benefits of vegetarian dietary practices has continued to generate relevant findings. The label *vegetarian* encompasses a heterogeneous group of dietary habits that range from eschewing all animal-derived foods (vegan) to including dairy and/or egg (lacto-ovo vegetarian) and fish (pesco-vegetarian) in the diet. In general, vegetarians avoid much of the dietary saturated fat found in animal foods and consume considerably higher quantities of cereal grains, legumes, vegetables, fruits, nuts, and seeds.

According to recent figures (Sacks et al., 2017), cardiovascular diseases are the leading global cause of death, accounting for 17.3 million, or 31%, of total global deaths in the year 2013. In the United States, the Centers for Disease Control estimates that diseases of the heart remain the primary cause of death and account for more than 610,000 deaths per year (Kochanek et al., 2016). In the past five decades, there have been age-adjusted declines in heart disease mortality, estimated at 55%–60%, but this decline has slowed (Jones and Greene, 2013) and efforts aimed at the prevention of this killer disease must continue.

Atherosclerotic cardiovascular disease (ASCVD), as defined by the American Heart Association/American College of Cardiology (AHA/ACA), includes coronary heart disease (CHD), heart attacks, peripheral vascular disease, and stroke. Dyslipidemia, particularly elevated blood concentrations of low-density lipoprotein cholesterol (LDL-C), is the underlying cause of the cardiovascular changes seen in these conditions. It is well established that current diets high in saturated fats are prime promoters of lipid abnormalities that lead to vascular changes and atherosclerosis (Mozaffarian et al., 2016). Atherosclerosis is a chronic inflammatory progressive disease that promotes narrowing of arteries due to the accumulation of macrophages filled with lipids. Pathological conditions, such as dyslipidemia, smoking, and high blood pressure, damage the endothelium, triggering endothelial permeability and activating it to express adhesion molecules. Various adhesion molecules bind monocytes and T-lymphocytes. These migrate into the intima of blood vessels, where they differentiate into macrophages. Oxidized lipoproteins extravasate through the leaky endothelium and are taken up by macrophages to form foam cells and subsequently atheromatous plaque. These lesions become cytotoxic, pro-inflammatory, and proliferative, leading to the progression of atherosclerotic lesions. Fatal events occur when thrombosis or ruptured and eroded plaques occur that occlude the blood vessels (Falk, 2006; Brown et al., 2017).

That dyslipidemia due largely to elevated blood concentrations of LDL-C is the major risk factor for ASCVD progression and mortality is well established. Also established is the fact that various dietary constituents modulate blood lipids and other risk factors. Saturated fat found in animal foods is the most potent dietary factor in raising LDL-C and the leading promoter of atherosclerosis (Sacks et al., 2017). The current AHA/ACA guideline for the prevention and management of heart disease is to reduce dietary saturated fat intake to 5% or 6% of kilocalories (Sacks et al., 2017). Such reductions cannot be obtained without dietary changes that involve major restrictions in the quantities of animal source foods. Vegetarian diets, with their emphasis on plants, provide an alternative healthier way of eating that incorporates not only reductions of dietary saturated fat but also a rich complement of protective components.

The purpose of this chapter is to review and discuss the scientific evidence related to the effect of vegetarian dietary practices on cardiovascular risk factors and on the prevention of atherosclerotic progression and its consequences. It focuses primarily on CHD, also known as ischemic heart disease (IHD), and addresses dietary influences on vascular changes involved in the atherosclerotic process.

4.2 CARDIOVASCULAR DISEASE RISK IN VEGETARIANS

Because vegetarian diets include more plant foods and exhibit a fatty acid profile lower in saturated fat than omnivore diets, there has been interest in how such dietary patterns influence cardiovascular risk factors. Decades of research have advanced our understanding of the benefits of vegetarian diets. The earlier studies were mostly cross-sectional and collected and analyzed data from small groups of representative individuals. Most, not all (Harman and Parnell, 1998), of these observational studies evaluating heart disease–related risk factors reported that plasma total cholesterol (total-C) concentrations are lower in vegetarians than in nonvegetarians (Hardinge and Stare, 1954; Sacks et al., 1975; Burslem et al., 1978; Fraser and Swannell, 1981). Lower blood lipids were shown in various ethnic groups of vegetarians, such as African Americans (Melby et al., 1994; Fraser et al., 2015), Hispanic Americans (Alexander et al., 1999), and Taiwanese women (Huang et al., 2014), to name a few. Compared with those who frequently consume meat and animal foods, individuals who adhere to vegetarian diets have lower body weight and body mass index (BMI) (Spencer et al., 2003), less type 2 diabetes (T2D) (Tonstad et al., 2009), and lower systolic blood pressure (Melby et al., 1994; Appleby et al., 2002).

In addition to observational findings of reduced ASCVD risk factors in vegetarians, considerable scientific evidence supports the cardiovascular advantages of plant-based diets. This evidence includes cohort studies, randomized controlled clinical trials (RCTs), systematic reviews, and meta-analyses, as well as medical case reports.

4.2.1 PROSPECTIVE COHORT STUDIES IN VEGETARIANS

Prospective cohort studies have provided valuable evidence of the protective effects of vegetarian diets in reducing cardiovascular disease mortality. The first cohort to report lower coronary disease mortality in vegetarians was the Seventh-day Adventists (SDAs) in California (Phillips et al., 1978) in the Adventist Mortality Study. Adventists are a conservative Christian denomination whose teachings emphasize healthful lifestyle practices as an important religious value and who promote adherence to vegetarian diets for spiritual and health reasons. The advantage of studying SDAs is the low incidence of confounding factors in the population, which, in addition to including many vegetarians, adheres to other healthful lifestyle practices, such as avoiding alcohol consumption, smoking, and illicit drug use. In the 6-year Adventist Mortality prospective study of approximately 24,000 California

SDAs, approximately one-half followed a lacto-ovo vegetarian diet. CHD mortality rates for ages 35–64 and 65+ were 28% and 50%, respectively, of the rates for the same age groups of the California population. The risk of fatal CHD among non-vegetarian males in the cohort's lower age group was almost three times greater than that of the vegetarian males.

Beginning in 1974–1976, the next cohort to enroll a large group of vegetarians was the Adventist Health Study-1 (AHS-1). Fraser (1999a) reported a 2.3-fold increased risk for fatal IHD in men who ate beef ≥3 times per week compared with vegetarian men. Also described in this study was a protective association between nut consumption and fatal and nonfatal IHD in both sexes. The risk of heart disease for subjects who ate nuts ≥5 times per week was 50% that of those who ate nuts <1 time per week.

Table 4.1 provides an overview of findings from selected Western prospective cohorts that have reported on CHD or IHD mortality according to vegetarian status and meat intake. Results from non-SDA Western cohorts that enrolled vegetarians are not entirely consistent. Some cohorts found a positive association between veg-etarian adherence and cardiovascular death rates and others did not. These discrep-ancies may be explained by the relatively small number of vegetarians in some of the cohorts and by the large variations in dietary and lifestyle practices of those who describe themselves as vegetarians that may not be limited to meat or animal food avoidance. For example, when analyzed separately, data obtained from studies on British vegetarians, such as the Health Food Shoppers Study, the Oxford Vegetarian Study, and the European Prospective Investigation into Cancer and Nutrition–Oxford (EPIC-Oxford), showed significant reductions in adjusted death rate ratios for overall mortality in vegetarians compared with omnivores, but reductions for IHD mortality were not significant (Key et al., 2003).

To obtain larger groups of vegetarians, combined analyses from two or more cohorts have been performed. Key et al. (1999) presented results from a combined analysis of five prospective cohort groups involving about 76,000 subjects from the United States, United Kingdom, and Germany. Death rates from IHD were 24% lower in vegetarians age <90 years ($p < 0.01$) and 45% lower in those age <65 years ($p < 0.05$) compared with regular meat eaters. The lower mortality from IHD in vegetarians was restricted to those who had followed the diet for >5 years, and there were no significant differences in mortality from cerebrovascular disease in this combined cohort. In a study of more than 44,000 participants of the EPIC-Oxford cohort who were followed for about 11.6 years, Crowe et al. (2013) reported that incident fatal and nonfatal IHD was 32% lower in vegetarians. A subsequent pooled analysis from the same group (Appleby et al., 2016) combined data on about 60,000 participants from two prospective studies, namely, the Oxford Vegetarian Study and EPIC-Oxford. Compared with regular meat eaters, vegetarians plus vegans showed reductions in death rates before age 90 for ischemic and cardiovascular causes, but the results were not significant.

The most recent Adventist Health Study-2 (AHS-2) recruited more than 95,000 par-ticipants from the United States and Canada. Orlich et al. (2013) reported on heart disease mortality from approximately 76,000 individuals who were followed for 5.8 years. In men, both IHD and cardiovascular disease death rates were 29% lower in vegetarians. Although risk ratios for these conditions were lower in vegetarian women,

TABLE 4.1

Overview of Selected Prospective Cohort Studies in Western Populations on Vegetarian Eating and Meat Intake and Cardiovascular Risk

Author (Date)	Name of Cohort (n)	Follow-Up (Years)	Comparison Variables	Results Hazard Ratio (95% CI)
Key et al. (1999)	Pooled analysis of five studies			Mortality
	Adventist Mortality (24,538)	5.6	Vegetarian vs. nonvegetarian	IHD 0.74 (0.63, 0.88)*
	Health Food Shopper (9,878)	18.4		IHD 0.97 (0.81, 1.16)
	AHS-1 (28,952)	11.1		IHD 0.62 (0.53, 0.73)*
	German Vegetarian (1,757)	9.9		IHD 0.45 (0.22, 0.95)
	Oxford Vegetarian (11,047)	13.7		IHD 0.90 (0.68, 1.20)
	Pooled results (76,172)	10.6		IHD 0.76 (0.62, 0.94)*
Orlich et al. (2013)	AHS-2 (73,308)	5.8	Vegetarian vs. nonvegetarian (men)	Mortality
				IHD 0.71 (0.51, 1.00)
				CVD 0.71 (0.57, 0.90)
			Vegetarian vs. nonvegetarian (women)	IHD 0.88 (0.65, 1.20)
				CVD 0.99 (0.83, 1.18)
Crowe et al. (2013)	EPIC-Oxford (44,561)	11.6	Vegetarian vs. nonvegetarian	Fatal and nonfatal
				IHD 0.68 (0.58–0.81)*
Appleby et al. (2016)	Pooled analysis of two studies (60,310)		Vegetarians plus vegans vs. regular meat eaters	Deaths before age 90
	Oxford Vegetarian Study			IHD 0.88 (0.70, 1.11)
	EPIC-Oxford			CVD 1.15 (0.87, 1.62)

(*Continued*)

TABLE 4.1 (CONTINUED)

Overview of Selected Prospective Cohort Studies in Western Populations on Vegetarian Eating and Meat Intake and Cardiovascular Risk

Author (Date)	Name of Cohort (n)	Follow-Up (Years)	Comparison Variables	Results Hazard Ratio (95% CI)
Sinha et al. (2009)	NIH-AARP Diet and Health Study (500,000)	10	Red meat intake (highest to lowest quintile)	Mortality
			Men	CVD 1.27 (1.20, 1.35)*
			Women	CVD 1.50 (1.37, 1.65)*
			Processed meat intake (highest to lowest quintile)	CVD 1.09 (1.03, 1.15)
			Men	CVD 1.38 (1.26, 1.51)*
			Women	
Pan et al. (2012a)	Pooled analysis of two studies (121,342) Health Professionals Follow-Up Study Nurses' Health Study	28	Red meat intake (1 serving/day increase) Processed meat intake (1 serving/day increase)	Mortality CVD 1.18 (1.13, 1.23) CVD 1.21 (1.13, 1.31)
Rohrmann et al. (2013)	EPIC-Europe (448,568)	12.7	Red meat intake (per 100 g/day) Processed meat intake (per 50 g/day)	Mortality CVD 1.09 (1.00, 1.18) CVD 1.30 (1.17, 1.45)*
Etemadi et al. (2017)	NIH-AARP Diet and Health Study (536,969)	16	Red meat intake (per 20 g/day increase)	Mortality CVD 1.13 (1.11, 1.15)*

Note: AARP = formerly American Association of Retired Persons; CVD = cardiovascular disease.
* Statistically significant $P < 0.05$.

they were not significant. Also, no significant associations with reduced ischemic or cardiovascular disease mortality were noted in the subcategories of vegetarian eating (vegan, lacto-ovo vegetarian, and pesco-vegetarian) when compared with nonvegetarians. One possible explanation may be that overall mortality in this cohort is low due to other healthy lifestyle habits of the group and the relatively short follow-up time. Other possible factors are the modest differences in lifestyle and in food and nutrient intake among the various dietary subgroups. Although some differences exist in the saturated fat, cholesterol, and fiber content of vegetarian diets compared with omnivore diets in the cohort, nonvegetarian Adventists on the whole consume substantially less meat, dairy, and eggs than the general U.S. population (Rizzo et al., 2013; Orlich et al., 2014). The average saturated fat intake of nonvegetarian AHS-2 participants is less than 10% of their kilocalories (Fraser, 2009). Health-conscious Adventists, whether vegetarian or not, consume little alcohol, avoid tobacco, and eat more whole grains, legumes, soy foods, vegetables, and fruits—all of which have benefits in reducing cardiovascular disease. Also, the study did not separately compute cardiovascular mortality in the younger age group of the cohort. In current medical practice, identification of cardiovascular risk factors in an individual generally leads to management of risk with statins and other medical procedures, which may attenuate dietary influences, and medical management is more likely to occur in older individuals.

Beneficial components of vegetarian diets vary across studies from diverse countries and sociocultural groups and are not always clearly identified. The only constant is the absence of meat, and examining the evidence linking meat intake to health outcomes can be valuable. Sinha et al. (2009) described results from the large prospective National Institutes of Health–AARP (NIH-AARP) Diet and Health Study in more than 500,000 participants. Comparing highest with lowest quintile of red meat intake, they found that rates of cardiovascular mortality were 27% higher in men and 50% higher in women. The quantity of red meat in the highest and lowest quintiles was approximately 4 ounces and <1 ounce, respectively, for a 2000 kcal/day diet. A follow-up study of the same cohort (Etemadi et al., 2017) calculated a 13% increase in cardiovascular death risk with every 20 g (0.7 ounce) intake of red meat per day. Comparable results were obtained by pooled analysis of two established Harvard University cohorts, the Health Professionals Follow-Up Study and the Nurses' Health Study (Pan et al., 2012a). Every one serving per day increase in unprocessed and processed red meat intake increased the risk of cardiovascular mortality by 18% and 21%, respectively. They estimated that 9.3% of deaths in men and 7.6% in women in their cohorts could be prevented if individuals had consumed fewer than 0.5 servings of red meat per day.

In general, prospective cohort studies show that CHD or IHD mortality rates are lower in vegetarians. Systematic reviews and meta-analyses corroborate the evidence that vegetarian dietary practices decrease cardiovascular risk and mortality. A recent meta-analysis showed that mortality from IHD was 29% lower in vegetarians than in omnivores (Huang et al., 2012). A potential weakness of cohort studies is in the accuracy and consistency of dietary intake assessment and quantification. In this regard, it is important to point out that studies with SDA vegetarians have documented the consistency and long-term reliability of dietary intake data (Singh et al., 2014; Teixeira Martins et al., 2015).

4.2.2 CLINICAL TRIALS IN VEGETARIANS

RCTs provide the most robust evidence for the benefits of vegetarian diets and are the cornerstone of evidence-based dietary guidelines for the control of modifiable risk conditions. A number of clinical trials have evaluated the effectiveness of vegetarian dietary interventions in reducing blood lipid concentrations and related cardiovascular risk factors. Table 4.2 provides an overview of the designs and results from a selected number of RCTs. Most of the trials were in free-living individuals, and participants exhibited good acceptance of and compliance with the vegetarian or vegan interventions. As shown in Table 4.2, these trials consistently reported reductions in total-C and LDL-C when individuals switched to vegetarian or vegan diets. The overall effect of the vegetarian diet on plasma lipid concentration varies and is dependent on the exact dietary pattern implemented, the length of the intervention, and the composition of the actual foods selected and consumed by participants, especially with respect to their content of saturated and unsaturated fatty acids.

Some unique features of the studies will be described in more detail. Barnard et al. (2000) evaluated a plant food low-fat vegan diet consisting of grains, vegetables, legumes, and fruits in premenopausal women with normal plasma lipid concentrations compared with the participants' customary diets. In 2 months, total-C, LDL-C, high-density lipoprotein cholesterol (HDL-C), and triglycerides decreased significantly, along with a significant reduction in body weight. Barnard et al. (2009) tested the same low-fat vegan diet in 99 obese individuals with T2D for 74 weeks. Participants assigned to the low-fat vegan diet compared with a diet based on the American Diabetes Association guidelines experienced substantially greater reductions in total-C and LDL.

Based on the fact that certain plant foods and their constituents possess considerable lipid-lowering properties, Jenkins et al. (2003) examined a vegetarian diet that included a portfolio of cholesterol-lowering foods. The portfolio foods included margarine fortified with plant sterols, plant protein, vegetables rich in soluble fibers (soybeans, oats, okra, and eggplant), and almonds. The portfolio diet was compared with a low-fat, lacto-ovo vegetarian diet and a low-fat lacto-ovo vegetarian diet plus statins. In 1 month, reductions in plasma LDL-C concentrations, as well as in the inflammatory biomarker C-reactive protein (CRP), on the portfolio diet were comparable to those obtained on the low-fat lacto-ovo vegetarian diet plus statins.

Vegetarian diets have also been shown to be effective in maintaining weight loss over time. A small RCT by Turner-McGrievy et al. (2007) demonstrated the efficacy of the vegan diet compared with conventional diets in long-term weight loss in postmenopausal women. After 1 year, participants showed a weight change of −4.9 kg versus −1.2 kg ($p = 0.02$), while at 2 years the weight change was −3.1 kg versus −0.8 kg ($p = 0.022$) on the vegan compared with the conventional diet, respectively.

The findings that vegetarian diets could effectively lower blood lipids have been substantiated by systematic reviews and meta-analysis studies (Ferdowsian and Barnard, 2009; Wang et al., 2015). Overall outcomes suggest that lacto-ovo vegetarian diets lower total-C or LDL-C by approximately 5%–10%, whereas exclusively plant diets lower lipids by 10%–20%. Plant diets with additional foods or modifications are effective in lowering lipids up to 30%, and greater reductions in dietary animal food consumption yield greater reductions in lipid levels.

TABLE 4.2
Overview of Selected Randomized Controlled Trials Evaluating the Effect of Vegetarian Diets on Risk Factors

Author (Year), Country	Treatment Diet	Control Diet	Participants[a]	Duration	Outcomes
Cooper et al. (1982), United States	LV (skim milk only)	Omnivore	$N = 15$ (5 F, 10 M) Age = 28 years Healthy weight	3 weeks	Treatment as percent change from control Total-C: ↓ 12.5% ($p < 0.05$) LDL-C: ↓ 14.7% ($p < 0.05$) Apolipoprotein B: ↓ 13.2% ($p < 0.05$)
Kestin et al. (1989), Australia	LOV	Omnivore (lean meat)	$N = 25$ (M) Age = 44 years BMI = 44 kg/m^2	6 weeks	Total-C: ↓ 10% treatment; ↓ 5% control ($p < 0.05$)
Nicholson et al. (1999), United States	Low-fat vegan	Low-fat omnivore (poultry, fish)	$N = 11$ (5 F, 6 M) Age = 34.3 years T2D	12 weeks	Weight: ↓ 7.2 kg treatment; ↓ 3.8 kg control ($p < 0.005$) Fasting glucose: ↓ 28% treatment; ↓ 12% control ($p < 0.05$) HDL-C: ↓ 0.02 mmol/L treatment; ↓ 0.20 mmol/L control ($p < 0.05$)
Barnard et al. (2000), United States	Low-fat (10% energy) vegan	Omnivore	$N = 35$ (F) Age = 36.1 years BMI = 25.5 kg/m^2 Premenopausal	2 months	Treatment as percent change from control Weight: ↓ 2.3% ($p < 0.001$) Total-C: ↓ 13.2% ($p < 0.001$) LDL-C: ↓ 16.9% ($p < 0.001$) HDL-C: ↓ 16.5% ($p < 0.001$) LDL/HDL ratio (not significant)

(Continued)

TABLE 4.2 (CONTINUED)
Overview of Selected Randomized Controlled Trials Evaluating the Effect of Vegetarian Diets on Risk Factors

Author (Year), Country	Treatment Diet	Control Diet	Participants[a]	Duration	Outcomes
Jenkins et al. (2003), Canada	Portfolio: Low-fat LOV plus portfolio foods[b]	Low-fat LOV or low-fat LOV plus statins	$N = 46$ (21 F, 25 M) Age = 59 years BMI = 27.6 kg/m^2	1 month	Change from baseline (%) LDL-C: ↓ 28.6% portfolio ($p < 0.001$); ↓ 8.0% control ($p = 0.002$); ↓ 30.9% control plus statins ($p < 0.001$) CRP: ↓ 28.2 portfolio ($p = 0.02$); ↓ 10.0 control; ↓ 33.3 control plus statins ($p = 0.002$)
Turner-McGrievy et al. (2007), United States	Low-fat vegan	NCEP step 2 guidelines	$N = 64$ (F) Age = 56 years BMI = 32 kg/m^2 Postmenopausal	1 and 2 years	Year 1 weight: ↓ 4.9 kg treatment; ↓ 1.8 kg control ($p < 0.05$) Year 2 weight: ↓ 3.1 kg treatment; ↓ 0.8 kg control ($p < 0.05$)
Barnard et al. (2009), United States	Low-fat vegan	American Diabetes Association	$N = 99$ (60 F, 39 M) Age = 55.6 years BMI = 34.9 kg/m^2 T2D	74 weeks	Weight: ↓ 4.4 kg treatment; ↓ 3.0 kg control (ns) Total-C: ↓ 20.4 mg/dL treatment; ↓6.8 mg/dL control ($p = 0.01$) LDL-C: ↓ 13.5 mg/dL treatment; ↓ 3.4 mg/dL control ($p = 0.03$) HbA$_{1c}$: ↓ 0.34% treatment; ↓ 0.14% control

(Continued)

TABLE 4.2 (CONTINUED)
Overview of Selected Randomized Controlled Trials Evaluating the Effect of Vegetarian Diets on Risk Factors

Author (Year), Country	Treatment Diet	Control Diet	Participants[a]	Duration	Outcomes
Kahleova et al. (2011), Czech Republic	Energy-restricted LV	Energy-restricted diabetic	$N = 74$ (39 F, 35 M) Age = 56.2 years BMI = 35 kg/m^2 T2D	24 weeks	Weight: ↓ 6.2 kg treatment; ↓ 3.2 kg control (p <0.001) Insulin sensitivity (as glucose clearance): ↑ 30% treatment; ↑ 20% control
Mishra et al. (2013), United States	Low-fat vegan	Habitual omnivore	$N = 291$ (241 F, 50 M) Age = 45.2 years BMI = 35.0 kg/m^2 Obese or T2D	18 weeks	Weight: ↓ 2.9 kg treatment; ↓ 0.06% control ($p < 0.001$) Total-C: ↓ 8.5 mg/dL treatment; ↓ 0.1 mg/dL control ($p < 0.01$) LDL-C: ↓ 8.1 mg/dL treatment; ↓ 0.9 mg/dL control ($p < 0.01$)
Jenkins et al. (2014), Canada	Eco-Atkins[c]	Energy-restricted, high-carbohydrate LOV	$N = 39$ (24 F, 15 M) BMI > 27 kg/m^2 Hyperlipidemic	1 month plus 6 months	Weight: ↓ 8.1 kg treatment; ↓ 5.9 kg control ($p = 0.047$) Total-C: ↓ 9.7% treatment, ↓ 3.9 control ($p < 0.001$) LDL-C: ↓ 10.4% treatment; none control ($p < 0.001$) Triglycerides: ↓ 32.7% treatment; ↓ 20.8% control ($p = 0.005$)

Note: LOV = lacto-ovo vegetarian; LV = lacto-vegetarian; NCEP = National Cholesterol Education Program.

[a] Age and BMI are mean values.

[b] Portfolio foods are sterol-enriched margarine, soy, almonds, and foods high in soluble fiber.

[c] Eco-Atkins is an energy-restricted, low-carbohydrate vegan diet.

In some of the clinical trials, low-fat vegetarian diets also reduced HDL-C (Barnard et al., 2000). This effect is not considered to be of consequence since the ratio of LDL-C to HDL-C is also reduced or unchanged and vegetarian diets are not associated with poor cardiovascular health.

Although clinical trials are important in providing evidence of benefits and in identifying effective preventive guidelines, the studies have limitations. Dietary effects on cardiovascular outcomes require many years because atherosclerotic changes take years to develop. Most clinical trials are of short duration and have limited sample sizes. There is a need for large high-quality clinical trials to test healthy vegetarian dietary patterns, similar to the intervention with the Mediterranean-style diet (Estruch et al., 2013).

4.2.3 REVERSING THE ATHEROSCLEROTIC PROCESS WITH VEGETARIAN DIETS

Studies utilizing vegetarian dietary interventions combined with other lifestyle changes are particularly effective in reducing cardiovascular risk. In the Life Style Heart Trial, Ornish et al. (1998) randomized 48 patients with moderate to severe CHD to either a low-fat (10% of energy) lacto-vegetarian diet combined with intensive lifestyle change that included aerobic exercise, smoking cessation, stress management, and psychological support, or the usual heart disease treatment. Seventy-one percent of patients in the experimental group maintained the lifestyle changes and completed the 5-year follow-up. Over the 5-year period, there were 2.5 times more cardiac events in the control group than the intervention group. Percent diameter stenosis of coronary vessels, a measure of atherosclerosis, decreased by 7.9% in the lifestyle group and progressed by 27.7% in the control group ($p < 0.001$). The lifestyle group experienced decreased frequency and duration of chest pain and a 39.8% drop in LDL-C concentrations that were similar to results obtained from those on lipid-lowering medications.

In a case series described by Esselstyn et al. (2014), 198 consecutive patients with established cardiovascular disease were enrolled in a low-fat entirely plant-based diet, along with the usual cardiovascular care. The prescribed diets were 10% energy as fat with no added oil, nuts or seeds, avocados, or olives. Of the enrolled patients, 89% were adherent to the diet for a mean of 3.7 years of follow-up. Of the adherent patients, 93% reported improvement in angina symptoms. Radiographic documentation of disease reversal was seen in 22% of adherent patients. Cardiac events, including myocardial infarcts, stroke, and death, were 2.2% in contrast to 62% in nonadherent patients ($p < 0.001$). Although the evidence to date is convincing that low-fat primarily or exclusively plant diets arrest and reverse the atherosclerotic process, clinical research efforts must continue in order to establish the most effective dietary guidelines for the prevention and management of heart disease.

4.3 VEGETARIAN DIETS AND ATHEROSCLEROTIC RISK FACTORS

Atherosclerosis is a persistent chronic condition, and current evidence indicates that its initiation and progression are influenced by lifestyle and dietary practices.

Individuals who consume plant-rich diets and avoid meat have been found to have reduced risk of cardiovascular disease. Much of the modifying effect of diet on heart disease risk is mediated through the effect of food and food components on the major risk factors of dyslipidemia, central adiposity, hypertension, and poor glycemic control. However, the consumption of plant foods may influence other aspects of cardiovascular physiology, such as endothelial function, oxidation, inflammation, and thrombosis.

4.3.1 DYSLIPIDEMIA

Risk factors for the development of cardiovascular diseases are multiple, and foremost among them is dyslipidemia. Elevated blood concentrations of LDL-C are the underlying cause of vascular endothelial cell injury and dysfunction that leads to atherosclerosis. Although much of the popular literature claims that saturated fat does not clog arteries and increase heart disease risk, findings from established cohorts continue to demonstrate increased mortality with increased consumption of saturated fat and *trans* fatty acids and reduced mortality with polyunsaturated fatty acids (Wang et al., 2016). As noted above, individuals adhering to vegetarian diets consistently exhibit lower blood lipids (Bradbury et al., 2014; Wang et al., 2015), and substantial reductions in total-C and LDL-C concentrations are achieved with vegetarian plant-rich dietary treatments (Ferdowsian and Barnard, 2009). Vegetarian diets reduce blood lipids through several mechanisms. Vegetarian and plant-rich diets are low in saturated fatty acids and cholesterol, leading to less absorption and conversion to blood cholesterol. Vegetarian diets tend to be rich in mono- and polyunsaturated fats, which are known to have strong LDL-C-lowering effects. Plant diets provide a high intake of soluble fiber, which increases cholesterol removal by binding bile salts and cholesterol and increasing their excretion from the body. Moreover, vegetarian diets provide a high intake of phytochemical constituents of plants, such as phytosterols, phenolics, carotenoids, and flavonoids (Cassidy et al., 2013, 2016). These influence cholesterol metabolism through a number of potential mechanisms, such as competing for its absorption or inhibiting its biosynthesis. In addition, some phytochemicals may have antioxidant and anti-inflammatory properties that attenuate vascular damage.

Nuts, a food with a favorable fatty acid profile, are consumed more frequently by vegetarians. In clinical trials, nuts have been shown to be effective in reducing total-C, LDL-C, and triglycerides when substituted for animal source foods (Sabaté et al., 1993; Sabaté and Fraser, 1994). The results from prospective cohorts and meta-analysis studies show an association between nut consumption and reduced risk of cardiovascular disease biomarkers and mortality (Fraser et al., 1992; Fraser, 1999b; Sabaté et al., 2010; Del Gobbo et al., 2015; Grosso et al., 2015).

Nuts and vegetable oils are rich sources of plant sterols. Plant sterols, or phytosterols, reduce intestinal cholesterol absorption by displacing cholesterol in the mixed micelle, thus inhibiting its absorption. It is estimated that plant sterols at 2 g/day significantly lower LDL-C concentration by approximately 8%–10% (Gylling and Simonen, 2015).

Vegetarians commonly substitute liquid vegetable oils for animal source fats. With the exception of the tropical oils (palm and coconut), vegetable oils contain a low proportion of saturated and more unsaturated fatty acids. Vegetable oils, such as corn, canola, soy, and sunflower, are high sources of polyunsaturated fat, which lowers LDL-C. The consumption of vegetable oils in place of partially hydrogenated margarine reduces exposure to *trans* fats, identified as one of the more potent dietary promoters of atherosclerosis (Wang et al., 2016). The use of extra-virgin olive oil may provide additional benefits due to its content of monounsaturated fat and polyphenols. When substituted for carbohydrates, monounsaturated fat lowers triglycerides and LDL-C and maintains HDL-C concentrations. Multiple cohort studies concluded that olive oil is associated with a reduced risk of cardiovascular mortality and stroke (Schwingshackl et al., 2015). In the Mediterranean-style diet study, extra-virgin olive oil and walnuts were emphasized and results confirmed their LDL-C-lowering and HDL-C-raising effects (Estruch et al., 2013). Unrefined olive oil contains the polyphenols oleuropein and hydroxytyrosol, which have been shown to stabilize HDL-C particles and increase their cholesterol efflux or removal capacity (Hernáez et al., 2016). Plant sources of the omega-3 essential fatty acid, alpha-linolenic acid, consumed by vegetarians, include walnuts, flaxseed, soy, and soy products. Higher alpha-linolenic acid intake is associated with a moderate decrease in cardiovascular risk, and there is no evidence of an increased risk in vegetarians due to their avoidance of marine omega-3 fats in their diets (Pan et al., 2012b).

4.3.2 CENTRAL ADIPOSITY

Excess body weight and central adiposity, along with their associated comorbidities of hypertension, dyslipidemia, and insulin resistance, contribute to cardiovascular disease dysfunction. Vegetarians have lower body weights than omnivores and a low incidence of obesity. In AHS-2, mean BMI (in kg/m^2) increased with increasing animal food consumption from 23.1 in vegan, to 25.5 in lacto-ovo vegetarian, to 25.7 in pesco-vegetarian, to 27.0 in semivegetarian, to 28.3 in nonvegetarian diet groups (Fraser, 2009).

A common disorder associated with central adiposity and excess body fat is chronic low-grade inflammation, which is a principal etiological agent of cardiovascular injury and dysfunction. Adipose tissue hypertrophy leads to infiltration of macrophages and T-cells and an inflammatory response characterized by the release of cytokines called adipocytokines. Adipocytokines exert many detrimental effects on vascular function and promote endothelial damage, plaque progression, and vulnerability (Liberale et al., 2017). Lifestyle change, which involves increased physical activity and plant-rich diets, may help reverse the process. Controlled clinical trials have demonstrated the efficacy of vegan and vegetarian diets in weight loss in both short-term (Nicholson et al., 1999; Barnard et al., 2000) and longer-term trials (Barnard et al., 2009; Mishra et al., 2013). Moreover, in a meta-analysis of 29 intervention studies with plant-based diets in obese individuals, the plant-rich diets were associated with improvements in the inflammatory profile (Eichelmann et al., 2016).

4.3.3   Type 2 Diabetes

Prospective epidemiological studies have shown that vegetarian diets protect against T2D. A significantly reduced incidence and prevalence of diabetes is shown in vegetarian AHS-2 participants compared with nonvegetarians (Fraser, 2009; Tonstad et al., 2009). Results from three established prospective cohorts of U.S. men and women also show lower incidence of T2D with plant-based dietary patterns (Satija et al., 2016). Plant-rich vegetarian diets support weight control since plant foods are generally low in energy density and provide adequate fullness satiety. Clinical dietary studies investigating the effect of vegetarian diets in diabetic patients have shown significant improvements in fasting blood sugar, hemoglobin (Hb) A_{1c} reduction, weight reduction, and improved insulin sensitivity (Barnard et al., 2009; Kahleova et al., 2011).

Vegetarian diets are characterized by greater consumptions of a variety of whole grains, legumes, vegetables, and fruits containing dietary fiber and phytochemicals. Soluble dietary fiber in oats and legumes is particularly effective in modulating blood sugar responses. Moreover, soluble fiber is fermented by intestinal bacteria to produce short-chain fatty acids, which modulate the glucose response, insulin signaling, and insulin sensitivity (Bach Knudsen, 2015).

4.3.4   Hypertension

High blood pressure is a strong, consistent, and independent risk factor for cardiovascular disease, stroke, heart failure, and kidney disease. Hypertension promotes endothelial injury and dysfunction, which progresses to atherosclerosis and cardiovascular dysfunction.

The incidence of hypertension appears to be lower in vegetarian populations. In the EPIC-Oxford study, Appleby et al. (2002) showed significant differences in age-adjusted mean values for self-reported hypertension across diet groups (meat eaters, fish eaters, vegetarians, and vegans), with the highest values in meat eaters and the lowest in vegans. Much of the variation in blood pressure was due to BMI, with vegan subjects tending to be leaner. Similarly, in a small substudy of 500 subjects of AHS-2 from which blood pressure measurements were obtained, covariate-adjusted analyses demonstrated that vegan and lacto-ovo vegetarians had lower systolic and diastolic blood pressure than omnivorous Adventists. The odds ratio of hypertension, defined as systolic blood pressure >139 mmHg, or the use of antihypertensive medication was 63% and 53% lower for vegan and lacto-ovo vegetarians, respectively, than for nonvegetarians (Pettersen et al., 2012). Dietary factors that effectively lower blood pressure are weight loss, reduced sodium intake, and increased potassium intake, all of which are more likely to occur in plant-rich diets.

4.3.5   Endothelial Dysfunction

The healthy endothelium is the major regulator of vascular function, maintaining the balance between vasodilation and constriction. A major function of the endothelium is vascular relation mediated by a number of endothelial systems, including nitric oxide, prostaglandins, and other factors. Nitric oxide is synthesized from L-arginine, an amino acid, by nitric oxide synthase. Nitric oxide is key to maintaining vascular wall integrity and inhibiting inflammation and thrombosis. Endothelial function is assessed in humans using a test called flow-mediated dilatation.

A number of dietary factors impact endothelial nitric oxide production. Foremost is saturated fat, which impairs flow-mediated dilatation compared with polyunsaturated fat, monounsaturated fat, or carbohydrates (Keogh et al., 2005). Ros et al. (2004) reported that supplementation of the diet with walnuts, a food rich in both omega-6 and omega-3 polyunsaturated fatty acids, enhanced flow-mediated dilatation and improved endothelial function.

Although L-arginine is a substrate for the endothelial nitric oxide synthesizing enzyme, L-arginine supplementation trials have not consistently shown a compelling effect on nitric oxide production (Alvarez et al., 2012). However, there is good evidence that dietary inorganic nitrate may contribute to nitric oxide production, improve endothelial function, and help control blood pressure in humans. Green leafy vegetables and beets are rich sources. Inorganic nitrate is absorbed from nitrate-rich foods and converted to nitrite by salivary bacteria and then to nitric oxide. These effects have been documented in the short term following consumption of leafy vegetables, beets, and beet juice and are not sustained when consumption ceases (Lara et al., 2016). Eating nitrate-containing plant foods at every meal is likely to prolong the beneficial effect.

In a prospective study of Australian older adult women (Blekkenhorst et al., 2017), dietary nitrate intake from vegetables was inversely associated with cardiovascular disease mortality. The observed effect was independent of lifestyle and cardiovascular risk and supports the concept of the beneficial effect of plant nitrates.

4.3.6 INFLAMMATION

The initial event in atherosclerosis is some form of endothelial injury brought about by dyslipidemia, high blood pressure, or other mechanisms resulting in an activated, leaky, and dysfunctional epithelium. The role of inflammation is central in the early development and progression of this pathophysiological process. Arterial injury and damage initiates leukocyte recruitment into the subendothelial space and the release of a cascade of inflammatory mediator chemokines and cytokines. This leads to the expression of adhesion molecules, lipid deposits, and smooth muscle proliferation. Further along, plaque instability, rupture, and thrombosis are also dependent in part on the inflammatory status of the plaque.

Inflammation is a normal process, and there are a large number of cells and mediators involved that may be used as indicators and biomarkers of the process. Currently, there is no consensus as to which of the many biomarkers best represent inflammation associated with cardiovascular disease. A commonly tested biomarker is high-sensitivity C-reactive protein (hsCRP), which is associated with endothelial dysfunction and has been shown to be a strong and independent predictor of future cardiovascular events. Another relevant biomarker is the cytokine interleukin (IL)-6. IL-6 is synthesized by macrophages and T-cells at the local injury site and also by adipocytes and is a one of the most important factors that promote the hepatic production of CRP. Serum concentrations of both hsCRP and IL-6 are elevated in obesity.

There is a substantial amount of evidence that nutrients modulate inflammation both acutely and chronically. Dietary fatty acids affect inflammatory processes indirectly through effects on body adipose tissue mass and directly via an impact on membrane and lipid raft composition and function. Inside cells, fatty acids influence inflammation by acting as transcription factors or as precursors for eicosanoids and related compounds. Although not always consistent, there is evidence for the pro-inflammatory effects of habitual saturated fat intake on fasting concentrations of cytokines. Stronger evidence exists for the postprandial impact of high-fat, high-saturated-fat meals on inflammatory biomarkers. In overweight men, plasma IL-6, tumor necrosis factor (TNF)-alpha, and soluble vascular adhesion molecule concentrations decreased after a polyunsaturated-rich meal and increased after a saturated-rich meal (Masson and Mensink, 2011). Inflammation in the postprandial state is relevant and contributes to the overall inflammatory state. Conversely, feeding studies with extra-virgin olive oil reduced inflammation and hsCRP and IL-6 concentrations (Schwingshackl et al., 2015).

A high intake of fruits, vegetables, plant foods, and vegetarian diets has a beneficial effect on the course of the inflammatory response. In the Multi-Ethnic Study of Atherosclerosis, the concentrations of a number of inflammatory biomarkers were assessed in more than 5000 nondiabetic participants. Using factor analysis, Nettleton et al. (2006) showed that a dietary pattern of whole grains, fruit, nuts, and green vegetables was inversely associated with CRP and IL-6. Similar findings were reported by other investigators and reported in a recent systematic review. The Healthy Food Pattern abundant in fruits and vegetables had a beneficial impact on endothelial function estimated by CRP, soluble intercellular adhesion molecule 1, soluble vascular adhesion molecule 1, and E-selectin molecule compared with patterns with higher intakes of processed meats, sweets, fried foods, and refined grains (Defago et al., 2014). Cross-sectional analysis of data from a subsample of participants in AHS-2 demonstrated an inverse association between vegetarian status and hsCRP concentration (Paalani et al., 2011).

Recently, Sutliffe et al. (2015) reported on a brief 3-week lifestyle intervention that tested a vegan diet in more than 600 individuals. Circulating hsCRP concentrations decreased and the baseline hsCRP concentration was an important indicator of the degree of improvement. Higher initial hsCRP concentrations resulted in greater declines after the plant diet intervention.

Although the underlying mechanisms are not clear, beneficial effects of plant-rich diets in reducing inflammation have also been attributed to their dietary polyphenol content. The association between dietary flavonoid polyphenol intake and serum hsCRP was examined among U.S. adults in the National Health and Nutrition Examination Survey (NHANES) 1999–2002 cohort. Dietary consumption of total flavonoids and individual flavonols, anthocyanidins, and isoflavones were inversely associated with serum hsCRP concentrations after adjusting for covariates such as gender, BMI, ethnicity, and lifestyle factors (Chun et al., 2008).

4.3.7 Oxidative Stress and LDL Oxidation

Oxidative stress refers to the imbalance between the body's beneficial production of reactive oxygen species and the system's ability to detoxify the oxidants and repair the damage. The role of oxidative processes in overall human health is complex, and many questions remain unanswered. However, the role of oxidative stress in atherogenesis is substantiated by the detection of oxidized lipids and proteins in vascular lesions and the fact that the degree of oxidation correlates with the severity of disease (Stocker and Keaney, 2005). Oxidized LDL promotes many of the proatherogenic processes of the vascular endothelium (Steinberg and Witztum, 2010).

Constituents of plant foods, particularly vitamins and phenolic substances, have the potential, when absorbed, to inhibit lipids and LDL-C from oxidative damage. When tested in feeding trials, some of the plant foods that have shown *in vivo* antioxidant protection include berries, red grapes and wine, cocoa, olive oil, and nuts (Haddad et al., 2014).

It is important to note that the large clinical trials that tested the effects of dietary supplements, such as vitamin E, beta-carotene, and selenium, on IHD outcomes showed no benefits. However, prospective cohort data clearly show that individuals with a high consumption of vegetables, fruits, and nuts, foods that naturally provide substantial food folate, vitamin E, vitamin C, beta-carotene, minerals, and polyphenols, experienced a decreased risk of cardiovascular disease and death (Mente et al., 2009). Data from a recent meta-analysis of prospective studies demonstrated an 8% decreased risk of cardiovascular disease and a 16% decreased risk of stroke with every 200 g increase in fruit and vegetable consumption (Aune et al., 2017).

4.4 POTENTIAL PROBLEMS WITH EATING ANIMAL SOURCE FOODS

It is generally accepted that some of the health benefits of vegetarian diets derive from the avoidance of meat and other animal source foods. Potential adverse health effects attributed to red and processed meat and full-fat dairy foods are primarily due to the high-saturated-fat content of these foods on the atherosclerotic process and disease progression. This fact is generally agreed on and consistently substantiated, as shown in this chapter. There are, however, several other potential mechanisms underlying the adverse effect of meat consumption on cardiovascular health that have received increased attention. Meat refers to animal flesh that is consumed as food, whereas red meat is beef, veal, pork, lamb, and mutton. Processed meat differs in that it undergoes treatment to extend its shelf life, such as smoking, curing, salting, or the addition of chemical preservatives. Processed meat typically contains more sodium, nitrites, nitrates, and additives to improve flavor and shelf life than unprocessed meat. All meats, poultry, and fish are nutrient-dense foods that tend to accumulate contaminants such as polychlorinated biphenyls (PCBs) and heavy metals from the environment (Lupton et al., 2017). Meat and animal foods may contain residues of antibiotics and hormones used during animal production (Jeong et al., 2010). At present, it is not known if these contaminants and residues impact cardiovascular health. More relevant are the products formed as a consequence of cooking or grilling meat. Grilling meat over an open flame produces benzo(a)pyrene, a form of polycyclic aromatic hydro-carbon (PAH). Moreover, cooking meat at high temperatures generates heterocy-clic amines (HCAs) and advanced glycation end (AGE) products, which have been shown to increase oxidative and inflammatory processes (Uribarri et al., 2015). Studies in humans have shown that diet-derived AGE products are associated with increased concentrations of CRP and other inflammatory and adhesion molecules in humans (Clarke et al., 2016).

The protein of meat and other animal foods contains a higher proportion of the branched-chain amino acids leucine, isoleucine, and valine. Branched-chain amino acids have been associated with insulin resistance. Data from the AHS-2 calibration study have shown that insulin resistance increases with increasing intake of animal protein and the animal-to-plant protein intake ratio (Azemati et al., 2017).

Adequate intake of iron is essential for human body growth and functioning, and its deficiencies are associated with anemia and poor performance. Meat is a source of heme iron, which is more readily absorbed (25%) than the nonheme iron in plant foods (5%–15%). This is generally considered to be a favorable effect but might not be entirely so. Increased dietary heme iron intake and increased stores of iron, as measured by serum ferritin concentration, are associated with a higher risk of chronic conditions. Iron is a pro-oxidant and participates in the production of reactive oxygen species that may contribute to cellular oxidative stress. Plasma concentrations of ferritin, a biomarker for body iron stores, are an identified risk factor for cardiovascular disease. Data from the prospective Multi-Ethnic Study of Atherosclerosis cohort indicated that dietary intakes of heme iron from red meat, but not from other sources, are associated with a greater risk of cardiovascular disease (De Oliveira Otto et al., 2012).

Another potential hazard found in meat and animal foods, such as eggs, is their high content of choline (eggs) and L-carnitine (meat). These substances are metab-olized by intestinal microbiota to produce trimethylamine and, subsequently, by a hepatic monooxygenase to produce trimethylamine N-oxide (TMAO). Increased plasma TMAO concentrations are related to vascular risk (Heianza et al., 2017). Plasma TMAO concentrations increase in response to the consumption of ani-mal foods and foods rich in choline and carnitine (Obeid et al., 2016). Due to the fact that vegetarian diets contain less choline or L-carnitine and more betaine, they may be less likely to form excessive TMAO. At present, evidence exists for the prothrombotic effect of elevated plasma TMAO concentrations, but the exact causal role of TMAO in cardiovascular disease remains to be determined (Zhu et al., 2017).

To enhance flavor and preservation, salt is a primary ingredient in the manufac-ture of processed meats. Dietary sodium increases cardiovascular risk through its effect on blood pressure. Excess salt in processed meat may be a factor underlying the observed linkage to increased blood pressure and stroke. Using dietary intake data from NHANES, Micha et al. (2017) estimated the top 10 dietary factors related to cardiovascular, stroke, and diabetes type 2 death. The factors that contributed to 9.2% and 8.2% of risk were excess sodium and processed meat intake, respectively.

Overall, and taking into account current scientific evidence, it is plausible to conclude that the consumption of red meat and processed meat is associated with an increased risk of cardiovascular disease and mortality. But as discussed above, the benefits of plant-based, vegan, and vegetarian diets in cardiovascular protection go beyond the absence of meat. Table 4.3 summarizes some of the beneficial effects of plant foods and their constituents on cardiovascular disease risk factors.

TABLE 4.3

Beneficial Effects of Plant Foods and Their Components on Cardiovascular Disease Risk Factors

Cardiovascular Disease Risk Factors	Plant Foods and Components That Reduce Risk
LDL-C	Vegetable oils (low saturated fat, high unsaturated fat)
	Nuts, avocados, olives (low saturated fat, high unsaturated fat)
	Whole grains and legumes (dietary fiber binds and promotes the excretion of bile acids and cholesterol)
	Nuts, vegetable oils (plant sterols inhibit cholesterol absorption)
	Extra-virgin olive oil (HDL-C efflux)
Triglycerides	Extra-virgin olive oil, nuts, seeds, whole-grain cereals, legumes (when substituted for refined starches and sugar)
Elevated blood pressure	Fruits and vegetable (high potassium, magnesium)
	Leafy vegetables (inorganic nitrate, calcium)
	Plant foods (low caloric density)
Central adiposity	Plant foods (low caloric density, low fat, high fiber)
Thrombotic tendency	Vegetable oils (low saturated fat, high unsaturated fat)
	Walnuts, flaxseed (omega-3 fatty acid, i.e., alpha-linolenic acid)
Endothelial injury and adhesion	Vegetable oils (low saturated fat, high unsaturated fat)
	Extra-virgin olive oil (polyphenols)
Systemic inflammation	Vegetable oils (low saturated fat, high unsaturated fat)
	Extra-virgin olive oil (polyphenols)
Elevated blood sugar and T2D	Legumes and soy (plant protein, arginine, low branched-chain amino acids)
	Legumes, soy, oats (dietary fiber, soluble fiber, low glycemic index)
	Whole grains, legumes, nuts (plant protein sources contain fiber and little saturated fat; linked to improved insulin sensitivity)
Oxidative stress, LDL-C oxidation	Vegetables, fruits, and berries (vitamin C, anthocyanins)
	Nuts, vegetable oil (vitamin E)
	Green and yellow vegetables (carotenoids, lutein)
	Cruciferous vegetables (sulforaphane, anthocyanin)
	Red grapes (resveratrol)
	Whole grains, legumes, nuts (plant protein sources with no heme iron or nitrosamines and little aromatic hydrocarbons, HCAs, or glycation products)

4.5 CONCLUSION

There is ample evidence that atherosclerotic vascular disease and its progression is largely a preventable condition. Adhering to a vegetarian diet can interrupt and reverse the process. However, the vegetarian diet is not a guarantee of lower risk. Other than the absence of meat, "heart-healthy" vegetarian diets need to incorporate a variety of whole grains, legumes, nuts, seeds, vegetables, and fruits. Modest amounts of liquid vegetable oils should substitute for animal fat, dairy fat, and hydrogenated products. In addition, a healthful dietary pattern must be low in refined breads and cereals and added sugars and salt.

REFERENCES

Alexander H, Lockwood LP, Harris MA, Melby CL. 1999. Risk factors for cardiovascular disease and diabetes in two groups of Hispanic Americans with differing dietary habits. *J Am Coll Nutr* 45:127–36.

Alvarez TS, Conte-Junior CA, Silva JT, Paschoalin VM. 2012. Acute L-arginine supplementation does not increase nitric oxide production in healthy subjects. *Nutr Metab (Lond)* 9:54. doi: 10.1186/1743-7075-9-54.

Appleby PN, Crowe FL, Bradbury KE, Travis RC, Key TJ. 2016. Mortality in vegetarians and comparable nonvegetarians in the United Kingdom. *Am J Clin Nutr* 103:218–30.

Appleby PN, Davey GK, Key TJ. 2002. Hypertension and blood pressure among meat eaters, fish eaters, vegetarians and vegans in EPIC-Oxford. *Public Health Nutr* 5:645–54.

Aune D, Giovannucci E, Boffetta P, Fadnes LT, Keum N, Norat T, Greenwood DC, Riboli E, Vatten LJ, Tonstad, S. 2017. Fruit and vegetable intake and the risk of cardiovascular disease, total cancer and all-cause mortality—A systematic review and dose-response meta-analysis of prospective studies. *Int J Epidemiol* 1–28. doi: 10.1093/ije/dyw319.

Azemati B, Rajaram S, Jaceldo-Siegl K, Sabate J, Shavlik D, Fraser GE, Haddad EH. 2017. Animal-protein intake is associated with insulin resistance in Adventist Health Study 2 (AHS-2) calibration substudy participants: A cross sectional analysis. *Curr Dev Nutr* 1:1–7.

Bach Knudsen KE. 2015. Microbial degradation of whole-grain complex carbohydrates and impact on short-chain fatty acids and health. *Adv Nutr* 6:206–13.

Barnard ND, Cohen J, Jenkins DJ, Turner-McGrievy G, Gloede L, Green A, Ferdowsian H. 2009. A low-fat vegan diet and a conventional diabetes diet in the treatment of type 2 diabetes: A randomized, controlled, 74-wk clinical trial. *Am J Clin Nutr* 89:1588s–96s.

Barnard ND, Scialli AR, Bertron P, Hurlock D, Edmonds K, Talev L. 2000. Effectiveness of a low-fat vegetarian diet in altering serum lipids in healthy premenopausal women. *Am J Cardiol* 85:969–72.

Blekkenhorst LC, Bondonno CP, Lewis JR, Devine A, Woodman RJ, Croft KD, Lim WH, Wong G, Beilin LJ, Prince RL, Hodgson JM. 2017. Association of dietary nitrate with atherosclerotic vascular disease mortality: A prospective cohort study of older adult women. *Am J Clin Nutr* 106:207–16.

Bradbury KE, Crowe FL, Appleby PN, Schmidt JA, Travis RC, Key TJ. 2014. Serum concentrations of cholesterol, apolipoprotein A-I and apolipoprotein B in a total of 1694 meat-eaters, fish-eaters, vegetarians and vegans. *Eur J Clin Nutr* 68:178–83.

Brown RA, Shantsila E, Varma C, Lip GY. 2017. Current understanding of atherogenesis. *Am J Med* 130:268–82.

Burslem J, Schonfeld G, Howald MA, Weidman SW, Miller JP. 1978. Plasma apoprotein and lipoprotein lipid levels in vegetarians. *Metabolism* 27:711–9.

Cassidy A, Bertoia M, Chiuve S, Flint A, Forman J, Rimm EB. 2016. Habitual intake of anthocyanins and flavanones and risk of cardiovascular disease in men. *Am J Clin Nutr* 104:587–94.

Cassidy A, Mukamal KJ, Liu L, Franz M, Eliassen AH, Rimm EB. 2013. High anthocyanin intake is associated with a reduced risk of myocardial infarction in young and middle-aged women. *Circulation* 127:188–96.

Chun OK, Chung SJ, Claycombe KJ, Song WO. 2008. Serum C-reactive protein concentrations are inversely associated with dietary flavonoid intake in U.S. adults. *J Nutr* 138:753–60.

Clarke RE, Dordevic AL, Tan SM, Ryan L, Coughlan MT. 2016. Dietary advanced glycation end products and risk factors for chronic disease: A systematic review of randomised controlled trials. *Nutrients* 8:125. doi: 10.3390/nu8030125.

Cooper RS, Goldberg RB, Trevisan M, Tsong Y, Liu K, Stamler J, Rubenstein A, Scanu AM. 1982. The selective lipid-lowering effect of vegetarianism on low density lipoproteins in a cross-over experiment. *Atherosclerosis* 44:293–305.

Crowe FL, Appleby PN, Travis RC, Key TJ. 2013. Risk of hospitalization or death from ischemic heart disease among British vegetarians and nonvegetarians: Results from the EPIC-Oxford cohort study. *Am J Clin Nutr* 97:597–603.

Defago MD, Elorriaga N, Irazola VE, Rubinstein AL. 2014. Influence of food patterns on endothelial biomarkers: A systematic review. *J Clin Hypertens (Greenwich)* 16:907–13.

Del Gobbo LC, Falk MC, Feldman R, Lewis K, Mozaffarian D. 2015. Effects of tree nuts on blood lipids, apolipoproteins, and blood pressure: Systematic review, meta-analysis, and dose-response of 61 controlled intervention trials. *Am J Clin Nutr D* 102:1347–56.

De Oliveira Otto MC, Alonso A, Lee DH, Delclos GL, Bertoni AG, Jiang R, Lima JA, Symanski E, Jacobs Jr. DR, Nettleton JA. 2012. Dietary intakes of zinc and heme iron from red meat, but not from other sources, are associated with greater risk of metabolic syndrome and cardiovascular disease. *J Nutr* 142:526–33.

Eichelmann F, Schwingshackl L, Fedirko V, Aleksandrova K. 2016. Effect of plant-based diets on obesity-related inflammatory profiles: A systematic review and meta-analysis of intervention trials. *Obes Rev* 17:1067–79.

Esselstyn Jr. CB, Gendy G, Doyle J, Golubic M, Roizen MF. 2014. A way to reverse CAD? *J Fam Pract* 63:356–64b.

Estruch R, Ros E, Martinez-Gonzalez MA. 2013. Mediterranean diet for primary prevention of cardiovascular disease. *N Engl J Med* 269:676–77.

Etemadi A, Sinha R, Ward MH, Graubard BI, Inoue-Choi M, Dawsey SM, Abnet CC. 2017. Mortality from different causes associated with meat, heme iron, nitrates, and nitrites in the NIH-AARP Diet and Health Study: Population based cohort study. *BMJ* 357:1957. doi: 10:1136/bmj/1957.

Falk E. 2006. Pathogenesis of atherosclerosis. *J Am Coll Cardiol* 47(8 Suppl.):C7–12.

Ferdowsian HR, Barnard ND. 2009. Effects of plant-based diets on plasma lipids. *Am J Cardiol* 104:947–56.

Fraser G, Katuli S, Anousheh R, Knutsen S, Herring P, Fan J. 2015. Vegetarian diets and cardiovascular risk factors in black members of the Adventist Health Study-2. *Public Health Nutr* 18:537–45.

Fraser GE. 1999a. Associations between diet and cancer, ischemic heart disease, and all-cause mortality in non-Hispanic white California Seventh-day Adventists. *Am J Clin Nutr* 70(3 Suppl.):532s–8s.

Fraser GE. 1999b. Nut consumption, lipids, and risk of a coronary event. *Clin Cardiol* 22(Suppl.):iii11–5.

Fraser GE. 2009. Vegetarian diets: What do we know of their effects on common chronic diseases? *Am J Clin Nutr* 89:1607s–12s.

Fraser GE, Sabate J, Beeson WL, Strahan TM. 1992. A possible protective effect of nut consumption on risk of coronary heart disease. The Adventist Health Study. *Arch Intern Med* 152:1416–24.

Fraser GE, Swannell RJ. 1981. Diet and serum cholesterol in Seventh-day Adventists: A cross-sectional study showing significant relationships. *J Chronic Dis* 34:487–501.

Grosso G, Yang J, Marventano S, Micek A, Galvano F, Kales SN. 2015. Nut consumption on all-cause, cardiovascular, and cancer mortality risk: A systematic review and meta-analysis of epidemiologic studies. *Am J Clin Nutr* 101:783–93.

Gylling H, Simonen P. 2015. Phytosterols, phytostanols, and lipoprotein metabolism. *Nutrients* 7:7965–77.

Haddad EH, Gaban-Chong N, Oda K, Sabate J. 2014. Effect of a walnut meal on postprandial oxidative stress and antioxidants in healthy individuals. *Nutr J* 13:4. doi: 10.1186/1475-2891-13-4.

Hardinge MG, Stare FJ. 1954. Nutritional studies of vegetarians. II. Dietary and serum levels of cholesterol. *J Clin Nutr* 2:83–8.

Harman SK, Parnell WR. 1998. The nutritional health of New Zealand vegetarian and non-vegetarian Seventh-day Adventists: Selected vitamin, mineral and lipid levels. *N Z Med J* 111:91–4.

Heianza Y, Ma W, Manson JE, Rexrode KM, Qi L. 2017. Gut microbiota metabolites and risk of major adverse cardiovascular disease events and death: A systematic review and meta-analysis of prospective studies. *J Am Heart Assoc* 6(7). doi: 10.1161/jaha.116.004947.

Hernáez A, Farras M, Fito M. 2016. Olive oil phenolic compounds and high-density lipoprotein function. *Curr Opin Lipidol* 27:47–53.

Huang T, Yang B, Zheng J, Li G, Wahlqvist ML, Li D. 2012. Cardiovascular disease mortality and cancer incidence in vegetarians: A meta-analysis and systematic review. *Ann Nutr Metab* 60:233–40.

Huang YW, Jian ZH, Chang HC, Nfor ON, Ko PC, Lung CC, Lin LY et al. 2014. Vegan diet and blood lipid profiles: A cross-sectional study of pre and postmenopausal women. *BMC Womens Health* 14:55. doi:10.1186/1472-6874-14-55.

Jenkins DJ, Kendall CW, Marchie A, Faulkner DA, Wong JM, de Souza R, Emam A et al. 2003. Effects of a dietary portfolio of cholesterol-lowering foods vs lovastatin on serum lipids and C-reactive protein. *JAMA* 290:502–10.

Jenkins DJ, Wong JM, Kendall CW, Esfahani A, Ng VW, Leong TC, Faulkner DA et al. 2014. Effect of a 6-month vegan low-carbohydrate ('Eco-Atkins') diet on cardiovascular risk factors and body weight in hyperlipidaemic adults: A randomised controlled trial. *BMJ Open* 4(2):e003505. doi: 10.1136/bmjopen-2013-003505.

Jeong SH, Kang D, Lim MW, Kang CS, Sung HJ. 2010. Risk assessment of growth hormones and antimicrobial residues in meat. *Toxicol Res* 26:301–13.

Jones DS, Greene JA. 2013. The decline and rise of coronary heart disease: Understanding public health catastrophism. *Am J Public Health* 103:1207–18.

Keogh JB, Grieger JA, Noakes M, Clifton PM. 2005. Flow-mediated dilatation is impaired by a high-saturated fat diet but not by a high-carbohydrate diet. *Arterioscler Thromb Vasc Biol* 25:1274–9.

Kestin M, Rouse IL, Correll RA, Nestel PJ. 1989. Cardiovascular disease risk factors in free-living men: Comparison of two prudent diets, one based on lactoovovegetarianism and the other allowing lean meat. *Am J Clin Nutr* 50:280–7.

Key TJ, Appleby PN, Davey GK, Allen NE, Spencer EA, Travis RC. 2003. Mortality in British vegetarians: Review and preliminary results from EPIC-Oxford. *Am J Clin Nutr* 78(3 Suppl.):533s–8s.

Key TJ, Fraser GE, Thorogood M, Appleby PN, Beral V, Reeves G, Burr ML et al. 1999. Mortality in vegetarians and nonvegetarians: Detailed findings from a collaborative analysis of 5 prospective studies. *Am J Clin Nutr* 70(3 Suppl.):516s–24s.

Kochanek KD, Murphy SL, Xu J, Tejada-Vera B. 2016. Deaths: Final data for 2014. *Natl Vital Stat Rep* 56(4):1–122.

Lara J, Ashor AW, Oggioni C, Ahluwalia A, Mathers JC, Siervo M. 2016. Effects of inorganic nitrate and beetroot supplementation on endothelial function: A systematic review and meta-analysis. *Eur J Nutr* 55:451–9.

Liberale L, Bonaventura A, Vecchie A, Matteo C, Dallegri F, Montecucco F, Carbone F. 2017. The role of adipocytokines in coronary atherosclerosis. *Curr Atheroscler Rep* 19(2):10. doi: 10.1007/s11883-017-0644-3.

Lupton SJ, O'Keefe M, Muniz-Ortiz JG, Clinch N, Basu P. 2017. Survey of polychlorinated dibenzo-p-dioxins, polychlorinated dibenzofurans, and non-ortho-polychlorinated biphenyls in U.S. meat and poultry from 2012–2013: Toxic equivalency levels, patterns, temporal trends, and implications. *Food Addit Contam Part A Chem Anal Control Expo Risk Assess.* doi: 10.1080/19440049.2017.1340674.

Masson CJ, Mensink RP. 2011. Exchanging saturated fatty acids for (n-6) polyunsaturated fatty acids in a mixed meal may decrease postprandial lipemia and markers of inflammation and endothelial activity in overweight men. *J Nutr* 141:816–21.

Melby CL, Toohey ML, Cebrick J. 1994. Blood pressure and blood lipids among vegetarian, semivegetarian, and nonvegetarian African Americans. *Am J Clin Nutr* 59:103–9.

Mente A, de Koning L, Shannon HS, Anand SS. 2009. A systematic review of the evidence supporting a causal link between dietary factors and coronary heart disease. *Arch Intern Med* 169:659–69.

Micha R, Penalvo JL, Cudhea F, Imamura F, Rehm CD, Mozaffarian D. 2017. Association between dietary factors and mortality from heart disease, stroke, and type 2 diabetes in the United States. *JAMA* 317:912–24.

Mishra S, Xu J, Agarwal U, Gonzales J, Levin S, Barnard ND. 2013. A multicenter randomized controlled trial of a plant-based nutrition program to reduce body weight and cardiovascular risk in the corporate setting: The GEICO study. *Eur J Clin Nutr* 67:718–24.

Mozaffarian D, Benjamin EJ, Go AS, Arnett DK, Blaha MJ, Cushman M, Das SR et al. 2016. Executive summary: Heart disease and stroke statistics—2016 update: A report from the American Heart Association. *Circulation* 133:447–54.

Nettleton JA, Steffen LM, Mayer-Davis EJ, Jenny NS, Jiang R, Herrington DM, Jacobs Jr. DR. 2006. Dietary patterns are associated with biochemical markers of inflammation and endothelial activation in the Multi-Ethnic Study of Atherosclerosis (MESA). *Am J Clin Nutr* 83:1369–79.

Nicholson AS, Sklar M, Barnard ND, Gore S, Sullivan R, Browning S. 1999. Toward improved management of NIDDM: A randomized controlled pilot intervention using a lowfat, vegetarian diet. *Prev Med* 29:87–91.

Obeid R, Awwad HM, Keller M, Geisel J. 2016. Trimethylamine-N-oxide and its biological variations in vegetarians. *Eur J Nutr.* doi: 10.1007/s00394-016-1295-9.

Orlich MJ, Jaceldo-Siegl K, Sabate J, Fan J, Singh PN, Fraser GE. 2014. Patterns of food consumption among vegetarians and non-vegetarians. *Br J Nutr* 112:1644–53.

Orlich MJ, Singh PN, Sabate J, Jaceldo-Siegl K, Fan J, Knutsen S, Beeson WL, Fraser GE. 2013. Vegetarian dietary patterns and mortality in Adventist Health Study 2. *JAMA Intern Med* 173:1230–8.

Ornish D, Brown SE, Scherwitz LW, Billings JH, Armstrong WT, Ports TA, McLanahan SM, Kirkeeide RL, Brand RJ, Gould KL. 1990. Can lifestyle changes reverse coronary heart disease? The Lifestyle Heart Trial. *Lancet* 336:129–33.

Ornish D, Scherwitz LW, Billings JH, Gould KL, Merritt TA, Sparler S, Armstrong WT, Ports TA, Kirkeeide RL, Hogeboom C, Brand RJ. 1998. Intensive lifestyle changes for reversal of coronary heart disease. *JAMA* 280:2001–7.

Paalani M, Lee JW, Haddad E, Tonstad S. 2011. Determinants of inflammatory markers in a bi-ethnic population. *Ethn Dis* 21:142–9.

Pan A, Chen M, Chowdhury R, Wu JH, Sun Q, Campos H, Mozaffarian D, Hu FB. 2012b. Alpha-linolenic acid and risk of cardiovascular disease: A systematic review and meta-analysis. *Am J Clin Nutr* 96:1262–73.

Pan A, Sun Q, Bernstein AM, Schulze MB, Manson JE, Stampfer MJ, Willett WC, Hu FB. 2012a. Red meat consumption and mortality: Results from 2 prospective cohort studies. *Arch Intern Med* 172:555–63.

Pettersen BJ, Anousheh R, Fan J, Jaceldo-Siegl K, Fraser GE. 2012. Vegetarian diets and blood pressure among white subjects: Results from the Adventist Health Study-2 (AHS-2). *Public Health Nutr* 15:1909–16.

Phillips RL, Lemon FR, Beeson WL, Kuzma JW. 1978. Coronary heart disease mortality among Seventh-day Adventists with differing dietary habits: A preliminary report. *Am J Clin Nutr* 31(10 Suppl.):s191–8.

Rizzo NS, Jaceldo-Siegl K, Sabate J, Fraser GE. 2013. Nutrient profiles of vegetarian and nonvegetarian dietary patterns. *J Acad Nutr Diet* 113:1610–9.

Rohrmann S, Overvad K, Bueno-de-Mesquita HB, Jakobsen MU, Egeberg R, Tjonneland A, Nailler L et al. 2013. Meat consumption and mortality—Results from the European Prospective Investigation into Cancer and Nutrition. *BMC Med* 11:63. doi: 10.1186/1741-7015-11-63.

Ros E, Nunez I, Perez-Heras A, Serra M, Gilabert R, Casals E, Deulofeu R. 2004. A walnut diet improves endothelial function in hypercholesterolemic subjects: A randomized crossover trial. *Circulation* 109:1609–14.

Sabaté J, Fraser GE. 1994. Nuts: A new protective food against coronary heart disease. *Curr Opin Lipidol* 5:11–16.

Sabaté J, Fraser GE, Burke K, Knutsen SF, Bennett H, Lindsted KD. 1993. Effects of walnuts on serum lipid levels and blood prssure in normal men. *N Engl J Med* 328:603–7.

Sabaté J, Oda K, Ros E. 2010. Nut consumption and blood lipid levels: A pooled analysis of 25 intervention trials. *Arch Intern Med* 170:821–7.

Sacks FM, Castelli WP, Donner A, Kass EH. 1975. Plasma lipids and lipoproteins in vegetarians and controls. *N Engl J Med* 292:1148–51.

Sacks FM, Lichtenstein AH, Wu JHY, Appel LJ, Creager MA, Kris-Etherton PM, Miller M et al. 2017. Dietary fats and cardiovascular disease: A presidential advisory from the American Heart Association. *Circulation*. doi: 10.1161/cir.0000000000000510.

Satija A, Bhupathiraju SN, Rimm EB, Spiegelman D, Chiuve SE, Borgi L, Willett WC, Manson JE, Sun Q, Hu FB. 2016. Plant-based dietary patterns and incidence of type 2 diabetes in US men and women: Results from three prospective cohort studies. *PLoS Med* 13(6):e1002039. doi: 10.1371/journal.pmed.1002039.

Schwingshackl L, Christoph M, Hoffmann G. 2015. Effects of olive oil on markers of inflammation and endothelial function—A systematic review and meta-analysis. *Nutrients* 7:7651–75.

Singh PN, Batech M, Faed P, Jaceldo-Siegl K, Martins M, Fraser GE. 2014. Reliability of meat, fish, dairy, and egg intake over a 33-year interval in Adventist Health Study 2. *Nutr Cancer* 66:1315–21.

Sinha, R, Cross AJ, Graubard BI, Leitzmann MF, Schatzkin A. 2009. Meat intake and mortality: A prospective study of over half a million people. *Arch Intern Med* 169:562–71.

Spencer EA, Appleby PN, Davey GK, Key TJ. 2003. Diet and body mass index in 38000 EPIC-Oxford meat-eaters, fish-eaters, vegetarians and vegans. *Int J Obes Relat Metab Disord* 27:728–34.

Steinberg D, Witztum JL. 2010. Oxidized low-density lipoprotein and atherosclerosis. *Arterioscler Thromb Vasc Biol* 30:2311–16.

Stocker R, Keaney Jr. JF. 2005. New insights on oxidative stress in the artery wall. *J Thromb Haemost* 3:1825–34.

Sutliffe JT, Wilson LD, de Heer HD, Foster RL, Carnot MJ. 2015. C-reactive protein response to a vegan lifestyle intervention. *Complement Ther Med* 23:32–37.

Teixeira Martins MC, Jaceldo-Siegl K, Fan J, Singh P, Fraser GE. 2015. Short- and long-term reliability of adult recall of vegetarian dietary patterns in the Adventist Health Study-2 (AHS-2). *J Nutr Sci* 4:e11. doi: 10.1017/jns.2014.67.

Tonstad S, Butler T, Yan R, Fraser GE. 2009. Type of vegetarian diet, body weight, and prevalence of type 2 diabetes. *Diabetes Care* 32:791–6.

Turner-McGrievy GM, Barnard ND, Scialli AR. 2007. A two-year randomized weight loss trial comparing a vegan diet to a more moderate low-fat diet. *Obesity (Silver Spring)* 15:2276–81.

Uribarri J, del Castillo MD, de la Maza MP, Filip R, Gugliucci A, Luevano-Contreras C, Macías-Cervantes MH et al. 2015. Dietary advanced glycation end products and their role in health and disease. *Adv Nutr* 6:461–73.

Wang DD, Li Y, Chiuve SE, Stampfer MJ, Manson JE, Rimm EB, Willett WC, Hu FB. 2016. Association of specific dietary fats with total and cause-specific mortality. *JAMA Intern Med* 176:1134–45.

Wang F, Zheng J, Yang B, Jiang J, Fu Y, Li D. 2015. Effects of vegetarian diets on blood lipids: A systematic review and meta-analysis of randomized controlled trials. *J Am Heart Assoc* 4(10):e002408. doi: 10.1161/jaha.115.002408.

Zhu W, Wang Z, Tang WH, Hazen SL. 2017. Gut microbe-generated trimethylamine N-oxide from dietary choline is prothrombotic in subjects. *Circulation* 135:1671–3. doi: 10.1161/circulationaha.116.025338.

5 Risk of Cancer in Vegetarians

Michael J. Orlich and Renae M. Thomas

CONTENTS

SUMMARY

Cancer is a diverse set of related diseases involving uncontrolled cell growth and division; consequently, risk factors for cancers may vary. Diet is an important potential risk factor for many cancers, and vegetarian diets have been hypothesized to reduce the risk of several common cancers. We review here the evidence of cancer risk among vegetarians compared with nonvegetarians, primarily based on the findings of several prospective cohort studies of vegetarians. We also review related evidence for associations of the consumption of meat, eggs, and dairy products to cancer risk and highlight selected evidence linking plant foods to reductions in cancer risk.

5.1 BACKGROUND

According to the World Health Organization (WHO), cancer is the second leading cause of death globally, with nearly one in six deaths attributable to cancer. In 2012, 14 million new cancer cases were diagnosed worldwide, a figure predicted to increase by approximately 70% over the next two decades (World Health Organization, 2017). The most commonly occurring cancers worldwide (excluding nonmelanoma skin cancers) are cancers of the lung, breast, colorectum, prostate, stomach, and liver (WCRF, 2012), and the leading causes of death from cancer worldwide are cancers of the lung, liver, colorectum, stomach, and breast (World Health Organization, 2017).

Cancer is a complex set of related diseases sharing many underlying mechanisms. The essential characteristic of cancers is the uncontrolled growth and division of a clone of cells. Carcinogenesis, or the initiation and formation of cancer, is a multistep process involving numerous molecular events, such as DNA damage and altered DNA repair mechanisms, aberrant activation of proto-oncogenes, inactivation of tumor suppressor genes, and impaired apoptosis (Kotecha et al., 2016). Given the pathophysiologic complexity and diversity of cancers, it is not surprising that risk factors for different cancers are similarly diverse and complex and, in many cases, still poorly understood. Diet represents a major, daily environmental exposure that varies greatly between persons. Thus, dietary variations have been the focus of extensive study as potential risk (or protective) factors for cancer.

Since 1982, the World Cancer Research Fund International (WCRF) and American Institute for Cancer Research (AICR) and their Continuous Update Project (CUP) have been analyzing global research on modifiable cancer risk factors, including the effects of diet on cancer risk and survival. WCRF/AICR currently estimates that approximately one-third of the most common cancers may be preventable through lifestyle (i.e., diet, weight, and physical activity) changes (WCRF/AICR, 2017c). Current WCRF/AICR guidelines recommend eating sufficient quantities of vegetables, fruits, legumes, and relatively unprocessed grains while limiting the intake of red meat and avoiding processed meat (WCRF, 2017). These recommendations are typical of many vegetarian diets, in which categories of animal-based foods (e.g., meats and sometimes dairy) are avoided. People adopt vegetarian diets for a variety of reasons, including religious and ethical beliefs, environmental concerns, and/or desires for perceived health benefits. In this chapter, we review the evidence relating vegetarian dietary patterns to cancer risk.

5.2 TYPES OF EVIDENCE

Conducting long-term controlled trials of diet and cancer risk is extremely difficult for many reasons. Hence, much of the evidence relevant to understanding the relationship of vegetarian diets to cancer is drawn from observational studies in human populations. These have traditionally included ecological studies (e.g., comparisons between countries), migration studies, and case-control studies, but these often have serious limitations and should be interpreted with caution. In this chapter, we focus primarily on evidence from large prospective cohort studies, where diet is assessed in advance for each study participant, and participants are then followed over time to compare cancer incidence and/or mortality. Such prospective studies are considered to be of higher quality and less subject to bias, though they may still have problems relating to imperfect measurement of diet and potential for confounding (where a related factor may be the true cause, rather than diet), despite best efforts to control for this.

5.3 COHORT STUDIES OF VEGETARIANS AND CANCER RISK

There have been several prospective observational cohort studies that have contributed much to our understanding of vegetarian diets and their relationship to health outcomes. These have mostly been studies of vegetarians in the United Kingdom or among Seventh-day Adventist populations in the United States, though there have been smaller studies in other populations. These studies have generally used food frequency questionnaires (FFQs) to divide participants into diet categories based on their intake of animal foods.

While the term *vegetarian* is commonly used and well recognized, studies have defined diets along a vegetarian spectrum in somewhat different ways. (See the below studies. Where not specified, groups consumed dairy and eggs in any amount. UK studies used the term *meat* to mean nonfish meat, that is, poultry or red meat.) These definitional inconsistencies must be borne in mind in interpreting the findings of such studies of vegetarian diets. We report the relevant findings from five major cohort studies below. In this section and onward, risk is generally reported as relative risk (RR) or the related measures of odds ratio (OR) or hazard ratio (HR), with ranges in parentheses indicating 95% confidence intervals, unless otherwise specified.

Adventist Health Study (AHS): A total of 34,192 participants were categorized into three groups: *vegetarians*, no meat, poultry, or fish (29.5%); *semivegetarians*, some fish and/or poultry but <1 time/week (21.2%); and *nonvegetarians* (all others) (49.2%) (Fraser, 1999).

Incident cancers of the colon (RR 1.88, 1.24–2.87) and prostate (RR 1.54, 1.05–2.26) were significantly more likely in nonvegetarians than in vegetarians (Fraser, 1999).

Adventist Health Study II (AHS-2): Approximately 96,000 participants were categorized into five groups: *vegans* (7.7%), red meat, poultry, fish, eggs, and dairy <1 time/month; *lacto-ovo vegetarians* (29.2%), red meat, poultry, and fish <1 time/month but eggs or dairy ≥1 time/month; *pesco-vegetarians* (9.9%), red meat and poultry <1 time/month but fish ≥1 time/month; *semivegetarians* (5.4%), red meat and poultry ≥1 time/month but all meats combined ≤1 time/week; and *nonvegetarians* (47.7%), red meat and poultry ≥1 time/month and all meats combined >1 time/week (Butler et al., 2008; Orlich and Fraser, 2014). Often, combined *vegetarians* (all vegans, lacto-ovo vegetarians, pesco-vegetarians, and semivegetarians) were compared with nonvegetarians.

In an analysis of all cancers, and cancers by organ system, all vegetarians combined had lower overall cancer risk (i.e., all cancers combined, excluding non-melanoma skin cancers) (HR 0.92, 0.85–0.99) and decreased risk of combined cancers of the gastrointestinal tract (HR 0.76, 0.63–0.90) (Tantamango-Bartley et al., 2013). In particular, vegans had a lower risk of all cancers (HR 0.84, 0.72–0.99) and combined female-specific cancers (HR 0.66, 0.47–0.92) (Tantamango-Bartley et al., 2013). However, in an analysis of all-cause and cause-specific mortality, cancer mortality was not significantly lower among vegetarian groups (Orlich et al., 2013).

Results have been published thus far examining the association of vegetarian dietary patterns with three major specific cancers: cancers of the colon and rectum, the prostate, and the female breast. Vegetarians combined had a lower risk of colorectal cancer (HR 0.78, 0.64–0.95) and specifically of colon cancer (HR 0.81, 0.65–1.00). In particular, pesco-vegetarians had a notably lower incidence of colorectal cancer (HR 0.57, 0.40–0.82) (Orlich et al., 2015). For prostate cancer, only vegans demonstrated a lower risk (HR 0.65, 0.49–0.85) (Tantamango-Bartley et al., 2016). For breast cancer, no vegetarian groups had a significantly lower risk, though point estimates of risk were nonsignificantly lower among vegans (HR 0.78, 0.58–1.05) (Penniecook-Sawyers et al., 2016).

Oxford Vegetarian Study (OVS): A total of 11,130 participants were categorized into two groups: *non–meat eaters* (including vegans, vegetarians, and fish eaters) (55%), meat <1 time/week, and *meat eaters* (45%), meat ≥1 time/week (Thorogood et al., 1994).

Initial analyses for this relatively small cohort were limited to comparisons of cancer mortality. There was decreased mortality from all cancers combined in non–meat eaters, with standardized mortality ratios (SMRs) of 80 (64–98) for meat eaters and 50 (39–62) for non–meat eaters, compared with the general population (i.e., 80% and 50% of the expected mortality rates, respectively). After adjusting for known risk factors, death rate ratios in non–meat eaters compared with meat eaters were 0.61 (0.44–0.84) for all cancers (Thorogood et al., 1994).

European Prospective Investigation into Cancer and Nutrition–Oxford (EPIC-Oxford): A total of 65,429 participants were categorized into four groups: *vegans* (4%), no animal products; *vegetarians* (29%), no meat or fish but consumed eggs and/or dairy; *fish eaters* (15%), fish but no meat; and *meat eaters* (52%), who consumed meat (Davey et al., 2003).

The EPIC-Oxford cohort was pooled together with the earlier OVS in publications examining comparative cancer incidence in vegetarians (including vegans) and nonvegetarians. Key and colleagues published initial findings from these cohorts in 2009 and updated findings in 2014. In the 2009 analysis, after adjusting for risk factors, the incidence rate ratio for all malignant neoplasms was 0.88 (0.81–0.96) for vegetarians and 0.82 (0.73–0.93) for fish eaters compared with meat eaters (Key et al., 2009). There were no significant differences by diet pattern in the risk of the three most common cancers: female breast cancer, prostate cancer, and colorectal cancer.

Updated results published 5 years later were similar, though increased statistical power allowed for examination of vegetarians and vegans separately for all cancers and for the most common cancers. For all cancers combined, compared with meat eaters, the adjusted risk for vegans was 0.82 (0.68–1.00); for vegetarians it was 0.90 (0.84–0.97); and for fish eaters it was 0.89 (0.81–0.98). For colorectal cancer, fish eaters had a lower risk than meat eaters (0.67, 0.48–0.92), whereas vegetarians and vegans did not. For female breast cancer, there were no significant differences between the diet patterns. For prostate cancer, there were also no significant differences, though effect estimates appeared lower for the non–meat eaters (vegans 0.61 [0.31–1.20], vegetarians 0.86 [0.66–1.11], and fish eaters 0.74 [0.51–1.08]). In both analyses, a few cancers occurred significantly less frequently among vegetarians than nonvegetarians (i.e., stomach, lymphatic/hematopoietic, and multiple myeloma), but these were based on very small numbers of incident cancers and should thus be considered quite preliminary findings (Key et al., 2014).

UK Women's Cohort Study: A total of 35,372 participants were categorized into four groups: *vegetarians* (19%), meat or fish <1 time/week; *fish eaters* (9%), fish ≥1 time/week but poultry and red meat <1 time/week; *poultry eaters* (13%), poultry ≥1 time/week but red meat <1 time/week; and *red meat eaters* (70%), red meat ≥1 time/week (Cade et al., 2010).

Vegetarians, fish eaters, and poultry eaters were compared with red meat eaters regarding their risk for breast cancer. For all breast cancer combined and for premenopausal breast cancers, there was no significant difference in risk between the diet groups. For postmenopausal breast cancer, in fully adjusted models, compared with red meat eaters, fish eaters had a lower risk (0.60, 0.38–0.96), but risk for vegetarians was not significantly lower (0.85, 0.58–1.25) (Cade et al., 2010).

In considering the results of the vegetarian-focused cohort studies as a whole, they seem to support the idea that vegetarians have a reduced overall cancer risk. The size of this risk reduction (~10%–15% lower) is modest, but would still result in the prevention of many cancers, assuming that the observed reduced risk was indeed caused by the vegetarian diet. However, the evidence regarding the risk of specific cancers (and cancer mortality) is limited and not entirely consistent at this point. Statistical power may still limit the ability to detect risk reductions of modest size. It should be noted that the nonvegetarians in these studies, which serve as the basis of comparison for the vegetarians, are generally health-conscious persons with relatively low meat intakes. Comparisons with a more average American (or British) nonvegetarian diet might look more favorable; however, such comparisons would be difficult to do while adequately addressing factors such as measurement error and confounding. A careful harmonization of the data and joint analysis of one of these cohorts (e.g., AHS-2) with another cohort having more heavy meat eaters may be helpful. Pesco-vegetarians, or fish eaters, often have risk estimates similar to those of vegetarians and lower than those of nonvegetarians, or meat eaters; so these diets as practiced may have similar benefits for cancer risk, perhaps due to eliminating or reducing red and processed meats. Vegans, in some cases, such as in prostate and breast cancer, may have lower risk estimates, but their smaller numbers make these estimates more uncertain. Longer follow-up in the AHS-2 and EPIC-Oxford should provide additional statistical power to clarify some of these uncertainties.

5.4 SYSTEMATIC REVIEWS AND META-ANALYSES OF VEGETARIAN DIETS AND CANCER

Systematic reviews and meta-analyses can be a helpful way of quantitatively summarizing many studies addressing a particular research question, though they cannot overcome the limitations of the individual studies included. Later in the chapter, we will often refer to meta-analyses as a helpful way to gain a sense of what the literature as a whole is saying about particular diet and cancer questions. Meta-analyses of the literature relating vegetarian dietary patterns to cancer have been limited by the small number of primary publications. A 2017 systematic review and meta-analysis yielded summary statistics as follows. Vegans had lower total cancer incidence (RR 0.85, 0.75–0.95; based on two studies of three cohorts). Vegetarians had a lower total cancer incidence (RR 0.92, 0.87–0.98; based on two studies of three cohorts), somewhat lower risk estimates (none statistically significant) for several major cancers, and no difference in cancer mortality (Dinu et al., 2017). A 2012 meta-analysis of seven cohort studies found an 18% lower total cancer incidence in vegetarians (RR 0.82, 0.67–0.97), though this contained several very early studies of lower quality, did not include AHS-2 findings, and mixed cancer mortality with cancer incidence (Huang et al., 2012).

5.5 DIETARY INTERVENTION STUDIES

While intervention studies of the effects of dietary changes on cancer progression are limited, there is some promising research in the area of prostate cancer. Because low-grade prostate cancer often progresses slowly, with relatively low metastatic potential, active surveillance, or "watchful waiting," is often a viable option (Matthes et al., 2017). Ornish and colleagues (2015) randomly assigned 93 men with prostate cancer (serum prostate-specific antigen [PSA] 4–10 ng/mL, Gleason scores <7), not undergoing conventional treatment, to an experimental group incorporating comprehensive lifestyle changes or to a usual-care control group. The experimental group followed a low-fat (10%) vegan diet with supplements of soy, fish oil, vitamin E, selenium, and vitamin C; engaged in moderate aerobic exercise; and attended stress management and group support sessions. After 12 months, none of the experimental group patients but six control patients underwent conventional treatment due to disease progression based on PSA or imaging (Ornish et al., 2005). The experimental group had PSA levels decline (average of 0.25 ng/mL, or 4% from baseline), whereas PSA increased (average of 0.38 ng/mL, or 6% from baseline) in the control group. Serum was tested on prostate cancer cell lines in vitro, with the experimental group inhibiting cell growth by 70%, compared with control inhibition of 9%. No significant changes in C-reactive protein, testosterone, or apoptosis were observed for either group (Ornish et al., 2005). At 2 years of follow-up, 27% of the control group but only 5% of the experimental group patients had undergone conventional treatment ($p < 0.05$) (Frattaroli et al., 2008). In the same study, investigators studied changes in gene expression in prostate tissue among 30 of the lifestyle intervention patients before and after 3 months of lifestyle intervention, finding significant modulation of genes responsible for tumorigenesis, including protein metabolism and modification, intracellular protein traffic, and protein phosphorylation (Ornish et al., 2008b). Similarly, telomerase activity (protects telomeres or chromosomes) was significantly enhanced in the peripheral blood mononuclear cells among 24 of the lifestyle intervention patients (Ornish et al., 2008a). Another small study among 10 men with biochemical recurrence after prostatectomy used a 4-month intervention combining mindfulness-based stress reduction and a low-saturated-fat, high-fiber, plant-based diet and found a decreased rate of rise in PSA in 8 of 10 men and a reduced median doubling time from 6.5 to 17.7 months ($p = 0.01$) (Saxe et al., 2001). Similarly, among 14 patients with recurrent prostate cancer, a 6-month intervention involving a plant-based diet and stress reduction decreased PSA doubling times (mean of 11.9 months [prestudy] to 112.3 months [postintervention]) (Saxe et al., 2006).

These interventions do not directly address primary prevention, because of the long timescales involved, but they do speak to how diet might modify the course of disease progression in existing prostate cancer cases. It is important to note that the interventions were not merely dietary, but included other lifestyle components; still, a healthy plant-based diet was a major feature of the interventions. These studies seem to provide evidence that, at least in low-grade prostate cancer, plant-based diets (and other lifestyle changes) may be able to delay disease progression for recurrence. It is possible that many mechanisms that could result in such delayed progression might also be relevant for primary prevention.

5.6 MEAT CONSUMPTION AND CANCER RISK

Comparative cancer risk has also been estimated in many studies related to meat consumption. While these studies do not examine vegetarian dietary patterns per se, they correlate cancer risk with meat consumption, providing findings relevant for dietary patterns with little or no meat (including red meat or processed meat), such as vegetarian diets. An exhaustive review of the literature of meat intake and cancer risk is beyond the scope of this chapter, but relevant evidence is highlighted related to several common cancers or where the evidence of a link seems stronger.

5.6.1 COLORECTAL CANCER

The strongest scientific evidence linking meat consumption to cancer risk is for cancers of the colon and rectum, for both processed meat and red meat. The 2017 WCRF/AICR report on diet and colorectal cancer categorizes the association as "strong evidence, convincing" for processed meat and "strong evidence, probable" for red meat (WCRF, 2017; WCRF/AICR, 2017b). In October 2015, the International Agency for Research on Cancer (IARC) of the World Health Organization classified processed meat as "carcinogenic to humans … based on sufficient evidence in humans that the consumption of processed meat causes colorectal cancer" (Bouvard et al., 2015). The IARC categorized red meat as "probably carcinogenic to humans … based on limited evidence that the consumption of red meat causes cancer in humans and strong mechanistic evidence supporting a carcinogenic effect. This association was observed mainly for colorectal cancer" (Bouvard et al., 2015).

In a 2011 meta-analysis, each 100 g/day increase in red meat consumption yielded an RR of 1.17 (1.05–1.31), with a similar RR of 1.18 (1.10–1.28) for 50 g/day of processed meat (Chan et al., 2011). While results, particularly for red meat, are not entirely consistent, findings from major studies, including the National Institutes of Health–American Association of Retired Persons (NIH-AARP) cohort (Cross et al., 2007) and the EPIC cohort (Norat et al., 2005), have generally supported these risk associations.

5.6.2 BREAST CANCER

The 2017 WCRF/AICR report on diet and breast cancer considers the evidence linking red and processed meat, poultry, or fish intake to breast cancer as limited and inconclusive for both premenopausal and postmenopausal breast cancer (WCRF, 2017; WCRF/AICR, 2017a). This is due to the inconsistent results of major prospective studies examining this relationship. For example, EPIC reported no significant association for high intake of red meat (RR 1.06, 0.98–1.14) and borderline significance for processed meat (RR 1.10, 1.00–1.20) (Pala et al., 2009). Findings from NIH-AARP have mostly showed no association of meat intake with breast cancer, though some subanalyses have highlighted possible relationships for specific types of postmenopausal breast cancer (Cross et al., 2007; Inoue-Choi et al., 2016). In the UK Women's Cohort Study, 50 g/day consumption of total meat was associated with increased premenopausal breast cancer (HR 1.12, 1.02–1.23) and postmenopausal breast cancer (HR 1.10, 1.01–2.20) (Taylor et al., 2007). A recent meta-analysis of 14 studies of red meat and 12 studies of processed meat estimated summary RRs of breast cancer as 1.11 (1.05–1.16) for each 120 g/day of red meat intake and 1.09 (1.03–1.16) for each 50 g/day of processed meat (Guo et al., 2015). It may be that meat intake at certain important life stages, such as adolescence, could be more important than later intake. The Nurses' Health Study II has linked adolescent consumption of red meat (but not poultry) to a higher risk of premenopausal (RR 1.43, 1.05–1.94) but not postmenopausal breast cancer (Farvid et al., 2015).

5.6.3 PROSTATE CANCER

As with breast cancer, the 2014 WCRF/AICR report on diet and prostate cancer considers the evidence linking red and processed meat, poultry, or fish intake to prostate cancer as limited and inconclusive (WCRF/AICR, 2014a). A 2010 meta-analysis of 15 studies of red meat and 11 studies of processed meat did not support an association with prostate cancer risk (Alexander et al., 2010). Similarly, a 2015 meta-analysis examining 26 publications from 19 cohort studies did not support an association of red or processed meat consumption (or of meat cooking methods or chemical compounds related to meat or meat processing) with prostate cancer, although there was a weak positive summary RR estimate for processed meat 1.05 (1.01–1.10) (Bylsma and Alexander, 2015). Finally, a 2016 pooled analysis from 15 cohort studies again mostly showed no significant association between meat intake and prostate cancer risk (Wu et al., 2016).

5.6.4 PANCREATIC CANCER

The 2012 WCRF/AICR report on diet and pancreatic cancer considers the evidence linking red and processed meat intake to pancreatic cancer as limited but suggestive of an adverse association, whereas the evidence for fish is limited and inconclusive (WCRF/AICR, 2012). A 2012 meta-analysis of 11 prospective studies reported a summary estimate of RR of 1.19 (1.04–1.36) for a 50 g/day increase in processed meat consumption; there was also a significant overall association for red meat, but only in men (Larsson and Wolk, 2012). The NIH-AARP study has reported a significant association for total meat intake (as well as for red meat, certain meat cooking methods, and heme iron from red meat) and pancreatic cancer (HR 1.20, 1.02–1.42) (Taunk et al., 2016). In contrast, the EPIC study found no significant association of either red meat or processed meat with pancreatic cancer, although there was an association with poultry (RR per 50 g/day: 1.72, 1.04–2.84) (Rohrmann et al., 2013a).

5.6.5 GASTRIC CANCER

The 2016 WCRF/AICR report on diet and gastric cancer indicates that there is strong evidence of a probable association of processed meat with a type of gastric cancer (noncardia), and that there is limited but suggestive evidence to link grilled (broiled) or barbecued (charbroiled) meat and fish consumption to stomach cancer (WCRF/AICR, 2016). A 2014 meta-analysis of 18 studies of red meat and gastric cancer showed a positive association, but with significant heterogeneity among studies, with case-control but not cohort studies supporting the association (Song et al., 2014). Another meta-analysis in 2013 of red and processed meat intake and gastric cancer examined 12 cohort and 30 case-control studies, showing positive associations for red and processed meats; again, case-control studies supported the association, but cohort studies did not (Zhu et al., 2013). Particularly significant findings linking meat intake to noncardia gastric cancers come from the EPIC study, with (calibrated) HRs for noncardia gastric cancers of 3.52 (1.96–6.34) per 100 g/day increase of total meat and 1.73 (1.03–2.88) and 2.45 (1.43–4.21) per 50 g/day increase of red and processed meats, respectively (Gonzalez et al., 2006).

5.6.6 LIVER CANCER

The 2015 WCRF/AICR report on diet and liver cancer points to limited evidence suggestive of a decreased risk for fish intake and limited and inconclusive evidence for an association with meat and poultry (WCRF/AICR, 2015). In the NIH-ARRP study, for cancers of the liver, highest versus lowest quintiles of red meat intake had an HR of 1.61 (1.12–2.31), but there was no significant association for processed meat (Cross et al., 2007); in a later analysis, for hepatocellular carcinoma (HCC) red meat was associated with higher risk (HR 1.74, 1.16–2.61), but white meat was associated with lower risk (Freedman et al., 2010). In the EPIC study, total meat, red or processed meat, and poultry were not associated with HCC, but fish intake was associated with lower risk (HR 0.80, 0.69–0.97, per 20 g/day increase) (Fedirko et al., 2013).

5.6.7 Cancer Mortality

While initial evaluation in AHS-2 did not reveal significantly lower cancer mortality among vegetarian groups than among nonvegetarians (Orlich et al., 2013), considerable evidence does link diets high in meat to higher cancer mortality. In a combined analysis of the Nurses' Health Study and the Health Professional's Follow-Up Study (NHS-HPFS), adjusted HRs for cancer mortality per one serving per day increase in processed red meat were 1.16 (1.09–1.23) and 1.10 (1.07–1.13) for unprocessed red meat (Pan et al., 2012). In a related analysis also in NHS-HPFS, a low-carbohydrate diet based on animal sources was associated with higher overall cancer mortality (HR 1.28, 1.02–1.60) (Fung et al., 2010). In the NIH-AARP study, higher cancer mortality was associated with higher intakes of red meat (HR 1.22, 1.16–1.29 in men; HR 1.20, 1.12–1.30 in women) and processed meat (HR 1.12, 1.06–1.19 in men; HR 1.11, 1.04–1.19 in women), whereas higher white meat intake was associated with lower cancer mortality (Sinha et al., 2009). In the EPIC study, red meat and poultry intakes were not associated with cancer mortality; however, higher processed meat was associated with higher cancer mortality (calibrate HR 1.11, 1.03–1.21 per 50 g/day) (Rohrmann et al., 2013b). A pooled analysis of Asian prospective cohorts revealed no significant association with total meat intake and cancer mortality in men or women but, perhaps surprisingly, showed a hazardous association with fish intake in men (HR 1.14, 1.04–1.26 for highest quintile) but protective associations in women for red meat (HR 0.85, 0.76–0.94) and poultry (HR 0.88, 0.79–0.97) (Lee et al., 2013). A 2016 meta-analysis of nine publications (involving 17 prospective cohorts) found a higher risk of cancer mortality for processed meat (RR 1.08, 1.06–1.11 per serving per day) and total red meat (RR 1.12, 1.10–1.14 per serving per day) but not unprocessed red meat (Wang et al., 2016).

5.7 DAIRY AND EGGS AND CANCER RISK

Although many vegetarians consume both eggs and dairy (lacto-ovo vegetarians), they often still consume lesser amounts than nonvegetarians (Orlich et al., 2014), and of course, vegan diets omit these foods. Thus, we briefly review evidence relating these animal products to cancer risk.

5.7.1 Eggs

For breast cancer, a 2015 meta-analysis found that compared with those consuming no eggs, women consuming five eggs per week (RR 1.04, 1.01–1.07) and those consuming about nine eggs per week (RR 1.09, 1.03–1.15) had an increased risk (Keum et al., 2015). A 2014 meta-analysis of 13 studies had similar findings (RR 1.04, 1.01–1.08) (Si et al., 2014).

For prostate cancer, a 2012 meta-analysis found no egg–prostate cancer association (Xie and He, 2012). In a 2015 meta-analysis, men consuming five eggs per week had an increased risk of fatal prostate cancer (RR 1.47, 1.01–2.14); however, no significant association was found for all incident prostate cancers with egg intake (Keum et al., 2015). In a 2016 pooled analysis of 15 prospective cohort studies, men eating ≥25 g/day of eggs (compared to <5 g/day; one egg is ~50 g) had a higher risk of advanced (RR 1.14, 1.01–1.28) and fatal (RR 1.14, 1.00–1.30) prostate cancers (Wu et al., 2016). In a study of the recurrence or progression of prostate cancer among 1294 men already diagnosed with prostate cancer, increased egg consumption was found to be associated with recurrence or progression (HR 2.02, 1.10–3.72, comparing extreme quintiles) (Richman et al., 2010). In the HPFS cohort, among 27,607 men without prostate cancer, those who consumed ≥2.5 eggs per week had a higher risk of developing fatal prostate cancer (HR 1.81, 1.13–2.89) than those consuming <0.5 eggs/week (Richman et al., 2011).

A 2014 meta-analysis of cohort and case-control studies found increased egg consumption to be associated with increased risk for gastrointestinal neoplasms (OR 1.15, 1.09–1.22), especially colon cancers (OR 1.29, 1.14–1.46) (Tse and Eslick, 2014). A 2013 meta-analysis of four cohort and nine case-control studies of egg consumption and bladder cancer found no association overall (Li et al., 2013).

5.7.2 DAIRY PRODUCTS

While evidence linking dairy consumption to most cancers is quite limited, it has tended to support a possible beneficial association of dairy consumption with colorectal cancer and, on the other hand, a possible adverse association of it with prostate cancer.

The 2017 WCRF/AICR CUP report concludes that "dairy product consumption probably protects against colorectal cancer" (WCRF, 2017; WCRF/AICR, 2017b). A 2012 systematic review and meta-analysis of 19 cohort studies found that for 400 g/day of total dairy product intake, there was a lower risk of colorectal cancer (RR 0.83, 0.78–0.88) (Aune et al., 2012). Subsequently, the EPIC study published broadly consistent findings (HR 0.93, 0.89–0.98 for 200 g/day milk consumption) (Murphy et al., 2013). A 2014 meta-analysis of 15 studies found a lower risk of colon cancer among men with a higher consumption of unfermented milk (RR 0.74, 0.60–0.91) but no significant association with rectal cancer, or with colon or rectal cancer in women, or with any outcome for fermented milk or cheese (Ralston et al., 2014). Dietary calcium intake has been associated with a lower risk of colorectal cancer (Keum et al., 2014), and this may help to explain the potential benefits of total dairy and milk consumption. In contrast to these findings, evidence for a possible adverse effect of early-life dairy consumption on colorectal cancer risk comes from an interesting study attempting to link childhood diet and adult cancer risk. This was a 65-year follow-up of a study of 4999 children living in England and Scotland between 1937 and 1939, whose family food consumption was measured by means of a 7-day household food inventory. When these were later matched with National Health Service cancer registries, it was found that high childhood household dairy intake was associated with a significantly increased risk of colorectal cancer (adjusted OR 2.90, 1.26–6.65) after adjustment for household meat, fruit, and vegetable intake and socioeconomic indicators (van der Pols et al., 2007).

For prostate cancer, there is concern for a possible adverse association with dairy. The 2014 WCRF/AICR CUP report categorizes dairy products (as well as diets high in calcium) as having limited evidence suggestive of an increased risk of prostate cancer (WCRF/AICR, 2014a). A 2015 meta-analysis of 32 studies estimated a summary RR per 400 g/day of total dairy consumed of 1.07 (1.02–1.12) for risk of all prostate cancers (Aune et al., 2015). A 2016 meta-analysis of 11 cohort studies of dairy products and cancer mortality found a linear dose–response relationship for whole-milk consumption and prostate cancer mortality (RR 1.43, 1.13–1.81 per serving per day) (Lu et al., 2016).

5.8 PLANT FOODS AND CANCER RISK

Although vegetarian dietary patterns are defined by the absence of animal foods, they also often differ with respect to the level of consumption of many plant foods, which might further affect the risk of cancer. Vegetarian dietary patterns often include higher levels of fruits, vegetables, legumes, whole grains, nuts, and soy foods (Orlich et al., 2014). A detailed review of the evidence relating these food groups to cancer risk is beyond the scope of this chapter. However, we will mention a few examples supporting such associations, to illustrate that varying the intake of plant foods might impact cancer risk among vegetarians.

5.8.1 FRUITS AND VEGETABLES

In the 1997 WCRF/AICR report, evidence for fruits and vegetables preventing many cancer types was considered convincing, based mainly on case-control studies; however, 10 years later in 2007, the report downgraded the evidence to "probable" for some cancers of the upper airway and digestive tract and "limited, suggestive" for a number of other cancers (Norat et al., 2014). Currently, WCRF/AICR rates the evidence as strong for fruits decreasing cancers of the mouth, pharynx, and larynx and of the lungs and for nonstarchy vegetables decreasing cancers of the mouth, pharynx, and larynx (WCRF/AICR, 2017c). It seems likely that direct preventive effects of fruit and vegetable intake may be quite modest for cancer as a whole. A 2017 systematic review and meta-analysis found a risk ratio, per 200 g/day consumption of fruits and vegetables combined, of 0.97 (0.95–0.99) for total cancer incidence and 0.93 (0.87–0.98) for highest versus lowest intakes (Aune et al., 2017). Interest continues in identifying specific compounds in fruits and vegetables that may have specific cancer-preventive activity.

A variety of dietary phytochemicals, found in commonly eaten fruits, vegetables, spices, and legumes, have been found (in cell culture studies and animal models) to modify various cellular mechanisms in cancer initiation and progression. A number of phytochemicals (such as genistein in soy, indole-3-carbinol and sulforaphane in cruciferous vegetables, and quercetin and various carotenoids in fruits and vegetables) that regulate cancer pathobiology are now being studied for their potential role as chemopreventive agents (Anand et al., 2008; Su et al., 2013; Shukla et al., 2014; Srivastava et al., 2015; Thakur et al., 2014; Yin et al., 2016; Mahadevappa and Kwok, 2017). Preliminary clinical trials involving curcumin (from turmeric) and resveratrol (from grapes) have shown potential in the treatment of colorectal cancer and other human cancers (Tan et al., 2014; Li et al., 2015).

5.8.2 Dietary Fiber and Whole Grains

The idea of dietary fiber's preventive potential for bowel cancers goes back many decades, at least to Denis Burkitt, yet the evidence has seemed to wax and wane. The WCRF/AICR 2017 CUP report has concluded that there is strong evidence of a probable decreased risk of colorectal cancer with consumption of foods containing dietary fiber and also specifically with consumption of whole grains (WCRF, 2017; WCRF/AICR, 2017b). A 2011 systematic review and meta-analysis (25 studies) reported an RR reduction of colorectal cancer, for each 10 g of daily total fiber, of 0.90 (0.86–0.94), with significance for cereal fiber specifically (RR 0.90, 0.83–0.97) (Aune et al., 2011). The same study estimated the RR of eating three additional servings per day of whole grains to be 0.83 (0.78–0.89) (Aune et al., 2011). A 2016 systematic review and meta-analysis of eight prospective studies of whole grains and cancer mortality found, per 50 g/day increase of whole grains, the risk ratio to be 0.82 (0.69–0.96) for total cancer mortality (Chen et al., 2016).

5.8.3 Soy

There has been much controversy around soy foods and the isoflavones they contain and breast cancer risk. Much of the literature, including several recent meta-analyses, has seemed to show a lower risk of breast cancer with increasing soy intake among Asian populations (where soy intakes are much higher), but not typically among Western populations (Dong and Qin, 2011; Chen et al., 2014; Liu et al., 2014). The 2017 WCRF/AICR CUP report classifies the evidence for soy and soy products as limited and inconclusive for both pre- and postmenopausal breast cancer incidence (WCRF, 2017; WCRF/AICR, 2017a). On the other hand, for breast cancer survival, a 2014 WCRF/AICR report classifies the evidence for foods containing soy in the diet after breast cancer diagnosis as limited, but suggestive of improving survival by reducing all-cause mortality (but not breast cancer mortality specifically) (WCRF/AICR, 2014b).

5.8.4 Nuts

A 2016 systematic review and meta-analysis of eight prospective studies found that per 28 g/day increase in nut consumption there was a decreased risk for all cancers combined (RR 0.85, 0.76–0.94) (Aune et al., 2016a). Another meta-analysis, which examined specific cancers but which had a very limited number of studies for each (and included case-control studies), found higher intakes of nuts to be associated with a decreased risk of colorectal cancer (RR 0.76, 0.61–0.96; three studies), endometrial cancer (RR 0.58, 0.43–0.79; two studies), pancreatic cancer (RR 0.68, 0.48–0.96; one study), and overall cancer incidence (RR 0.85, 0.76–0.95) (Wu et al., 2015). Higher intakes of nuts have also been associated with decreased cancer-specific mortality, with a 2015 meta-analysis finding an RR of 0.86 (0.75–0.98) for cancer mortality (Grosso et al., 2015).

5.9 POTENTIALLY RELEVANT MECHANISMS LINKING DIET TO CANCER RISK

Nutritional epidemiology traditionally has sought to detect statistical associations between diet and the occurrence of disease, such as cancer, while attempting to control for any potential confounding factors. While detecting such associations is very important, causality is often hard to firmly establish by such associational evidence alone; hence, there is great interest in identifying particular molecular compounds that might provide a plausible mechanistic link between foods and cancer biology.

5.9.1 CHEMICALS ASSOCIATED WITH MEAT AND ITS PREPARATION

A number of such compounds present in meat or related to meat cooking or processing, such as heterocyclic amines (HCAs), polyaromatic hydrocarbons (PAHs), nitrites and N-nitroso compounds (NOCs), and heme iron, have been proposed as being potentially related to cancer risk. See Abid et al. (2014) for a review of the evidence of several of these compounds and their association with cancer risk.

5.9.2 HORMONAL MECHANISMS SUCH AS IGF-1

Other attempts at mechanistic explanations link changes in the levels of hormones or other signaling molecules to dietary patterns. An example is insulin-like growth factor 1 (IGF-1), a hormone that can stimulate cell proliferation and inhibit cell death and which may be increased with high intakes of proteins rich in essential amino acids (often concentrated in animal foods) (Allen et al., 2002). In the EPIC-Oxford cohort, vegan participants had significantly lower serum IGF-1 concentrations, 13% lower in women (Allen et al., 2002) and 9% in men (Allen et al., 2000).

5.9.3 VEGETARIAN DIETS, OBESITY, AND CANCER RISK

A thorough discussion of vegetarian diets and overweight and obesity can be found in Chapter 7 in this book. However, to summarize, both lacto-ovo vegetarian and vegan diets are consistently associated with lower rates of obesity, with mean body mass index (BMI) often increasing in a stepwise fashion as animal product consumption increases. These differences are more dramatic in the Adventist studies, but also clearly present in the British vegetarian studies (Fraser, 1999; Spencer et al., 2003; Tonstad et al., 2009). Assuming that this association is causal (i.e., that vegetarian diets lead to lower BMI levels), this reduced adiposity could then be considered an important mechanism, or intermediate state, by which vegetarian diets might lead to a lower risk of several cancers. This is because being overweight or obese has been linked to an increased risk for several cancers (and the list has been growing). The WRCF identifies 11 cancers linked to high BMI. A 2016 systematic review and meta-analysis of 230 cohort studies found that adiposity is an established risk factor for at least 10 different cancers, including cancers of the esophagus, liver, gallbladder, colorectum, pancreas, kidney, prostate (advanced), breast (postmenopausal), endometrium, and ovaries, and also potentially a risk factor for thyroid cancers, leukemia, multiple myeloma, and lymphomas (Aune et al., 2016b). A lower survival after a cancer diagnosis and increased cancer-specific mortality rates have also been associated with higher BMIs (Aune et al., 2016b).

5.10 CHALLENGES AND CONCLUSIONS

It is very difficult to conclusively link specific dietary choices to the risk of specific cancers. This is partly because diet is a complex and highly variable exposure that is hard to measure accurately. It can thus be very challenging to try to assess the long-term exposure to a particular dietary component and disentangle its possible effects from the other aspects of diet. It is also difficult to conclusively link dietary choices to the risk of cancer, because cancer is a complex and varied set of diseases that develops over years and decades. In some sense, every single cancer (in every individual) is somewhat different and has a unique set of causes related to inherited risk, chance, and environmental exposures throughout life. For a simple and very strong environmental risk factor, such as tobacco smoke (where the RR for lung cancer may be on the order of 10- to 20-fold), it is easier to cut through the complexity and define the increased risk with certainty. However, with diet, the RRs may be an increase or decrease of only 10%–30%. Such modest risk is much more prone to be missed (or to be seen when not really there) due to measurement error or uncontrolled confounding.

For these reasons, one will notice a substantial amount of uncertainty in the literature reviewed in this chapter. Given this, what conclusions can we reasonably draw about the risk of cancer in vegetarians, given the current evidence? First, from the cohort studies of vegetarians, such as AHS-2 and EPIC-Oxford, there is fairly good evidence to suggest a modest reduction in risk for vegetarians for any cancer (i.e., all cancers combined), on the order of 8%–15% less risk, possibly with the risk for vegans being somewhat lower. Mainly based on research regarding red and processed meat intake, vegetarian diets seem likely to offer some protection against colorectal cancer, although findings from studies of vegetarians are inconsistent. Also based on evidence regarding meat (mainly red and processed meat) consumption and cancer mortality, vegetarians may have a lower overall risk of dying of cancer, although again, evidence from studies of vegetarians does not yet clearly support this. Beyond this, it is difficult to conclude much about the risk of vegetarians for other cancers. Vegans may have some protection against prostate cancer, which may partly be due to their reduced dairy product consumption.

It is important to remember that not all vegetarian (or vegan) diets are equal, and that cancer risk due to diet may thus vary considerably among vegetarians. Vegetarians would be advised to take care to eat a healthful and balanced diet, beyond their avoidance of particular animal foods. Generally, emphasizing a wide variety of whole foods in a less refined state would seem advisable. Specifically, following the recommendations of WCRF/AICR could be a good dietary strategy based on current evidence. For nonvegetarians, reducing or eliminating the consumption of red meat, especially processed meat, would be a good dietary improvement. Nondietary lifestyle choices and related risk factors are also important. In particular, avoiding obesity or excess weight gain, or attempting to return to a normal body weight if overweight or obese, may be more important for lowering cancer risk than many specific dietary choices. Engaging in regular exercise and maintaining physical fitness is also likely to be helpful in cancer prevention. Of course, avoiding tobacco is an extremely high priority, and alcohol consumption has been linked to an increased risk for multiple cancers, including breast cancer and colorectal cancer.

It is important to recognize that the odds of anyone ending up as a cancer patient are significant, and we should not have unrealistic expectations about the ability of diet to prevent cancer. A healthy lifestyle, including a healthy vegetarian diet, can help to reduce the chance of cancer. In addition, continuing a healthy diet and lifestyle may help improve the survival of a cancer patient.

REFERENCES

Abid Z, Cross AJ, Sinha R. 2014. Meat, dairy, and cancer. *Am J Clin Nutr* 100(Suppl. 1): 386S–93S. doi: 10.3945/ajcn.113.071597.

Alexander DD, Mink PJ, Cushing CA, Sceurman B. 2010. A review and meta-analysis of prospective studies of red and processed meat intake and prostate cancer. *Nutr J* 9:50. doi: 10.1186/1475-2891-9-50.

Allen NE, Appleby PN, Davey GK, Kaaks R, Rinaldi S, Key TJ. 2002. The associations of diet with serum insulin-like growth factor I and its main binding proteins in 292 women meat-eaters, vegetarians, and vegans. *Cancer Epidemiol Biomarkers Prev* 11(11):1441–8.

Allen NE, Appleby PN, Davey GK, Key TJ. 2000. Hormones and diet: Low insulin-like growth factor-I but normal bioavailable androgens in vegan men. *Br J Cancer* 83(1):95–7.

Anand P, Kunnumakara AB, Sundaram C, Harikumar KB, Tharakan ST, Lai OS, Sung B, Aggarwal BB. 2008. Cancer is a preventable disease that requires major lifestyle changes. *Pharm Res* 25(9):2097–116. doi: 10.1007/s11095-008-9661-9.

Aune D, Chan DSM, Lau R, Vieira R, Greenwood DC, Kampman E, Norat T. 2011. Dietary fibre, whole grains, and risk of colorectal cancer: Systematic review and dose-response meta-analysis of prospective studies. *BMJ* 343:d6617.

Aune D, Giovannucci E, Boffetta P, Fadnes LT, Keum N, Norat T, Greenwood DC, Riboli E, Vatten LJ, Tonstad S. 2017. Fruit and vegetable intake and the risk of cardiovascular disease, total cancer and all-cause mortality—A systematic review and dose-response meta-analysis of prospective studies. *Int J Epidemiol* 46(3):1029–56.

Aune D, Keum N, Giovannucci E, Fadnes LT, Boffetta P, Greenwood DC, Tonstad S, Vatten LJ, Riboli E, Norat T. 2016a. Nut consumption and risk of cardiovascular disease, total cancer, all-cause and cause-specific mortality: A systematic review and dose-response meta-analysis of prospective studies. *BMC Med* 14:207.

Aune D, Lau R, Chan DSM, Vieira R, Greenwood DC, Kampman E, Norat T. 2012. Dairy products and colorectal cancer risk: A systematic review and meta-analysis of cohort studies. *Ann Oncol* 23(1):37–45.

Aune D, Navarro Rosenblatt DA, Chan DS, Vieira AR, Vieira R, Greenwood DC, Vatten LJ, Norat T. 2015. Dairy products, calcium, and prostate cancer risk: A systematic review and meta-analysis of cohort studies. *Am J Clin Nutr* 101:87–117. doi: 10.3945/ajcn.113.067157.

Aune D, Sen A, Prasad M, Norat T, Janszky I, Tonstad S, Romundstad P, Vatten LJ. 2016b. BMI and all cause mortality: Systematic review and non-linear dose-response meta-analysis of 230 cohort studies with 3.74 million deaths among 30.3 million participants. *BMJ* 353:i2156.

Bouvard V, Loomis D, Guyton KZ, Grosse Y, Ghissassi FE, Benbrahim-Tallaa L, Guha N, Mattock H, Straif K, International Agency for Research on Cancer Monograph Working Group. 2015. Carcinogenicity of consumption of red and processed meat. *Lancet Oncol* 16:1599–600. doi: 10.1016/S1470-2045(15)00444-1.

Butler TL, Fraser GE, Beeson WL, Knutsen SF, Herring RP, Chan J, Sabaté J et al. 2008. Cohort profile: The Adventist Health Study-2 (AHS-2). *Int J Epidemiol* 37(2):260–5.

Bylsma LC, Alexander DD. 2015. A review and meta-analysis of prospective studies of red and processed meat, meat cooking methods, heme iron, heterocyclic amines and prostate cancer. *Nutr J* 14:125. doi: 10.1186/s12937-015-0111-3.

Cade JE, Taylor EF, Burley VJ, Greenwood DC. 2010. Common dietary patterns and risk of breast cancer: Analysis from the United Kingdom Women's Cohort Study. *Nutr Cancer* 62:300–6. doi: 10.1080/01635580903441246.

Chan DS, Lau R, Aune D, Vieira R, Greenwood DC, Kampman E, Norat T. 2011. Red and processed meat and colorectal cancer incidence: Meta-analysis of prospective studies. *PLoS One* 6:e20456. doi: 10.1371/journal.pone.0020456.

Chen G-C, Tong X, Xu J-Y, Han S-F, Wan Z-X, Qin J-B, Qin L-Q. 2016. Whole-grain intake and total, cardiovascular, and cancer mortality: A systematic review and meta-analysis of prospective studies. *Am J Clin Nutr* 104(1):164–72.

Chen M, Rao Y, Zheng Y, Wei S, Li Y, Guo T, Yin P. 2014. Association between soy isoflavone intake and breast cancer risk for pre- and post-menopausal women: A meta-analysis of epidemiological studies. *PLoS One* 9:e89288. doi: 10.1371/journal.pone.0089288.

Cross AJ, Leitzmann MF, Gail MH, Hollenbeck AR, Schatzkin A, Sinha R. 2007. A prospective study of red and processed meat intake in relation to cancer risk. *PLoS Med* 4(12):e325.

Davey GK, Spencer EA, Appleby PN, Allen NE, Knox KH, Key TJ. 2003. EPIC–Oxford: Lifestyle characteristics and nutrient intakes in a cohort of 33 883 meat-eaters and 31 546 non meat-eaters in the UK. *Public Health Nutr* 6(3):259–68.

Dinu M, Abbate R, Gensini GF, Casini A, Sofi F. 2017. Vegetarian, vegan diets and multiple health outcomes: A systematic review with meta-analysis of observational studies. *Crit Rev Food Sci Nutr* 57(17):3640–9.

Dong JY, Qin LQ. 2011. Soy isoflavones consumption and risk of breast cancer incidence or recurrence: A meta-analysis of prospective studies. *Breast Cancer Res Treat* 125(2):315–23.

Farvid MS, Cho E, Chen WY, Eliassen AH, Willett WC. 2015. Adolescent meat intake and breast cancer risk. *Int J Cancer* 136:1909–20. doi: 10.1002/ijc.29218.

Fedirko V, Trichopoulou A, Bamia C, Duarte-Salles T, Trepo E, Aleksandrova K, Nothlings U et al. 2013. Consumption of fish and meats and risk of hepatocellular carcinoma: The European Prospective Investigation into Cancer and Nutrition (EPIC). *Ann Oncol* 24:2166–73. doi: 10.1093/annonc/mdt168.

Fraser GE. 1999. Associations between diet and cancer, ischemic heart disease, and all-cause mortality in non-Hispanic white California Seventh-day Adventists. *Am J Clin Nutr* 70(3):532S–8S.

Frattaroli J, Weidner G, Dnistrian AM, Kemp C, Daubenmier JJ, Marlin RO, Crutchfield L, Yglecias L, Carroll PR, Ornish D. 2008. Clinical events in prostate cancer lifestyle trial: Results from two years of follow-up. *Urology* 72:1319–23. doi: 10.1016/j.urology.2008.04.050.

Freedman ND, Cross AJ, McGlynn KA, Abnet CC, Park Y, Hollenbeck AR, Schatzkin A, Everhart JE, Sinha R. 2010. Association of meat and fat intake with liver disease and hepatocellular carcinoma in the NIH-AARP cohort. *J Natl Cancer Inst* 102(17):1354–65.

Fung TT, van Dam RM, Hankinson SE, Stampfer M, Willett WC, Hu FB. 2010. Low-carbohydrate diets and all-cause and cause-specific mortality: Two cohort studies. *Ann Intern Med* 153(5):289–98.

Gonzalez CA, Jakszyn P, Pera G, Agudo A, Bingham S, Palli D, Ferrari P et al. 2006. Meat intake and risk of stomach and esophageal adenocarcinoma within the European Prospective Investigation into Cancer and Nutrition (EPIC). *J Natl Cancer Inst* 98(5):345–54.

Grosso G, Yang J, Marventano S, Micek A, Galvano F, Kales SN. 2015. Nut consumption on all-cause, cardiovascular, and cancer mortality risk: A systematic review and meta-analysis of epidemiologic studies. *Am J Clin Nutr* 101(4):783–93.

Guo J, Wei W, Zhan L. 2015. Red and processed meat intake and risk of breast cancer: A meta-analysis of prospective studies. *Breast Cancer Res Treat* 151:191–8. doi: 10.1007/s10549-015-3380-9.

Huang T, Yang B, Zheng J, Li G, Wahlqvist ML, Li D. 2012. Cardiovascular disease mortality and cancer incidence in vegetarians: A meta-analysis and systematic review. *Ann Nutr Metab* 60(4):233–40.

Inoue-Choi M, Sinha R, Gierach GL, Ward MH. 2016. Red and processed meat, nitrite, and heme iron intakes and postmenopausal breast cancer risk in the NIH-AARP Diet and Health Study. *Int J Cancer* 138:1609–18. doi: 10.1002/ijc.29901.

Keum N, Aune D, Greenwood DC, Ju W, Giovannucci EL. 2014. Calcium intake and colorectal cancer risk: Dose-response meta-analysis of prospective observational studies. *Int J Cancer* 135:1940–8. doi: 10.1002/ijc.28840.

Keum N, Lee DH, Marchand N, Oh H, Liu H, Aune D, Greenwood DC, Giovannucci EL. 2015. Egg intake and cancers of the breast, ovary and prostate: A dose-response meta-analysis of prospective observational studies. *Br J Nutr* 114(7):1099–107.

Key TJ, Appleby PN, Crowe FL, Bradbury KE, Schmidt JA, Travis RC. 2014. Cancer in British vegetarians: Updated analyses of 4998 incident cancers in a cohort of 32,491 meat eaters, 8612 fish eaters, 18,298 vegetarians, and 2246 vegans. *Am J Clin Nutr* 100(1):378S–85S.

Key TJ, Appleby PN, Spencer EA, Travis RC, Roddam AW, Allen NE. 2009. Cancer incidence in vegetarians: Results from the European Prospective Investigation into Cancer and Nutrition (EPIC-Oxford). *Am J Clin Nutr* 89(5):1620S–6S.

Kotecha R, Takami A, Espinoza JL. 2016. Dietary phytochemicals and cancer chemoprevention: A review of the clinical evidence. *Oncotarget* 7(32):52517–29.

Larsson SC, Wolk A. 2012. Red and processed meat consumption and risk of pancreatic cancer: Meta-analysis of prospective studies. *Br J Cancer* 106:603–7. doi: 10.1038/bjc.2011.585.

Lee JE, McLerran DF, Rolland B, Chen Y, Grant EJ, Vedanthan R, Inoue M et al. 2013. Meat intake and cause-specific mortality: A pooled analysis of Asian prospective cohort studies. *Am J Clin Nutr* 98:1032–41. doi: 10.3945/ajcn.113.062638.

Li F, Zhou Y, Hu RT, Hou LN, Du YJ, Zhang XJ, Olkkonen VM, Tan WL. 2013. Egg consumption and risk of bladder cancer: A meta-analysis. *Nutr Cancer* 65:538–46. doi: 10.1080/01635581.2013.770041.

Li YH, Niu YB, Sun Y, Zhang F, Liu CX, Fan L, Mei QB. 2015. Role of phytochemicals in colorectal cancer prevention. *World J Gastroenterol* 21(31):9262–72.

Liu XO, Huang YB, Gao Y, Chen C, Yan Y, Dai HJ, Song FJ, Wang YG, Wang PS, Chen KX. 2014. Association between dietary factors and breast cancer risk among Chinese females: Systematic review and meta-analysis. *Asian Pac J Cancer Prev* 15(3):1291–8.

Lu W, Chen H, Niu Y, Wu H, Xia D, Wu Y. 2016. Dairy products intake and cancer mortality risk: A meta-analysis of 11 population-based cohort studies. *Nutr J* 15(1):91. Review. PubMed PMID: 27765039; PubMed Central PMCID: PMC5073921.

Mahadevappa R, Kwok HF. 2017. Phytochemicals—A novel and prominent source of anti-cancer drugs against colorectal cancer. *Comb Chem High Throughput Screen* 20(5):376–94. doi: 10.2174/1386207320666170112141833.

Matthes KL, Limam M, Dehler S, Korol D, Rohrmann S. 2017. Primary treatment choice over time and relative survival of prostate cancer patients: Influence of age, grade, and stage. *Oncol Res Treat* 40(9):484–9.

Murphy N, Norat T, Ferrari P, Jenab M, Bueno-de-Mesquita B, Skeie G, Olsen A et al. 2013. Consumption of dairy products and colorectal cancer in the European Prospective Investigation into Cancer and Nutrition (EPIC). *PLoS One* 8:e72715. doi: 10.1371/journal .pone.0072715.

Norat T, Aune D, Chan D, Romaguera D. 2014. Fruits and vegetables: Updating the epidemiologic evidence for the WCRF/AICR lifestyle recommendations for cancer prevention. *Cancer Treat Res* 159:35–50. doi: 10.1007/978-3-642-38007-5_3.

Norat T, Bingham S, Ferrari P, Slimani N, Jenab M, Mazuir M, Overvad K et al. 2005. Meat, fish, and colorectal cancer risk: The European Prospective Investigation into cancer and nutrition. *J Natl Cancer Inst* 97(12):906–16.

Orlich MJ, Fraser GE. 2014. Vegetarian diets in the Adventist Health Study 2: A review of initial published findings. *Am J Clin Nutr* 100 Suppl 1:353S–8S. doi: 10.3945/ajcn.113 .071233.

Orlich MJ, Jaceldo-Siegl K, Sabaté J, Fan J, Singh PN, Fraser GE. 2014. Patterns of food consumption among vegetarians and non-vegetarians. *Br J Nutr* 112(10):1644–53.

Orlich MJ, Singh PN, Sabaté J, Fan J, Sveen L et al. 2015. Vegetarian dietary patterns and the risk of colorectal cancers. *JAMA Intern Med* 175:767–76. doi: 10.1001/jamainternmed .2015.59.

Orlich MJ, Singh PN, Sabaté J, Jaceldo-Siegl K, Fan J, Knutsen S, Beeson WL, Fraser GE. 2013. Vegetarian dietary patterns and mortality in Adventist Health Study 2. *JAMA Intern Med* 173(13):1230–8.

Ornish D, Lin J, Daubenmier J, Weidner G, Epel E, Kemp C, Magbanua MJ, Marlin R, Yglecias L, Carroll PR, Blackburn EH. 2008a. Increased telomerase activity and comprehensive lifestyle changes: A pilot study. *Lancet Oncol* 9:1048–57. doi: 10.1016 /S1470-2045(08)70234-1.

Ornish D, Magbanua MJM, Weidner G, Weinberg V, Kemp C, Green C, Mattie MD, Marlin R, Simko J, Shinohara K, Haqq CM, Carroll PR. 2008b. Changes in prostate gene expression in men undergoing an intensive nutrition and lifestyle intervention. *Proc Natl Acad Sci U S A* 105(24):8369–74.

Ornish D, Weidner G, Fair WR, Marlin R, Pettengill EB, Raisin CJ, Dunn-Emke S et al. 2005. Intensive lifestyle changes may affect the progression of prostate cancer. *J Urol* 174(3):1065–9; discussion 1069–70.

Pala V, Krogh V, Berrino F, Sieri S, Grioni S, Tjonneland A, Olsen A et al. 2009. Meat, eggs, dairy products, and risk of breast cancer in the European Prospective Investigation into Cancer and Nutrition (EPIC) cohort. *Am J Clin Nutr* 90:602–12. doi: 10.3945 /ajcn.2008.27173.

Pan A, Sun Q, Bernstein AM, Schulze MB, Manson JE, Stampfer MJ, Willett WC, Hu FB. 2012. Red meat consumption and mortality: Results from 2 prospective cohort studies. *Arch Intern Med* 172(7):555–63.

Penniecook-Sawyers JA, Jaceldo-Siegl K, Fan J, Beeson L, Knutsen S, Herring P, Fraser GE. 2016. Vegetarian dietary patterns and the risk of breast cancer in a low-risk population. *Br J Nutr* 115:1790–7. doi: 10.1017/S0007114516000751.

Ralston RA, Truby H, Palermo CE, Walker KZ. 2014. Colorectal cancer and nonfermented milk, solid cheese, and fermented milk consumption: A systematic review and meta-analysis of prospective studies. *Crit Rev Food Sci Nutr* 54(9):1167–79.

Richman EL, Kenfield SA, Stampfer MJ, Giovannucci EL, Chan JM. 2011. Egg, red meat, and poultry intake and risk of lethal prostate cancer in the prostate-specific antigen-era: Incidence and survival. *Cancer Prev Res (Phila)* 4(12):2110–21.

Richman EL, Stampfer MJ, Paciorek A, Broering JM, Carroll PR, Chan JM. 2010. Intakes of meat, fish, poultry, and eggs and risk of prostate cancer progression. *Am J Clin Nutr* 91(3):712–21.

Rohrmann S, Linseisen J, Nothlings U, Overvad K, Egeberg R, Tjonneland A, Boutron-Ruault MC et al. 2013a. Meat and fish consumption and risk of pancreatic cancer: Results from the European Prospective Investigation into Cancer and Nutrition. *Int J Cancer* 132:617–24. doi: 10.1002/ijc.27637.

Rohrmann S, Overvad K, Bueno-de-Mesquita HB, Jakobsen MU, Egeberg R, Tjonneland A, Nailler L et al. 2013b. Meat consumption and mortality—Results from the European Prospective Investigation into Cancer and Nutrition. *BMC Med* 11:63. doi: 10.1186/1741-7015-11-63.

Saxe GA, Hebert JR, Carmody JF, Kabat-Zinn J, Rosenzweig PH, Jarzobski D, Reed GW, Blute RD. 2001. Can diet in conjunction with stress reduction affect the rate of increase in prostate specific antigen after biochemical recurrence of prostate cancer? *J Urol* 166(6):2202–7.

Saxe GA, Major JM, Nguyen JY, Freeman KM, Downs TM, Salem CE. 2006. Potential attenuation of disease progression in recurrent prostate cancer with plant-based diet and stress reduction. *Integr Cancer Ther* 5(3):206–13.

Shukla S, Meeran SM, Katiyar SK. 2014. Epigenetic regulation by selected dietary phytochemicals in cancer chemoprevention. *Cancer Lett* 355(1):9–17. doi: 10.1016/j.canlet.2014.09.017.

Si R, Qu K, Jiang Z, Yang X, Gao P. 2014. Egg consumption and breast cancer risk: A meta-analysis. *Breast Cancer* 21:251–61. doi: 10.1007/s12282-014-0519-1.

Sinha R, Cross AJ, Graubard BI, Leitzmann MF, Schatzkin A. 2009. Meat intake and mortality: A prospective study of over half a million people. *Arch Intern Med* 169:562–71. doi: 10.1001/archinternmed.2009.6.

Song P, Lu M, Yin Q, Wu L, Zhang D, Fu B, Wang B, Zhao Q. 2014. Red meat consumption and stomach cancer risk: A meta-analysis. *J Cancer Res Clin Oncol* 140:979–92. doi: 10.1007/s00432-014-1637-z.

Spencer EA, Appleby PN, Davey GK, Key TJ. 2003. Diet and body mass index in 38000 EPIC-Oxford meat-eaters, fish-eaters, vegetarians and vegans. *Int J Obes Relat Metab Disord* 27:728–34. doi: 10.1038/sj.ijo.0802300.

Srivastava SK, Arora S, Averett C, Singh S, Singh AP. 2015. Modulation of microRNAs by phytochemicals in cancer: Underlying mechanisms and translational significance. *Biomed Res Int* 2015:848710. doi: 10.1155/2015/848710.

Su ZY, Shu L, Khor TO, Lee JH, Fuentes F, Kong AN. 2013. A perspective on dietary phytochemicals and cancer chemoprevention: Oxidative stress, nrf2, and epigenomics. *Top Curr Chem* 329:133–62. doi: 10.1007/128_2012_340.

Tan HK, Moad AIH, Tan ML. 2014. The mTOR signalling pathway in cancer and the potential mTOR inhibitory activities of natural phytochemicals. *Asian Pac J Cancer Prev* 15(16):6463–75.

Tantamango-Bartley Y, Jaceldo-Siegl K, Fan J, Fraser GE. 2013. Vegetarian diets and the incidence of cancer in a low-risk population. *Cancer Epidemiol Biomarkers Prev* 22:286–94. doi: 10.1158/1055-9965.EPI-12-1060.

Tantamango-Bartley Y, Knutsen SF, Knutsen R, Jacobsen BK, Fan J, Beeson WL, Sabate J et al. 2016. Are strict vegetarians protected against prostate cancer? *Am J Clin Nutr* 103(1):153–60.

Taunk P, Hecht E, Stolzenberg-Solomon R. 2016. Are meat and heme iron intake associated with pancreatic cancer? Results from the NIH-AARP diet and health cohort. *Int J Cancer* 138:2172–89. doi: 10.1002/ijc.29964.

Taylor EF, Burley VJ, Greenwood DC, Cade JE. 2007. Meat consumption and risk of breast cancer in the UK Women's Cohort Study. *Br J Cancer* 96(7):1139–46.

Thakur VS, Deb G, Babcook MA, Gupta S. 2014. Plant phytochemicals as epigenetic modulators: Role in cancer chemoprevention. *AAPS J* 16(1):151–63. doi: 10.1208/s12248-013-9548-5.

Thorogood M, Mann J, Appleby P, McPherson K. 1994. Risk of death from cancer and ischaemic heart disease in meat and non-meat eaters. *BMJ* 308(6945):1667–70.

Tonstad S, Butler T, Yan R, Fraser GE. 2009. Type of vegetarian diet, body weight, and prevalence of type 2 diabetes. *Diabetes Care* 32:791–6. doi: 10.2337/dc08-1886.

Tse G, Eslick GD. 2014. Egg consumption and risk of GI neoplasms: Dose-response meta-analysis and systematic review. *Eur J Nutr* 53(7):1581–90.

van der Pols JC, Bain C, Gunnell D, Smith GD, Frobisher C, Martin RM. 2007. Childhood dairy intake and adult cancer risk: 65-y follow-up of the Boyd Orr cohort. *Am J Clin Nutr* 86(6):1722–9.

Wang X, Lin X, Ouyang YY, Liu J, Zhao G, Pan A, Hu FB. 2016. Red and processed meat consumption and mortality: Dose-response meta-analysis of prospective cohort studies. *Public Health Nutr* 19:893–905. doi: 10.1017/S1368980015002062.

WCRF (World Cancer Research Fund International). 2012. Cancer facts and figures: Worldwide data. Available at http://www.wcrf.org/int/cancer-facts-figures/worldwide-data (accessed September 1, 2017).

WCRF (World Cancer Research Fund International). 2017. Our cancer prevention recommendations. Available at http://www.wcrf.org/int/research-we-fund/cancer-prevention-recommendations/plant-foods (accessed September 1, 2017).

WCRF/AICR (World Cancer Research Fund International/American Institute for Cancer Research). 2012. Continuous Update Project report: Diet, nutrition, physical activity and pancreatic cancer. Available at wcrf.org/cupreports.

WCRF/AICR (World Cancer Research Fund International/American Institute for Cancer Research). 2014a. Continuous Update Project report: Diet, nutrition, physical activity and prostate cancer. Available at wcrf.org/prostate-cancer-2014. All CUP reports are available at wcrf.org/cupreports.

WCRF/AICR (World Cancer Research Fund International/American Institute for Cancer Research). 2014b. Continuous Update Project report: Diet, nutrition, physical activity and breast cancer survivors. Available at www.wcrf.org/sites/default/files/Breast-Cancer-Survivors-2014-Report.pdf.

WCRF/AICR (World Cancer Research Fund International/American Institute for Cancer Research). 2015. Continuous Update Project report: Diet, nutrition, physical activity and liver cancer. Available at wcrf.org/sites/default/files/Liver-Cancer-2015-Report.pdf. All CUP reports are available at wcrf.org/cupreports.

WCRF/AICR (World Cancer Research Fund International/American Institute for Cancer Research). 2016. Continuous Update Project report: Diet, nutrition, physical activity and stomach cancer. Available at wcrf.org/stomach-cancer-2016. All CUP reports are available at wcrf.org/cupreports.

WCRF/AICR (World Cancer Research Fund International/American Institute for Cancer Research). 2017a. Continuous Update Project report: Diet, nutrition, physical activity and breast cancer. Available at wcrf.org/breast-cancer-2017. All CUP reports are available at wcrf.org/cupreports.

WCRF/AICR (World Cancer Research Fund International/American Institute for Cancer Research). 2017b. Continuous Update Project report: Diet, nutrition, physical activity and colorectal cancer. Available at wcrf.org/colorectal-cancer-2017. All CUP reports are available at wcrf.org/cupreports.

WCRF/AICR (World Cancer Research Fund International/American Institute for Cancer Research). 2017c. Continuous Update Project summary report. Available at http://www.wcrf.org/sites/default/files/CUP_Summary_Report_Sept17.pdf.

World Health Organization. 2017. Cancer—Fact sheet. Available at http://www.who.int/mediacentre/factsheets/fs297/en/ (modified February 2017).

Wu K, Spiegelman D, Hou T, Albanes D, Allen NE, Berndt SI, van den Brandt PA et al. 2016. Associations between unprocessed red and processed meat, poultry, seafood and egg intake and the risk of prostate cancer: A pooled analysis of 15 prospective cohort studies. *Int J Cancer* 138:2368–82. doi: 10.1002/ijc.29973.

Wu L, Wang Z, Zhu J, Murad AL, Prokop LJ, Murad MH. 2015. Nut consumption and risk of cancer and type 2 diabetes: A systematic review and meta-analysis. *Nutr Rev* 73(7):409–25.

Xie B, He H. 2012. No association between egg intake and prostate cancer risk: A meta-analysis. *Asian Pac J Cancer Prev* 13:4677–81.

Yin TF, Wang M, Qing Y, Lin YM, Wu D. 2016. Research progress on chemopreventive effects of phytochemicals on colorectal cancer and their mechanisms. *World J Gastroenterol* 22(31):7058–68.

Zhu H, Yang X, Zhang C, Zhu C, Tao G, Zhao L, Tang S et al. 2013. Red and processed meat intake is associated with higher gastric cancer risk: A meta-analysis of epidemiological observational studies. *PLoS One* 8:e70955. doi: 10.1371/journal.pone.0070955.

6 Plant-Based Diets and Risk of Osteoporosis

Kelly Virecoulon Giudici and Connie M. Weaver

CONTENTS

SUMMARY

Plant-based diets often contain low amounts of calcium, vitamin D, and protein, and also insufficient contents of other nutrients related to bone metabolism, such as vitamin B12, zinc, and n-3 fatty acids. In accordance, bone mineral density (BMD) may be negatively impacted and the risk of osteoporosis increased. However, most studies have shown that vegetarians are not at a higher risk of developing osteoporosis than people following nonvegetarian diets. This may be explained by the fact that plant-based diets include dairy products and also have nutritional factors that could contribute to the accretion and maintenance of adequate bone, such as the low acid load and the high intake of potassium and polyphenols. Vegans who do not include dairy products are at a higher risk for osteoporosis. Nutritional recommendations include the use of fortified foods and supplements to supply adequate amounts of nutrients related to bone health.

6.1 INTRODUCTION

Although bone is a living tissue requiring all essential nutrients, specific nutrients are known to have a major role in bone metabolism (Mangels, 2014; Weaver, 2017), acting on the growth and development of the skeleton, collagen and cartilage formation, and regulation of calcium and phosphate homeostasis (Prentice et al., 2006). Accordingly, people consuming specific diets that restrict any group of foods should carefully consider ways to keep optimal bone maintenance. Bone mass is built and preserved majorly by metabolic pathways depending on nutrients that are more commonly found in animal sources (e.g., calcium, vitamin D, and protein) (Heaney, 2000; Ilich et al., 2003; Sutton and MacDonald, 2003). Thus, being vegetarian or vegan might potentially impair bone metabolism and increase the risk for osteoporosis. There are, however, typical factors of plant-based diets that may partially counterbalance the negative effects of nutrient deficiency, promoting a protective influence over bone metabolism.

Most intake of calcium usually comes from dairy products (Heaney, 2000). Nonvegan vegetarians are those consuming dairy products (lacto-vegetarians), eggs (ovo-vegetarians), or both (lacto-ovo vegetarians), and they consistently have higher calcium and protein intakes than vegans (Burckhardt, 2016). For this reason, lacto-vegetarians and lacto-ovo vegetarians are not at a specific risk of calcium deficiency. On the other hand, people following vegan diets can be considered a risk group. When daily calcium intake is lower than 800 mg, the risk of hip fracture increases significantly (Warensjö et al., 2011), as also occurs when protein intake is below 1.2 g/kg of body weight (Munger et al., 1999). In contrast, other studies have shown different and even lower protein intake thresholds associated with impaired bone health, that is, 0.8 g/kg of body weight (Kurpad and Vaz, 2000; Darling et al., 2009). Vegetarians, especially vegans, usually present with lower intakes of both (Kohlenberg-Mueller and Raschka, 2003; Ho-Pham et al., 2009a; Crowe et al., 2011; Knurick et al., 2015; Burckhardt, 2016).

The evident modifications in plant-based diets, compared with omnivorous diets, usually result in alterations in macronutrient and micronutrient intakes and ratios. Two studies evaluating large cohorts compared nutrient intakes among vegetarians and nonvegetarians. The European Prospective Investigation into Cancer and Nutrition (EPIC) study, including 43,993 omnivorous, 18,840 lacto-ovo vegetarians or lacto-vegetarians, and 2,596 vegans from the United Kingdom, found lower protein intake among vegetarians and vegans than omnivores. In addition, vegans presented the lowest intakes of calcium, vitamin D, vitamin B12, and zinc (Davey et al., 2003). On the other hand, the Adventist Health Study-2, evaluating 33,634 omnivorous, 21,799 lacto-ovo vegetarians, and 5,694 vegans from United States and Canada, did not observe differences in protein, calcium, vitamin B12, and zinc intake among groups. However, vitamin D intake was lower among vegans (Rizzo et al., 2013).

Several smaller studies have also shown that vegetarians often consume lower amounts of vitamin D (Outila et al., 2000; Crowe et al., 2011), vitamin B12 (Herrmann et al., 2003; Krivosíková et al., 2010; Shridhar et al., 2014), and zinc (Hunt, 2003; Shridhar et al., 2014), nutrients also related to bone metabolism (Mangels, 2014). Therefore, assuming that plant-based diets affect the consumption of nutrients importantly recognized as key elements to bone metabolism, the investigation of bone mineral density (BMD) and the risk of osteoporosis among vegetarians and vegans has become highly newsworthy in recent years.

6.2 BONE MINERAL DENSITY AND FRACTURE RISK AMONG PEOPLE FOLLOWING VEGETARIAN AND VEGAN DIETS

Low BMD favors the development of osteoporosis and is considered a consistent predictor of the risk of fracture (Bagger et al., 2006). Studies evaluating BMD in vegetarians and vegans yielded discrepant results, but in several studies, vegetarians had lower BMD than nonvegetarians (Chiu et al., 1997; Lau et al., 1998; Fontana et al., 2005; Welch et al., 2005; Ho-Pham et al., 2009a). A meta-analysis of nine studies with 2749 subjects demonstrated lower BMD at the femoral neck and lumbar spine among vegetarian and vegan subjects than among omnivores, and showed that vegans had a lower BMD than lacto-vegetarians, which the authors attributed to their lower protein and calcium intake (Ho-Pham et al., 2009a). Similar results were observed by Smith (2006) in a review study, who concluded that findings consistently support the hypothesis that vegans have lower BMD than their nonvegan counterparts. Indeed, in an earlier study, vegans had a 3.9 times higher risk for osteopenia than lacto-ovo vegetarians or omnivores (95% confidence interval [CI] 1.2–12.8) (Chiu et al., 1997). Moreover, a higher risk of wrist fracture was identified among vegetarian women (Thorpe et al., 2008). In this study, vegetarians who consumed the least vegetable protein intake were at highest risk for fracture. However, increasing levels of plant-based high-protein foods decreased wrist fracture risk, with a 68% reduction in risk (CI 0.13–0.79) in the highest intake group.

In contrast, other studies have not reported differences in bone loss and/or BMD between omnivores and vegetarians (Lloyd et al., 1991; Reed et al., 1994; Siani et al., 2003; Kim et al., 2007; Wang et al., 2008; Ho-Pham et al., 2012). A review concluded that lacto-ovo vegetarians did not have lower BMD than omnivores, in spite of their lower protein and calcium intake (New, 2004). Another review from the same author concluded that vegetarianism was not a risk for osteoporotic fractures (Lanham-New, 2009). A possible explanation for the discrepancy between studies that do and do not show lower BMD in vegetarians compared with nonvegetarians is the fact that demonstration of bone loss is not a quickly responding metabolic activity (Riggs et al., 1998). People following plant-based diets do not usually start before adolescence (Worsley and Skrzypiec, 1998), the critical period for bone development and growth (Saggese et al., 2002). Choosing vegetarianism or veganism with inadequate protein and calcium intake in adulthood will not change BMD rapidly. In addition, inconsistencies between studies may be driven by differences in the classification of vegetarians, small sample sizes, and failure in controlling for confounding factors, such as nutrient intake, body mass index, and physical activity level.

Fracture risk (measured by self-reporting) was examined in the EPIC-Oxford study, including more than 34,000 adults (aged 20–89 years) and a follow-up of 5.2 years. In this study, vegans presented a higher fracture risk; however, adjustments for alcohol intake and nondietary factors, such as age, smoking, and physical activity, have attenuated the findings (Appleby et al., 2007). Subjects were then reevaluated according to their estimated average requirement (EAR) for calcium, and no differences in fracture incidence were found among subjects with adequate calcium intake. No significant higher fracture risk among vegetarians and vegans was observed in another study that evaluated Vietnamese postmenopausal women (Ho-Pham et al., 2012). In summary, individuals following plant-based diets generally do not present important BMD deficits or a large difference in fracture rates when calcium and protein intakes are adequate.

6.3 OSTEOPOROSIS PREVALENCE AMONG VEGETARIANS AND VEGANS COMPARED WITH NONVEGETARIANS

Osteoporosis is a chronic disease characterized by loss of bone mass, leading to low BMD, skeletal fragility, and increased risk of fracture. Such a condition develops gradually and, consequently, is more frequently observed among the elderly (Riggs et al., 1998). Bone is constantly remodeling, through the balance of resorption (done by osteoclasts) and formation (performed by osteoblasts) (Teitelbaum, 2000). In the first decades of life, bone formation rates exceed bone resorption, allowing growth until reaching the peak of bone mass in early adulthood. Despite the fact that nutrition has a major impact on bone metabolism (Prentice et al., 2006; Mangels, 2014), nonnutritional factors also influence BMD, such as genetics (Seeman et al., 1996) and circulating levels of estrogen, a hormone found in high levels among females in reproductive age (Riggs et al., 1998). For this reason, older women are naturally at a higher risk for osteoporosis, since estrogen levels become much lower following menopause (Leboime et al., 2010). The rate of bone turnover also depends on parathyroid hormone (PTH) circulating levels, which increase in response to low calcium intake in order to maintain circulating calcium levels in the normal range (Adami et al., 2008).

In spite of the number of studies evaluating BMD among people following plant-based diets, information about the prevalence of the diagnosis of osteoporosis is scarce in this population. A study with a cohort of 1865 adults from Taiwan has found a prevalence of approximately 5% of osteoporosis among vegetarian men and about 30% among vegetarian women; however, this was not different from that in nonvegetarians (Wang et al., 2008). In another study, the prevalence of osteoporosis at the femoral neck in vegan Mahayana Buddhist nuns was 17.1%, also not different from the prevalence of 14.3% observed among omnivorous women (Ho-Pham et al., 2009b). Thus, the prevalence of osteoporosis in vegetarians and vegans does not seem to be higher than the prevalence observed among omnivores, in spite of the differences in nutrient intakes. This can be explained, in part, by the fact that plant-based diets naturally include both risk factors and protective factors for the loss of bone mass (more extensively described hereafter), and the balance among them depends on individual food choices and also on the presence or absence of other—nonnutritional—risk factors (e.g., gender, age, and hormone variations). Vegan diets, however, should be more carefully developed to avoid a higher risk for osteoporosis, since vegan subjects tend to present lower calcium intake (Burckhardt, 2016).

6.4 NUTRITIONAL ACID LOAD IN VEGETARIAN AND VEGAN DIETS AND ITS IMPACT ON BONE HEALTH

The low prevalence of osteoporosis or low BMD among vegetarians is thought by some to be partly due to the low acid load of these diets (Burckhardt, 2016). Nutritional acid load is based, generally but not only, on the quantity of protein and potassium that is consumed (Frassetto et al., 1998) and negatively correlates with BMD (New et al., 2004; MacDonald et al., 2005; Remer et al., 2014). Indeed, a significant lower net acid excretion was observed after 6 months of potassium citrate supplementation among adults >55 years old (Moseley et al., 2013). Taken together with other studies (Lemann et al., 1989; Sebastian et al., 1994; Frassetto et al., 2005), these findings suggest that organic salts of potassium (such as occurs in fruits and vegetables) in doses sufficient to effectively neutralize net renal acid excretion can improve calcium balance. Accordingly, a diet rich in fruits and vegetables corresponds to a high intake of potassium, which favors a low acid load (Ferraro et al., 2016). Metabolic mechanisms, however, remain unclear, given the fact that the benefit of potassium salts may be independent of changes in net renal acid excretion (Weaver, 2013).

For such reasons, the total nutritional acid load on vegetarian and vegan diets has gained special attention and was recently assessed in several studies, which found very low or absent values (Ausman et al., 2008; Ströhle et al., 2011; Gunn et al., 2015; Knurick et al., 2015). A study with young American adults found an acid load of −1.5 mEq/day in lacto-ovo vegetarians and −15.2 mEq/day in vegans (Knurick et al., 2015). Findings from another study with American women observed acid loads of 31.3 mEq/day among vegetarians and 17.3 mEq/day among vegans (Ausman et al., 2008), while the strongly alkalizing value of −39 mEq/day was identified among German strict vegans (Ströhle et al., 2011). In general, findings suggest that the more vegetarian a diet, the lower its acid load (Ströhle et al., 2010).

Meanwhile, the typical Western diet of omnivores was shown to produce approximately 30–52 mEq of acid daily, majorly due to the substantial intake of meats, which promotes an excess of protein consumption (MacDonald et al., 2005). Such a high acid load could, then, stimulate bone resorption. Indeed, the negative effect of the nutritional acid load on BMD has been demonstrated by several studies (New et al., 2004; MacDonald et al., 2005; Remer et al., 2014). Moreover, the neutralization of the Western diet with salt supplements administered in gelatin capsules was shown to inhibit bone resorption independently of potassium intake (Maurer et al., 2003).

The absence of meat consumption associated with the abundant intake of vegetables and fruits, typical of plant-based diets, therefore promotes a good acid–basic balance that could be useful for bone health, by decreasing bone resorption and increasing bone formation (Lanham-New, 2008; Knurick et al., 2015). The alkalizing attribute of plant-based diets could even compensate the typical nutritional deficiency of calcium and protein of vegetarians and vegans (Knurick et al., 2015). Consequently, the low acid load of regular vegetarian and vegan diets might be an important factor protecting against the development of osteoporosis. One cannot dismiss, however, the remarkable importance of protein intake on adequate bone maintenance. Dietary proteins are known to enhance insulin-like growth factor 1 (IGF-1), a factor that exerts positive activity on skeletal development and bone formation, while deficiency in dietary proteins contributes to marked deterioration in bone mass, microarchitecture, and strength (Bonjour, 2005). Therefore, the positive effect of the low acid load of plant-based diets should not be accompanied by a neglected protein intake.

6.5   VITAMIN D ADEQUACY IN VEGETARIAN AND VEGAN DIETS

Vitamin D plays an important role in bone metabolism, regulating active calcium absorption and controlling normal mineralization of bones (Sutton and MacDonald, 2003). Despite the lack of consensus on the reference ranges proposed in the literature to classify vitamin D status (Dawson-Hughes et al., 2005), vitamin D deficiency and insufficiency are prevalent conditions affecting many different populations all over the world, independent of the type of diet (Holick, 2007). Few foods naturally contain good quantities of calciferol, and fortified foods are not widely available in many countries yet. Therefore, endogenous skin production of vitamin D, after exposure to UV-B radiation from sunlight, corresponds to about 90% of circulating levels of 25-hydroxyvitamin D (Hollick, 2003). It has been shown that vitamin D status is affected by several factors, including latitude, season of the year, use of sunscreen, skin pigmentation, clothing coverage, and food intake (Kull et al., 2009; Nakamura et al., 2015). In this scenario, vegetarian and vegan diets may be additional factors contributing to vitamin D insufficiency or deficiency, since most natural, and in some countries fortified, sources of this vitamin are from animal origin (fish, oysters, milk, and eggs). However, given that dietary intake corresponds to a minor proportion of circulating 25-hydroxyvitamin D, vitamin D status may be improved with other alternatives, as with the habit of regular but safe sun exposure.

Several studies have examined vitamin D intake and vitamin D status among people following plant-based diets (Outila et al., 2000; Chan et al., 2009; Crowe et al., 2011; Ho-Pham et al., 2012). Low vitamin D intake and low plasma 25-hydroxyvitamin D concentrations were reported in vegan and vegetarian participants of the EPIC-Oxford study, with vegans presenting the lowest mean 25-hydroxyvitamin D concentrations (55.8 nmol/L) (Crowe et al., 2011). In accordance, lacto-vegetarians had significantly lower vitamin D intakes and lower plasma 25-hydroxyvitamin D concentrations than did nonvegetarians in a Finnish study (Outila et al., 2000), while lower dietary vitamin D intake was observed among non-Hispanic white vegetarians but not among black vegetarians in the Adventist Health Study-2 (Chan et al., 2009).

6.6   STRATEGIES TO ACHIEVE AN ADEQUATE INTAKE OF CALCIUM, PROTEIN, AND VITAMIN D IN VEGETARIAN AND VEGAN DIETS

Given the risks for low bone mass associated with impaired intakes of calcium, protein, and vitamin D, providing adequate intake of these nutrients is of major importance for subjects following plant-based diets. In the case of calcium, a normal intake can be achieved with no special difficulties by lacto-vegetarians and lacto-ovo vegetarians, with regular consumption of milk and dairy products. For ovo-vegetarians and vegans, in turn, specific strategies might be considered. Giving preference to vegetables with a higher bioavailability of calcium (e.g., Chinese mustard greens and Chinese cabbage flower leaves) (Weaver et al., 1997) provides some help in achieving daily recommendations. Calcium-fortified foods tend to be more expensive than their regular versions and are not still widely available in many regions of the world. If possible, however, the intake of food products fortified with calcium should be encouraged for people following plant-based diets, especially for vegans.

Regarding vitamin D, not many foods naturally contain much of it, and most of them are from animal origin (oysters, beef liver, milk, fish, and eggs). Sun-exposed (UV-treated) mushrooms, however, can be considered a good vegetarian or vegan source of this vitamin (Simon et al., 2013). Adequate content of vitamin D can also be achieved with fortified products. Food products more often fortified with vitamin D are milk and yogurts. However, other fortified options include orange juices and "plant" milks, a relatively recent innovation in the food industry.

Moreover, for promoting an adequate vitamin D status among people following plant-based diets, the dietary approach must be combined with usual sun exposure, given that the amount of vitamin D from the food supply is limited (Hollick, 2003). A regular exposure to sunlight—in safe hours, avoiding the hours of the day when the incidence of UV radiation is the highest—has been shown to be more effective in improving vitamin D status than dietary intake (Wolpowitz and Gilchrest, 2006). Still, supplemental vitamin D may be needed. It must be noted, however, that vitamin D3 (cholecalciferol) supplements are mostly made from lanolin from sheep's wool (Holick, 2009) or from fish liver oils (Holick, 2003); that is, they are not suitable for vegans, while a vegan form of vitamin D3 has been isolated from lichen (Wang et al., 2001). Vitamin D2 (ergocalciferol), on the other hand, is a vegan source of vitamin D, being found in UV-treated mushrooms (Simon et al., 2013). At short-term supplementation (11 weeks) and in low doses (1000 IU/day), vitamins D2 and D3 appear to be equivalent (Holick et al., 2008; Biancuzzo et al., 2013), but at long-term supplementation (25 weeks) (Logan et al., 2013) or in higher doses (Tripkovic et al., 2012), vitamin D2 appears to be less effective than vitamin D3.

To achieve the adequate daily recommendation of protein, the intake of vegetables with higher content of this nutrient should be encouraged. In this matter, legumes are the food group most relevant in plant-based diets, including all kinds of beans, soy, lentils, peas, chickpeas, lupini, and peanuts. It should be noted, however, that peanuts have a high content of fatty acids and a consequently lower amount of protein. Similarly, nuts (e.g., hazelnuts, Brazilian nuts, almonds, and macadamias) can also provide good quantities of protein, in spite of their high content of fatty acids (Brufau et al., 2006). Also, products made from textured soy protein have become a good alternative to animal proteins, since they can imitate meat semblance and presentation, being used in recipes replacing original meat ingredients. In addition to legumes and products made of soy protein, protein-enriched beverages—also known as "plant" milks, made from oat, almond, rice, soy, and sweet chestnut—could also be considered when planning plant-based diets.

6.7 BIOACTIVE COMPOUNDS IN FOODS AND BONE HEALTH

Similar to other chronic diseases, increasing evidence has associated the development of osteoporosis with inflammatory metabolic responses (Vassalle and Mazzone, 2016; Zhao et al., 2016). In this scenario, the anti-inflammatory properties of phytochemicals as flavonoids—a class of polyphenols—could play a role in protecting against bone loss, especially among people following plant-based diets. As shown by a large observational study with more than 3000 Scottish women, flavonol, catechin, and total flavonoid intakes were positively associated with femoral neck BMD and with an increase in BMI of the spine and hip (Hardcastle et al., 2011).

Vegetarians often use soy products as substitutes of food from animal origin. The impact of soy products on bone health is still uncertain (Taku et al., 2011), although findings suggest that soy isoflavones have a protective effect on the risk of fracture (Zhang et al., 2005; Koh et al., 2009) and osteoporosis (Ho et al., 2003) among women. Studies with Asian populations have shown an absence of low BMD in vegetarians, which could be possibly explained, in part, by the high consumption of phytoestrogens from soy (Kim et al., 2007; Wang et al., 2008). Isoflavones are biologically active compounds mainly synthesized in leguminous plants, such as soybeans, and considered a nonnutritive subcategory of flavonoids with structural similarities to estrogen and with the capacity to bind to estrogen receptors and consequently affect estrogen-regulated gene products (Kuiper et al., 1998). On the other hand, randomized controlled trials evaluating the effects of isoflavone supplements observed positive effects of isoflavones on bone only in high doses, considerably above the usual intakes from soy foods (Morabito et al., 2002; Weaver et al., 2009; Shedd-Wise et al., 2011), while others showed minor (Wong et al., 2009) or no bone-sparing effect of extracted soy isoflavones (Alekel et al., 2010; Levis et al., 2011).

Olive oil and olive polyphenols have also shown beneficial effects on the maintenance of BMD, which could be attributed to their ability to reduce oxidative stress and inflammation and to their capacity to enhance preosteoblast proliferation, differentiate osteoblasts, and decrease the formation of osteoclast-like cells (Chin and Ima-Nirwana, 2016). Other types of polyphenols associated with bone health include quercetin, resveratrol, catechins, anthocyanins, and proanthocyanidins (Cantos et al., 2002; Xu et al., 2011), which can be found in good quantities in grapes (and consequently in grape juices and wine, especially in the red variations). Several of the polyphenols from grapes were shown to benefit bone health in animal models. Quercetin (Siddiqui et al., 2011), kaempferol (Trivedi et al., 2008), resveratrol (Liu et al., 2005), and catechins (Shen et al., 2008) protected against bone loss in ovariectomized rats. In calcium-depleted rats, adding grape seed proanthocyanidin extract to a calcium-replete diet restored bone mineral content to a greater extent than a calcium-replete diet alone (Yahara et al., 2005). In ovariectomized Sprague Dawley rats, a 10-day treatment with dietary grape extract and grapeseed extract decreased urinary N-terminal telopeptide (NTx), a marker of bone resorption, whereas resveratrol significantly improved bone ^{45}Ca retention (Pawlowski et al., 2014). A 2-month grape-enriched diet containing 25% dried grapes increased bone calcium retention as well as cortical bone structure and strength in rats, although no significant effects on femoral BMD, trabecular bone microarchitecture, or tissue-level material properties were observed (Hohman and Weaver, 2015).

Findings from studies with humans have also shown positive relationships of flavonoids with bone health. Total flavonoid, anthocyanin, flavonol, and flavonoid polymer intakes were positively associated with spine BMD, and anthocyanin intake was positively associated with hip BMD in women aged 18–79 years (Welch et al., 2012). In men only, red wine consumption was positively associated with change in lumbar spine BMD over 2 years (Yin et al., 2011). Since polyphenols are found in nonanimal sources, their consumption should be encouraged for people following plant-based diets. Thus, soy, olive, and grape-enriched diets could be an additional device conferring benefits to bone health and calcium metabolism for vegetarians and vegans.

6.8   OTHER FACTORS THAT MAY AFFECT BONE HEALTH

In addition to the nutrients and bioactive compounds already mentioned, other dietary factors commonly found in plant-based diets have been shown to enhance bone mass. In contrast, other constituents have been shown to interfere with calcium absorption and retention, thereby promoting a negative effect on BMD.

6.8.1   PHYTATES AND OXALATES

All seeds, such as cereals, peas, nuts, oilseeds, and legumes, contain phytate (myo-inositol-hexaphosphate) (Reddy et al., 1982), which negatively affects the absorption of many essential elements, including calcium and zinc. A study with Swiss adults showed that the addition of 100 mg or more of phytate-P to a meal significantly decreased calcium retention compared with meals with no added phytate, and concluded that the inhibitory effect of phytate on the absorption of zinc and the retention of calcium was dose dependent (Fredlund et al., 2006). Studies using radioisotope techniques found significantly higher calcium absorption among subjects fed low-phytate diets than those fed high-phytate diets (Heaney et al., 1991; Weaver et al., 1991, 1993).

Another nutritional compound commonly present in plant foods is oxalate, which is the most potent inhibitor of calcium absorption in plants. In general, calcium absorption is inversely proportional to the oxalic acid content of the food. Thus, calcium bioavailability is high from low-oxalate vegetables such as kale, broccoli, and bok choy; intermediate from sweet potatoes; and low from both American and Chinese varieties of spinach and rhubarb. Exceptionally, soy products have relatively high calcium bioavailability, although soybeans are rich in both oxalate and phytate (Weaver et al., 1993, 1997).

Thus, the negative effect of phytate and oxalate on BMD among people following plant-based diets may be prevented by encouraging a liberal consumption of dairy products (in the case of lacto-vegetarians and lacto-ovo vegetarians) and by increasing the intake of foods with higher absorbable calcium. For many people, however, the quantity of vegetables required to reach sufficient calcium intake can make an exclusively plant-based diet impractical, unless fortified foods or supplements are included (Weaver et al., 1999).

6.8.2 VITAMIN B12

Inadequate vitamin B12 status has been related to low BMD, increased fracture risk, and osteoporosis (Dhonukshe-Rutten et al., 2005; Morris et al., 2005; Tucker et al., 2005; McLean et al., 2008; Herrmann et al., 2009). Vitamin B12 is almost exclusively naturally found in animal products, such as meat, milk, egg yolk, fish, and shellfish (Watanabe, 2007). Thus, it is presumed that vegetarians and vegans are at a higher risk for impaired vitamin B12 status. In accordance, a high prevalence of inadequacy for dietary vitamin B12 was observed among vegans in the EPIC-Oxford study (Sobiecki et al., 2016). Another European study comparing lacto-ovo vegetarians and vegans with nonvegetarians found a prevalence of low vitamin B12 status (holotranscobalamin II < 35 pmol/L) of 11% in omnivores, 77% in lacto-ovo vegetarians, and 92% in vegans (Herrmann et al., 2003). The impact of this vitamin on bone seems to be through the action of homocysteine (whose plasma concentrations are a hallmark of vitamin B12 deficiency), but direct effects on bone are also suggested, as the stimuli in cell proliferation and alkaline phosphatase activity in human bone marrow stromal osteoprogenitor cells (hBMSCs) and UMR106 osteoblastic cells (Kim et al., 1996). Homocysteine, in turn, was shown to stimulate osteoclasts, inhibit osteoblasts, and disturb collagen crosslinking (Herrmann et al., 2009). A meta-analysis with eight studies evaluating a total of 11,511 individuals found a 4% greater fracture risk for each millimole per liter increase in homocysteine concentration (RR 1.04, 95% CI 1.02–1.07) (van Wijngaarden et al., 2013).

Several studies have evaluated vitamin B12 concentrations and bone metabolism (Dhonukshe-Rutten et al., 2003; Stone et al., 2004; van Wijngaarden et al., 2013; Bailey et al., 2015). In a study from the Netherlands, the prevalence of osteoporosis was reported to be almost seven times higher in women with serum vitamin B12 concentrations <210 pmol/L than those with concentrations >320 pmol/L (Dhonukshe-Rutten et al., 2003), while a longitudinal study of 42 months evaluating American elderly women showed a significantly greater decline in total hip BMD with vitamin B12 concentrations below 280 pg/mL (Stone et al., 2004). A meta-analysis including four prospective studies and a total of 7475 individuals found a 4% lower fracture risk for each 50 pmol/L increase in vitamin B12 concentration (RR 0.96, 95% CI 0.92–1.00) (van Wijngaarden et al., 2013). On the other hand, a study with a nationally representative population of 2806 North American women ≥50 years old with high exposure to B vitamins through food fortification and dietary supplements observed serum total homocysteine, but not vitamin B12, to be significantly associated with lumbar and total body BMD (Bailey et al., 2015). In turn, studies evaluating the relationship of vitamin B12 deficiency and bone outcomes among people following plant-based diets are not numerous. Vegetarians have been shown to have lower vitamin B12 and higher homocysteine concentrations than nonvegetarians (Krivosíková et al., 2010). Also, vegetarians with low vitamin B12 concentrations were shown to present greater bone remodeling, which may accelerate bone loss (Herrmann et al., 2009).

Strategies to guarantee vitamin B12 intake among people following plant-based diets may include the consumption of egg yolk (in the case of ovo-vegetarians and lacto-ovo vegetarians) and fortified food products, such as soy products, nutritional yeast, and breakfast cereals. Supplements are also indicated, especially in the case of vegans, to ensure vitamin B12 adequacy (Tucker, 2014).

6.8.3 Zinc

Zinc is another mineral normally associated with meat intake, given that its natural sources include oysters, beef, beef liver, dark meat of poultry, and egg yolk (Murphy et al., 1975). Although zinc is also available in nuts, beans, and whole grains, the phytate content in these foods reduces its bioavailability, compared with animal-based sources, making higher total zinc intakes from these foods necessary to meet requirements. Consequently, zinc intake is frequently inadequate in plant-based diets (Hunt, 2003; Shridhar et al., 2014; Foster and Samman, 2015). A systematic review and meta-analysis evaluating the zinc status of vegetarians during pregnancy concluded that pregnant vegetarian women had lower zinc intakes than nonvegetarian control populations, and that both groups consumed lower than recommended amounts (Foster et al., 2015). In the EPIC-Oxford study, vegans of both sexes and vegetarian men had a high estimated prevalence of zinc inadequacy (>55%) (Sobiecki et al., 2016).

Considering the high inadequacy of zinc intake among vegetarians and vegans, the Food and Nutrition Board recommends at least 50% more zinc for those who obtain it from vegetarian sources (Food and Nutrition Board, Institute of Medicine, 2001). Given that lower serum and bone zinc have been observed in patients with osteoporosis (Atik, 1983), efforts to ensure an adequate intake of this mineral among vegetarians and vegans should be encouraged. Ways of limiting the effects of phytates on zinc availability in vegetal sources are also worthy, such as soaking, heating, sprouting, fermenting, and leavening processes (Saunders et al., 2013). In addition, fortified foods, such as breakfast cereals, may be an option for increasing zinc intake among vegetarians and vegans.

6.8.4 n-3 Fatty Acids

Polyunsaturated fatty acids may influence bone metabolism through several complex pathways, including the modulation of prostaglandin E2 production (Watkins et al., 2001, 2003), the enhancement of calcium transport and retention (Coetzer et al., 1994; Baggio et al., 2000), and effects on inflammatory cytokines (Kettler, 2001; Albertazzi and Coupland, 2002). In the Rancho Bernardo Study, higher intake ratios of n-6 to n-3 fatty acids were associated with lower hip BMD (Weiss et al., 2005). Whereas plant-based diets tend to have a high content of n-6 fatty acids, the exclusion of fish from the diet implies low intakes of n-3 fatty acids, particularly of docosahexaenoic acid (DHA) and eicosapentaenoic acid (EPA), which are the most biologically active forms. Some nonanimal foods, however, also contain n-3 fatty acids. Vegetarian sources of n-3 fatty acids include walnuts, flaxseeds, canola oil, and certain algae, but most of them provide n-3 fatty acids in the form of α-linoleic acid (ALA). Although ALA can be converted to EPA and DHA in the body, this conversion seems to be inefficient (Poulsen et al., 2007). Still, dietary ALA intakes have been shown to protect against hip fracture in the Framingham Osteoporosis Study (Farina et al., 2011).

Supplements of EPA and DHA are usually made from fish oil and, thus, are avoided by vegetarians and vegans. However, supplements from algae can also provide DHA (Doughman et al., 2007). Research on the effect of n-3 fatty acid supplementation on the risk of fracture has brought contradictory findings (Kruger et al., 1998; Bassey et al., 2000; Terano, 2001). Supplementation with fish oil was shown to be protective in postmenopausal women (Kruger et al., 1998; Terano, 2001), but another study found no differences in women supplemented for 12 months with fish oil and calcium compared with calcium alone (Bassey et al., 2000). Although further studies are needed, the importance of n-3 fatty acids on bone health is apparent, which highlights the need for improving their consumption among people following plant-based diets.

6.9   CONCLUSIONS

In this chapter, it is shown that particularities of plant-based diets may affect bone metabolism. Vegetarians, and principally vegans, often consume lower quantities of many nutrients importantly related to metabolic pathways involved with bone health, including calcium, protein, vitamin D, vitamin B12, zinc, and n-3 fatty acids.

Most studies evaluating BMD and risk of osteoporosis among vegetarian and vegan subjects have shown a relatively small but higher risk to this population group—especially vegans—compared with nonvegetarians. Despite the inadequate intake of key nutrients to bone metabolism, the increased intake of potassium and the low acid load of plant-based diets seem to positively contribute to bone health. Nevertheless, further research is needed to better understand the long-term effect of plant-based diets on BMD and the consequent risk of osteoporosis. In this scenario, prospective studies with long follow-up periods and larger samples could contribute to clarify questions that remain unclear.

Considering their particularities, plant-based diets are able to provide adequate amounts of the key nutrients for maintaining bone health. Although the literature still presents some inconsistencies, the risk for low BMD, osteoporosis, and fracture is higher among vegans. Specific dietary recommendations can support adequate function of bone metabolism, fight low BMD, and reduce the risk of fracture in this specific population. With adequate nutritional support and periodic health examinations, opting for plant-based diets does not represent a harm to bone health. Recommendations include the frequent consumption of large and diverse amounts of fruits and vegetables, adequate intake of protein from vegetable sources, regular but safe sun exposure, and—especially in the case of vegans—intake of food products fortified with calcium, vitamin D, zinc, and vitamin B12, and/or use of supplements from nonanimal origins.

REFERENCES

Adami S, Viapiana O, Gatti D, Idolazzi L, Rossini M. 2008. Relationship between serum parathyroid hormone, vitamin D sufficiency, age, and calcium intake. *Bone* 42(2):267–70.

Albertazzi P, Coupland K. 2002. Polyunsaturated fatty acids. Is there a role in postmenopausal osteoporosis prevention? *Maturitas* 42(1):13–22.

Alekel DL, Van Loan MD, Koehler KJ, Hanson LN, Stewart JW, Hanson KB, Kurzer MS, Peterson CT. 2010. The soy isoflavones for reducing bone loss (SIRBL) study: A 3-y randomized controlled trial in postmenopausal women. *Am J Clin Nutr* 91(1):218–30.

Appleby P, Roddam A, Allen N, Key T. 2007. Comparative fracture risk in vegetarians and nonvegetarians in EPIC-Oxford. *Eur J Clin Nutr* 61(12):1400–6.

Atik OS. 1983. Zinc and senile osteoporosis. *J Am Geriatr Soc* 31(12):790–1.

Ausman LM, Oliver LM, Goldin BR, Woods MN, Gorbach SL, Dwyer JT. 2008. Estimated net acid excretion inversely correlates with urine pH in vegans, lacto-ovo vegetarians, and omnivores. *J Ren Nutr* 18(5):456–65.

Bagger YZ, Tankó LB, Alexandersen P, Hansen HB, Qin G, Christiansen C. 2006. The long-term predictive value of bone mineral density measurements for fracture risk is independent of the site of measurement and the age at diagnosis: Results from the Prospective Epidemiological Risk Factors study. *Osteoporos Int* 17(3):471–7.

Baggio B, Budakovic A, Nassuato MA, Vezzoli G, Manzato E, Luisetto G, Zaninotto M. 2000. Plasma phospholipid arachidonic acid content and calcium metabolism in idiopathic calcium nephrolithiasis. *Kidney Int* 58(3):1278–84.

Bailey RL, Looker AC, Lu Z, Fan R, Eicher-Miller HA, Fakhouri TH, Gahche JJ, Weaver CM, Mills JL. 2015. B-Vitamin status and bone mineral density and risk of lumbar osteoporosis in older females in the United States. *Am J Clin Nutr* 102(3):687–94.

Bassey EJ, Littlewood JJ, Rothwell MC, Pye DW. 2000. Lack of effect of supplementation with essential fatty acids on bone mineral density in healthy pre- and postmenopausal women: Two randomized controlled trials of Efacal v. calcium alone. *Br J Nutr* 83(6):629–35.

Biancuzzo RM, Clarke N, Reitz RE, Travison TG, Holick MF. 2013. Serum concentrations of 1,25-dihydroxyvitamin D2 and 1,25-dihydroxyvitamin D3 in response to vitamin D2 and vitamin D3 supplementation. *J Clin Endocrinol Metab* 98(3):973–9.

Bonjour JP. 2005. Dietary protein: An essential nutrient for bone health. *J Am Coll Nutr* 24(6 Suppl.):526S–36S.

Brufau G, Boatella J, Rafecas M. 2006. Nuts: Source of energy and macronutrients. *Br J Nutr* 96(Suppl. 2):S24–8.

Burckhardt P. 2016. The role of low acid load in vegetarian diet on bone health: A narrative review. *Swiss Med Wkly* 146:w14277.

Cantos E, Espín JC, Tomás-Barberán FA. 2002. Varietal differences among the polyphenol profiles of seven table grape cultivars studied by LC-DAD-MS-MS. *J Agric Food Chem* 50(20):5691–6.

Chan J, Jaceldo-Siegl K, Fraser GE. 2009. Serum 25-hydroxyvitamin D status of vegetarians, partial vegetarians, and nonvegetarians: The Adventist Health Study-2. *Am J Clin Nutr* 89(5):1686S–92S.

Chin KY, Ima-Nirwana S. 2016. Olives and bone: A green osteoporosis prevention option. *Int J Environ Res Public Health* 13(8):E755. doi: 10.3390/ijerph13080755.

Chiu JF, Lan SJ, Yang CY, Wang PW, Yao WJ, Su LH, Hsieh CC. 1997. Long-term vegetarian diet and bone mineral density in postmenopausal Taiwanese women. *Calcif Tissue Int* 60(3):245–9.

Coetzer H, Claassen N, van Papendorp DH, Kruger MC. 1994. Calcium transport by isolated brush border and basolateral membrane vesicles: Role of essential fatty acid supplementation. *Prostaglandins Leukot Essent Fatty Acids* 50(5):257–66.

Crowe FL, Steur M, Allen NE, Appleby PN, Travis RC, Key TJ. 2011. Plasma concentrations of 25-hydroxyvitamin D in meat eaters, fish eaters, vegetarians and vegans: Results from the EPIC-Oxford study. *Public Health Nutr* 14(2):340–6.

Darling AL, Millward DJ, Torgerson DJ, Hewitt CE, Lanham-New SA. 2009. Dietary protein and bone health: A systematic review and meta-analysis. *Am J Clin Nutr* 90(6):1674–92.

Davey GK, Spencer EA, Appleby PN, Allen NE, Knox KH, Key TJ. 2003. EPIC-Oxford: Lifestyle characteristics and nutrient intakes in a cohort of 33,883 meat-eaters and 31,546 non meat-eaters in the UK. *Public Health Nutr* 6(3):259–69.

Dawson-Hughes B, Heaney RP, Holick MF, Lips P, Meunier PJ, Vieth R. 2005. Estimates of optimal vitamin D status. *Osteoporos Int* 16(7):713–6.

Dhonukshe-Rutten RA, Pluijm SM, de Groot LC, Lips P, Smit JH, van Staveren WA. 2005. Homocysteine and vitamin B12 status relate to bone turnover markers, broadband ultrasound attenuation, and fractures in healthy elderly people. *J Bone Miner Res* 20(6):921–9.

Dhonukshe-Rutten RAM, Lips M, de Jong N, Chin A, Paw MJM, Hiddink GJ, van Dusseldorp M, De Groot LC, van Staveren WA. 2003. Vitamin B-12 status is associated with bone mineral content and bone mineral density in frail elderly women but not in men. *J Nutr* 133(3):801–7.

Doughman SD, Krupanidhi S, Sanjeevi CB. 2007. Omega-3 fatty acids for nutrition and medicine: Considering microalgae oil as a vegetarian source of EPA and DHA. *Curr Diabetes Rev* 3(3):198–203.

Farina EK, Kiel DP, Roubenoff R, Schaefer EJ, Cupples LA, Tucker KL. 2011. Dietary intakes of arachidonic acid and alpha-linolenic acid are associated with reduced risk of hip fracture in older adults. *J Nutr* 141(6):1146–53.

Ferraro PM, Mandel EI, Curhan GC, Gambaro G, Taylor EN. 2016. Dietary protein and potassium, diet-dependent net acid load, and risk of incident kidney stones. *Clin J Am Soc Nephrol* 11(10):1834–44. doi: 10.2215/CJN.01520216.

Fontana L, Shew JL, Holloszy JO, Villareal DT. 2005. Low bone mass in subjects on a long-term raw vegetarian diet. *Arch Intern Med* 165(6):684–9.

Food and Nutrition Board, Institute of Medicine. 2001. Dietary Reference Intakes for vitamin A, vitamin K, arsenic, boron, chromium, copper, iodine, iron, manganese, molybdenum, nickel, silicon, vanadium, and zinc. Washington, DC: National Academies Press.

Foster M, Herulah UN, Prasad A, Petocz P, Samman S. 2015. Zinc status of vegetarians during pregnancy: A systematic review of observational studies and meta-analysis of zinc intake. *Nutrients* 7(6):4512–25.

Foster M, Samman S. 2015. Vegetarian diets across the lifecycle: Impact on zinc intake and status. *Adv Food Nutr Res* 74:93–131.

Frassetto L, Morris Jr. RC, Sebastian A. 2005. Long-term persistence of the urine calcium-lowering effect of potassium bicarbonate in postmenopausal women. *J Clin Endocrinol Metab* 90(2):831–4.

Frassetto LA, Todd KM, Morris Jr. RC, Sebastian A. 1998. Estimation of net endogenous noncarbonic acid production in humans from diet potassium and protein contents. *Am J Clin Nutr* 68(3):576–83.

Fredlund K, Isaksson M, Rossander-Hulthén L, Almgren A, Sandberg AS. 2006. Absorption of zinc and retention of calcium: Dose-dependent inhibition by phytate. *J Trace Elem Med Biol* 20(1):49–57.

Gunn CA, Weber JL, McGill A-T, Kruger MC. 2015. Increased intake of selected vegetables, herbs and fruit may reduce bone turnover in post-menopausal women. *Nutrients* 7(4):2499–517.

Hardcastle AC, Aucott L, Reid DM, MacDonald HM. 2011. Associations between dietary flavonoid intakes and bone health in a Scottish population. *J Bone Miner Res* 26(5):941–7. doi: 10.1002/jbmr.285.

Heaney RP. 2000. Calcium, dairy products and osteoporosis. *J Am Coll Nutr* 19(2 Suppl.):83S–99S.

Heaney RP, Weaver CM, Fitzsimmons ML. 1991. Soybean phytate content: Effect on calcium absorption. *Am J Clin Nutr* 53:745–7.

Herrmann W, Obeid R, Schorr H, Hübner U, Geisel J, Sand-Hill M, Ali N, Herrmann N. 2009. Enhanced bone metabolism in vegetarians—The role of vitamin B12 deficiency. *Clin Chem Lab Med* 47(11):1381–7.

Herrmann W, Schorr H, Obeid R, Geisel J. 2003. Vitamin B-12 status, particularly holotranscobalamin II and methylmalonic acid concentrations, and hyperhomocysteinemia in vegetarians. *Am J Clin Nutr* 78(1):131–6.

Ho SC, Woo J, Lam S, Chen Y, Sham A, Lau J. 2003. Soy protein consumption and bone mass in early postmenopausal Chinese women. *Osteoporos Int* 14(10):835–42.

Hohman EE, Weaver CM. 2015. A grape-enriched diet increases bone calcium retention and cortical bone properties in ovariectomized rats. *J Nutr* 145(2):253–9.

Holick MF. 2003. Vitamin D: A millennium perspective. *J Cell Biochem* 88(2):296–307.

Holick MF. 2007. Vitamin D deficiency. *New Engl J Med* 357:266–81.

Holick MF. 2009. Vitamin D status: Measurement, interpretation, and clinical application. *Ann Epidemiol* 19(2):73–8.

Holick MF, Biancuzzo RM, Chen TC, Klein EK, Young A, Bibuld D, Reitz R, Salameh W, Ameri A, Tannenbaum AD. 2008. Vitamin D2 is as effective as vitamin D3 in maintaining circulating concentrations of 25-hydroxyvitamin D. *J Clin Endocrinol Metab* 93(3):677–81.

Ho-Pham LT, Nguyen ND, Nguyen TV. 2009a. Effect of vegetarian diets on bone mineral density: A Bayesian meta-analysis. *Am J Clin Nutr* 90(4):943–50.

Ho-Pham LT, Nguyen PL, Le TT, Doan TA, Tran NT, Le TA, Nguyen TV. 2009b. Veganism, bone mineral density, and body composition: A study in Buddhist nuns. *Osteoporos Int* 20(12):2087–93.

Ho-Pham LT, Vu BQ, Lai TQ, Nguyen ND, Nguyen TV. 2012. Vegetarianism, bone loss, fracture and vitamin D: A longitudinal study in Asian vegans and non-vegans. *Eur J Clin Nutr* 66(1):75–82.

Hunt JR. 2003. Bioavailability of iron, zinc, and other trace minerals from vegetarian diets. *Am J Clin Nutr* 78(3 Suppl.):633S–9S.

Ilich JZ, Brownbill RA, Tamborini L. 2003. Bone and nutrition in elderly women: Protein, energy, and calcium as main determinants of bone mineral density. *Eur J Clin Nutr* 57(4):554–65.

Kettler DB. 2001. Can manipulation of the ratios of essential fatty acids slow the rapid rate of postmenopausal bone loss? *Altern Med Rev* 6(1):61–77.

Kim GS, Kim CH, Park JY, Lee KU, Park CS. 1996. Effects of vitamin B12 on cell proliferation and cellular alkaline phosphatase activity in human bone marrow stromal osteoprogenitor cells and UMR106 osteoblastic cells. *Metabolism* 45(12):1443–6.

Kim M-H, Choi M-K, Sung C-J. 2007. Bone mineral density of Korean postmenopausal women is similar between vegetarians and nonvegetarians. *Nutr Res* 27(10):612–7.

Knurick JR, Johnston CS, Wherry SJ, Aguayo I. 2015. Comparison of correlates of bone mineral density in individuals adhering to lacto-ovo, vegan, or omnivore diets: A cross-sectional investigation. *Nutrients* 7(5):3416–26.

Koh W-P, Wu AH, Wang R, Ang L-W, Heng D, Yuan J-M, Yu MC. 2009. Gender-specific associations between soy and risk of hip fracture in the Singapore Chinese Health Study. *Am J Epidemiol* 170(7):901–9.

Kohlenberg-Mueller K, Raschka L. 2003. Calcium balance in young adults on a vegan and lactovegetarian diet. *J Bone Miner Metab* 21(1):28–33.

Krivosíková Z, Krajcovicová-Kudlácková M, Spustová V, Stefíková K, Valachovicová M, Blazícek P, Nemcova C. 2010. The association between high plasma homocysteine levels and lower bone mineral density in Slovak women: The impact of vegetarian diet. *Eur J Nutr* 49(3):147–53.

Kruger MC, Coetzer H, de Winter R, Gericke G, van Papendorp DH. 1998. Calcium, gammalinolenic acid and eicosapentaenoic acid supplementation in senile osteoporosis. *Aging* (Milano) 10(5):385–94.

Kuiper GG, Lemmen JG, Carlsson B, Corton JC, Safe SH, van der Saag PT, van der Burg B, Gustafsson JA. 1998. Interaction of estrogenic chemicals and phytoestrogens with estrogen receptor beta. *Endocrinology* 139(10):4252–63.

Kull M, Kallikorm R, Lember M. 2009. Body mass index determines sunbathing habits: Implications on vitamin D levels. *Intern Med J* 39(4):256–8.

Kurpad AV, Vaz M. 2000. Protein and amino acid requirements in the elderly. *Eur J Clin Nutr* 54(Suppl. 3):S131–42.

Lanham-New SA. 2008. The balance of bone health: Tipping the scales in favor of potassium-rich, bicarbonate-rich foods. *J Nutr* 138(1):172S–7S.

Lanham-New SA. 2009. Is "vegetarianism" a serious risk factor for osteoporotic fracture? *Am J Clin Nutr* 90(4):910–1.

Lau EM, Kwok T, Woo J, Ho SC. 1998. Bone mineral density in Chinese elderly female vegetarians, vegans, lacto-vegetarians and omnivores. *Eur J Clin Nutr* 52(1):60–4.

Leboime A, Confavreux CB, Mehsen N, Paccou J, David C, Roux C. 2010. Osteoporosis and mortality. *Joint Bone Spine* 77(Suppl. 2):S107–12.

Lemann Jr. J, Gray RW, Pleuss JA. 1989. Potassium bicarbonate, but not sodium bicarbonate, reduces urinary calcium excretion and improves calcium balance in healthy men. *Kidney Int* 35(2):688–95.

Levis S, Strickman-Stein N, Ganjei-Azar P, Xu P, Doerge DR, Krischer J. 2011. Soy isoflavones in the prevention of menopausal bone loss and menopausal symptoms: A randomized, double-blind trial. *Arch Intern Med* 171(15):1363–9.

Liu ZP, Li WX, Yu B, Huang J, Sun J, Huo JS, Liu CX. 2005. Effects of trans-resveratrol from *Polygonum cuspidatum* on bone loss using the ovariectomized rat model. *J Med Food* 8(1):14–9.

Lloyd T, Schaeffer JM, Walker MA, Demers LM. 1991. Urinary hormonal concentrations and spinal bone densities of premenopausal vegetarian and nonvegetarian women. *Am J Clin Nutr* 54(6):1005–10.

Logan VF, Gray AR, Peddie MC, Harper MJ, Houghton LA. 2013. Long-term vitamin D3 supplementation is more effective than vitamin D2 in maintaining serum 25-hydroxyvitamin D status over the winter months. *Br J Nutr* 109(6):1082–8.

MacDonald HM, New SA, Fraser WD, Campbell MK, Reid DM. 2005. Low dietary potassium intakes and high dietary estimates of net endogenous acid production are associated with low bone mineral density in premenopausal women and increased markers of bone resorption in postmenopausal women. *Am J Clin Nutr* 81(4):923–33.

Mangels AR. 2014. Bone nutrients for vegetarians. *Am J Clin Nutr* 100(Suppl. 1):469S–75S.

Maurer M, Riesen W, Muser J, Hulter HN, Krapf R. 2003. Neutralization of Western diet inhibits bone resorption independently of K intake and reduces cortisol secretion in humans. *Am J Physiol Renal Physiol* 284(1):F32–40.

McLean E, de Benoist B, Allen LH. 2008. Review of the magnitude of folate and vitamin B12 deficiencies worldwide. *Food Nutr Bull* 29(2 Suppl.):S38–51.

Morabito N, Crisafulli A, Vergara C, Gaudio A, Lasco A, Frisina N, D'Anna R et al. 2002. Effects of genistein and hormone-replacement therapy on bone loss in early postmenopausal women: A randomized double-blind placebo-controlled study. *J Bone Miner Res* 17(10):1904–12.

Morris MS, Jacques PF, Selhub J. 2005. Relation between homocysteine and B-vitamin status indicators and bone mineral density in older Americans. *Bone* 37(2):234–42.

Moseley KF, Weaver CM, Appel L, Sebastian A, Sellmeyer DE. 2013. Potassium citrate supplementation results in sustained improvement in calcium balance in older men and women. *J Bone Miner Res* 28(3):497–504.

Munger RG, Cerhan JR, Chiu BC. 1999. Prospective study of dietary protein intake and risk of hip fracture in postmenopausal women. *Am J Clin Nutr* 69(1):147–52.

Murphy EW, Willis BW, Watt BK. 1975. Provisional tables on the zinc content of foods. *J Am Diet Assoc* 66(4):345–55.

Nakamura K, Kitamura K, Takachi R, Saito T, Kobayashi R, Oshiki R, Watanabe Y, Tsugane S, Sasaki A, Yamazaki O. 2015. Impact of demographic, environmental, and lifestyle factors on vitamin D sufficiency in 9084 Japanese adults. *Bone* 74:10–7.

New SA. 2004. Do vegetarians have a normal bone mass? *Osteoporos Int* 15(9):679–88.

New SA, MacDonald HM, Campbell MK, Martin JC, Garton MJ, Robins SP, Reid DM. 2004. Lower estimates of net endogenous non-carbonic acid production are positively associated with indexes of bone health in premenopausal and perimenopausal women. *Am J Clin Nutr* 79(1):131–8.

Outila TA, Kärkkäinen MU, Seppänen RH, Lamberg-Allardt CJ. 2000. Dietary intake of vitamin D in premenopausal, healthy vegans was insufficient to maintain concentrations of serum 25-hydroxyvitamin D and intact parathyroid hormone within normal ranges during the winter in Finland. *J Am Diet Assoc* 100(4):434–41.

Pawlowski JW, Martin BR, McCabe GP, Ferruzzi MG, Weaver CM. 2014. Plum and soy aglycon extracts superior at increasing bone calcium retention in ovariectomized Sprague Dawley rats. *J Agric Food Chem* 62(26):6108–17.

Poulsen RC, Moughan PJ, Kruger MC. 2007. Long-chain polyunsaturated fatty acids and the regulation of bone metabolism. *Exp Biol Med (Maywood)* 232(10):1275–88.

Prentice A, Schoenmakers I, Laskey MA, de Bono S, Ginty F, Goldberg GR. 2006. Nutrition and bone growth and development. *Proc Nutr Soc* 65(4):348–60.

Reddy NR, Sathe SK, Salunkhe DK. 1982. Phytates in legumes and cereals. *Adv Food Res* 28:1–92.

Reed JA, Anderson JJ, Tylavsky FA, Gallagher PN. 1994. Comparative changes in radial-bone density of elderly female lacto-ovovegetarians and omnivores. *Am J Clin Nutr* 59(5 Suppl.):1197S–202S.

Remer T, Krupp D, Shi L. 2014. Dietary protein's and dietary acid load's influence on bone health. *Crit Rev Food Sci Nutr* 54(9):1140–50.

Riggs BL, Khosla S, Melton LJ 3rd. 1998. A unitary model for involutional osteoporosis: Estrogen deficiency causes both type I and type II osteoporosis in postmenopausal women and contributes to bone loss in aging men. *J Bone Miner Res* 13(5):763–73.

Rizzo NS, Jaceldo-Siegl K, Sabate J, Fraser GE. 2013. Nutrient profiles of vegetarian and nonvegetarian dietary patterns. *J Acad Nutr Diet* 113(12):1610–9.

Saggese G, Baroncelli GI, Bertelloni S. 2002. Puberty and bone development. *Best Pract Res Clin Endocrinol Metab* 16(1):53–64.

Saunders AV, Craig WJ, Baines SK. 2013. Zinc and vegetarian diets. *Med J Aust* 199(4 Suppl.):S17–21.

Sebastian A, Harris ST, Ottaway JH, Todd KM, Morris Jr. RC. 1994. Improved mineral balance and skeletal metabolism in postmenopausal women treated with potassium bicarbonate. *N Engl J Med* 330(25):1776–81.

Seeman E, Hopper JL, Young NR, Formica C, Goss P, Tsalamandris C. 1996. Do genetic factors explain associations between muscle strength, lean mass, and bone density? A twin study. *Am J Physiol* 270(2 Pt. 1):E320–7.

Shedd-Wise KM, Alekel DL, Hofmann H, Hanson KB, Schiferl DJ, Hanson LN, Van Loan MD. 2011. The soy isoflavones for reducing bone loss study: 3-yr effects on pQCT bone mineral density and strength measures in postmenopausal women. *J Clin Densitom* 14(1):47–57.

Shen C-L, Wang P, Guerrieri J, Yeh JK, Wang J-S. 2008. Protective effect of green tea polyphenols on bone loss in middle-aged female rats. *Osteoporos Int* 19(7):979–90.

Shridhar K, Dhillon PK, Bowen L, Kinra S, Bharathi AV, Prabhakaran D, Reddy KS, Ebrahim S. 2014. Nutritional profile of Indian vegetarian diets—The Indian Migration Study (IMS). *Nutr J* 13:55. doi: 10.1186/1475-2891-13-55.

Siani V, Mohamed EI, Maiolo C, Di Daniele N, Ratiu A, Leonardi A, Lorenzo A. 2003. Body composition analysis for healthy Italian vegetarians. *Acta Diabetol* 40(Suppl. 1):S297–8.

Siddiqui JA, Sharan K, Swarnkar G, Rawat P, Kumar M, Manickavasagam L, Maurya R, Pierroz D, Chattapadhyay. 2011. Quercetin-6-C-β-D-glucopyranoside isolated from *Ulmus wallichiana* Planchon is more potent than quercetin in inhibiting osteoclastogenesis and mitigating ovariectomy-induced bone loss in rats. *Menopause* 18(2):198–207.

Simon RR, Borzelleca JF, DeLuca HF, Weaver CM. 2013. Safety assessment of the post-harvest treatment of button mushrooms (*Agaricus bisporus*) using ultraviolet light. *Food Chem Toxicol* 56:278–89.

Smith AM. 2006. Veganism and osteoporosis: A review of the current literature. *Int J Nurs Pract* 12(5):302–6.

Sobiecki JG, Appleby PN, Bradbury KE, Key TJ. 2016. High compliance with dietary recommendations in a cohort of meat eaters, fish eaters, vegetarians, and vegans: Results from the European Prospective Investigation into Cancer and Nutrition-Oxford study. *Nutr Res* 36(5):464–77.

Stone KL, Bauer DC, Sellmeyer D, Cummings SR. 2004. Low serum vitamin B-12 levels are associated with increased hip bone loss in older women: A prospective study. *J Clin Endocrinol Metab* 89(3):1217–21.

Ströhle A, Hahn A, Sebastian A. 2010. Estimation of the diet-dependent net acid load in 229 worldwide historically studied hunter-gatherer societies. *Am J Clin Nutr* 91(2):406–12.

Ströhle A, Waldmann A, Koschizke J, Leitzmann C, Hahn A. 2011. Diet-dependent net endogenous acid load of vegan diets in relation to food groups and bone health-related nutrients: Results from the German Vegan Study. *Ann Nutr Metab* 59(2–4):117–26.

Sutton AL, MacDonald PN. 2003. Vitamin D: More than a "bone-a-fide" hormone. *Mol Endocrinol* 17:177–91.

Taku K, Melby MK, Nishi N, Omori T, Kurzer MS. 2011. Soy isoflavones for osteoporosis: An evidence-based approach. *Maturitas* 70(4):333–8.

Teitelbaum SL. 2000. Bone resorption by osteoclasts. *Science* 289:1504–8.

Terano T. 2001. Effect of omega 3 polyunsaturated fatty acid ingestion on bone metabolism and osteoporosis. *World Rev Nutr Diet* 88:141–7.

Thorpe DL, Knutsen SF, Beeson WL, Rajaram S, Fraser GE. 2008. Effects of meat consumption and vegetarian diet on risk of wrist fracture over 25 years in a cohort of peri- and postmenopausal women. *Public Health Nutr* 11(6):564–72.

Tripkovic L, Lambert H, Hart K, Smith CP, Bucca G, Penson S, Chope G, Hyppönen E, Berry J, Vieth R, Lanham-New S. 2012. Comparison of vitamin D2 and vitamin D3 supplementation in raising serum 25-hydroxyvitamin D status: A systematic review and meta-analysis. *Am J Clin Nutr* 95(6):1357–64.

Trivedi R, Kumar S, Kumar A, Siddiqui JA, Swarnkar G, Gupta V, Kendurker A et al. 2008. Kaempferol has osteogenic effect in ovariectomized adult Sprague-Dawley rats. *Mol Cell Endocrinol* 289(1–2):85–93.

Tucker KL. 2014. Vegetarian diets and bone status. *Am J Clin Nutr* 100(Suppl. 1):329S–35S.

Tucker KL, Hannan MT, Qiao N, Jacques PF, Selhub J, Cupples LA, Kiel DP. 2005. Low plasma vitamin B12 is associated with lower BMD: The Framingham Osteoporosis Study. *J Bone Miner Res* 20(1):152–8.

van Wijngaarden JP, Doets EL, Szczecińska A, Souverein OW, Duffy ME, Dullemeijer C, Cavelaars AE et al. 2013. Vitamin B12, folate, homocysteine, and bone health in adults and elderly people: A systematic review with meta-analyses. *J Nutr Metab* 2013:486186. doi: 10.1155/2013/486186.

Vassalle C, Mazzone A. 2016. Bone loss and vascular calcification: A bi-directional interplay? *Vascul Pharmacol* 86:77–86.

Wang T, Bengtsson G, Kärnefelt I, Björn LO. 2001. Provitamins and vitamins D_2 and D_3 in *Cladina* spp. over a latitudinal gradient: Possible correlation with UV levels. *J Photochem Photobiol B* 62(1–2):118–22.

Wang Y-F, Chiu J-S, Chuang M-H, Chiu J-E, Lin C-L. 2008. Bone mineral density of vegetarian and non-vegetarian adults in Taiwan. *Asia Pac J Clin Nutr* 17(1):101–6.

Warensjö E, Byberg L, Melhus H, Gedeborg R, Mallmin H, Wolk A, Michaelsson K. 2011. Dietary calcium intake and risk of fracture and osteoporosis: Prospective longitudinal cohort study. *BMJ* 342:d1473. doi: 10.1136/bmj.d1473.

Watanabe F. 2007. Vitamin B12 sources and bioavailability. *Exp Biol Med (Maywood)* 232(10):1266–74.

Watkins BA, Li Y, Lippman HE, Feng S. 2003. Modulatory effect of omega-3 polyunsaturated fatty acids on osteoblast function and bone metabolism. *Prostaglandins Leukot Essent Fatty Acids* 68(6):387–98.

Watkins BA, Lippman HE, Le Bouteiller L, Li Y, Seifert MF. 2001. Bioactive fatty acids: Role in bone biology and bone cell function. *Prog Lipid Res* 40(1–2):125–48.

Weaver CM. 2013. Potassium and health. *Adv Nutr* 4(3):368S–77S.

Weaver CM. 2017. Nutrition and bone health. *Oral Dis* 23(4):412–5. doi: 10.1111/odi.12515.

Weaver CM, Heaney RP, Martin BR, Fitzsimmons ML. 1991. Human calcium absorption from whole-wheat products. *J Nutr* 121:1769–75.

Weaver CM, Heaney RP, Nickel KP, Packard PI. 1997. Calcium bioavailability from high oxalate vegetables: Chinese vegetables, sweet potatoes and rhubarb. *J Food Sci* 62:524–5.

Weaver CM, Heaney RP, Proulx WR, Hinders SM, Packard PT. 1993. Absorbability of calcium from common beans. *J Food Sci* 58:1401–3.

Weaver CM, Martin BR, Jackson GS, McCabe GP, Nolan JR, McCabe LD, Barnes S, Reinwald S, Boris ME, Peacock M. 2009. Antiresorptive effects of phytoestrogen supplements compared with estradiol or risedronate in postmenopausal women using (41) Ca methodology. *J Clin Endocrinol Metab* 94(10):3798–805.

Weaver CM, Proulx WR, Heaney R. 1999. Choices for achieving adequate dietary calcium with a vegetarian diet. *Am J Clin Nutr* 70(3 Suppl.):543S–8S.

Weiss LA, Barrett-Connor E, von Mühlen D. 2005. Ratio of n-6 to n-3 fatty acids and bone mineral density in older adults: The Rancho Bernardo Study. *Am J Clin Nutr* 81(4):934–8.

Welch A, Bingham S, Camus J, Dalzell N, Reeve J, Day N, Khaw KT. 2005. Calcaneum broadband ultrasound attenuation relates to vegetarian and omnivorous diets differently in men and women: An observation from the European Prospective Investigation into Cancer in Norfolk (EPIC-Norfolk) population study. *Osteoporos Int* 16(6):590–6.

Welch A, MacGregor A, Jennings A, Fairweather-Tait S, Spector T, Cassidy A. 2012. Habitual flavonoid intakes are positively associated with bone mineral density in women. *J Bone Miner Res* 27(9):1872–8. doi: 10.1002/jbmr.1649.

Wolpowitz D, Gilchrest BA. 2006. The vitamin D questions: How much do you need and how should you get it? *J Am Acad Dermatol* 54(2):301–17.

Wong WW, Lewis RD, Steinberg FM, Murray MJ, Cramer MA, Amato P, Young RL et al. 2009. Soy isoflavone supplementation and bone mineral density in menopausal women: A 2-y multicenter clinical trial. *Am J Clin Nutr* 90(5):1433–9.

Worsley A, Skrzypiec G. 1998. Teenage vegetarianism: Prevalence, social and cognitive contexts. *Appetite* 30(2):151–70.

Xu Y, Simon JE, Welch C, Wightman JD, Ferruzzi MG, Ho L, Pasinetti GM, Wu Q. 2011. Survey of polyphenol constituents in grapes and grape-derived products. *J Agric Food Chem* 59(19):10586–93. doi: 10.1021/jf202438d.

Yahara N, Tofani I, Maki K, Kojima K, Kojima Y, Kimura M. 2005. Mechanical assessment of effects of grape seed proanthocyanidins extract on tibial bone diaphysis in rats. *J Musculoskelet Neuronal Interact* 5(2):162–9.

Yin J, Winzenberg T, Quinn S, Giles G, Jones G. 2011. Beverage-specific alcohol intake and bone loss in older men and women: A longitudinal study. *Eur J Clin Nutr* 65(4):526–32.

Zhang X, Shu X-O, Li H, Yang G, Li Q, Gao YT, Zheng W. 2005. Prospective cohort study of soy food consumption and risk of bone fracture among postmenopausal women. *Arch Intern Med* 165(16):1890–5.

Zhao HX, Huang YX, Tao JG. 2016. ST1926 attenuates steroid-induced osteoporosis in rats by inhibiting inflammation response. *J Cell Biochem*. doi: 10.1002/jcb.25812.

7 The Role of Vegetarian Diets in Weight Management

Celine E. Heskey

CONTENTS

SUMMARY

Historically, observational studies have set the foundation for a relationship between plant-based dietary patterns and healthy weight status. Vegetarians, especially vegans, tend to weigh less than nonvegetarians and have a lower prevalence of overweight or obesity. Multiple studies, utilizing vegan and vegetarian dietary interventions, have demonstrated that plant-based diets may be successfully utilized in weight management treatment of overweight or obese individuals. Reduced energy, fat, and animal protein intake, and increased carbohydrate, fiber, whole grain, fruit, vegetable, and phytochemical intake, help to explain some of the weight management benefits of these patterns.

7.1 INTRODUCTION

7.1.1 OVERWEIGHT AND OBESITY

Overweight and obesity are global issues with significant health implications. Excess body weight has been linked to increased risk of chronic diseases, including cardiovascular disease and diabetes mellitus (Bastien et al., 2014). Excess abdominal fat, particularly visceral adipose tissue, contributes to the etiological pathway of cardiometabolic risk factor aberrations, including insulin resistance, dyslipidemia, and hypertension (HTN) (Bastien et al., 2014).

The definition of adiposity based on body mass index (BMI) (kg/m^2), in most adult populations, is as follows: (1) underweight, <18.5 kg/m^2; normal weight, 18.5–24.9 kg/m^2; (2) overweight, 25–29.9 kg/m^2; and (3) obese, ≥30 kg/m^2 (CDC, 2016d; WHO, 2016). Abdominal obesity can be assessed by measuring waist circumference. Individuals are considered to have abdominal obesity if their waist circumference is >88 cm for women or >102 cm for men (Bastien et al., 2014). Waist-to-hip ratio has also been used to assess disease risk, as it relates to abdominal obesity, but this measurement has been found to be a poor predictor of chronic disease in women (Lee and Nieman, 2013). Waist-to-hip ratios that are linked to increased disease risk are ≥0.8 for women and ≥0.9 for men (Lee and Nieman, 2013). Other ways that researchers can measure or estimate body composition (including excess adiposity) include using skinfold thickness measurements, air displacement plethysmography, bioelectrical impedance analysis (BIA), dual-energy x-ray absorptiometry (DXA), and magnetic resonance imaging (MRI), to determine percent body fat, fat mass, and fat-free mass (Lee and Nieman, 2013; CDC, 2016d). In regard to percent body fat, the ideal ranges are 6%–24% for men and 9%–31% for women (Lee and Nieman, 2013).

7.1.1.1 Prevalence

According to the Centers for Disease Control (CDC), the prevalence of obesity in the United States is 36.5% in adults and 17% in children and adolescents (CDC, 2016a, 2016b). Worldwide the prevalence of overweight and obesity in adults is 39% and 18%, respectively (WHO, 2016).

7.1.1.2 Link to Morbidity and Mortality

Overweight and obesity are risk factors for several of the top 10 causes of death in the United States, including heart disease, certain cancers, stroke, and diabetes

(CDC, 2016c, 2017). Other health conditions that have been linked to obesity include dyslipidemia, HTN, gallbladder disease, osteoarthritis, and sleep apnea. Additionally, obesity contributes to increased disability or reduced quality of life, either directly or indirectly through previously mentioned diseases, or by increasing the occurrence of pain, decreasing mobility, and increasing risk of depression and other psychiatric illnesses (CDC, 2016c). It has been estimated that the cost in the United States to treat obesity is approximately \$147 billion (2008) (CDC, 2016c).

Obesity is also linked to an increased risk for early mortality. Overweight individuals have a 11% higher risk of all-cause mortality than normal weight individuals (combined analysis of cohorts from North America, Europe, Asia, Australia, and New Zealand) (Global BMI Mortality Collaboration et al., 2016). In this same study, the hazard ratios (HRs) and 95% confidence intervals (CIs) were as follows: for grade 1 obesity (30.0–34.9 kg/m^2), 1.44 (1.41, 1.47); for grade 2 obesity (35.0–39.9 kg/m^2), 1.92 (1.86, 1.98); and for grade 3 obesity (40.0–59.9 kg/m^2), 2.71 (2.55, 2.86), with normal weight as the reference (Global BMI Mortality Collaboration et al., 2016).

7.1.2 WEIGHT MANAGEMENT

7.1.2.1 Current Recommendations

Realistic weight loss goals recommended by the Academy of Nutrition and Dietetics (AND) include 10% of baseline body weight over approximately 6–12 months (AND, 2014b). As little as 3%–5% of sustained weight loss can have cardiometabolic benefits, including improved triglycerides and blood glucose control. Greater losses have beneficial effects on blood pressure and cholesterol (AND, 2014b; Jensen et al., 2014; Raynor and Champagne, 2016). The current AND goal for weight loss is 5%–10% over 6 months (Raynor and Champagne, 2016). These goals are important to consider when evaluating the effectiveness of various dietary patterns for weight management. It should also be noted that the most effective weight management strategies include a combination of diet, physical activity, and behavior modification techniques (Raynor and Champagne, 2016).

According to AND recommendations, it is essential for dietary weight loss interventions to be hypocaloric (Raynor and Champagne, 2016). In its evidence analysis library, AND lists a hypocaloric lacto-ovo vegetarian diet as one of a multitude of dietary patterns or manipulations that may be effective for reducing excess weight (AND, 2014a). The 2013 American Heart Association/American College of Cardiology/The Obesity Society (AHA/ACC/TOS) recommendations for managing overweight and obesity in adults also includes hypocaloric lacto-ovo vegetarian and vegan diets as dietary treatment options for reducing weight (Jensen et al., 2014). The *2015–2020 Dietary Guidelines for Americans* also includes a "Healthy Vegetarian Eating Pattern" as one of the healthy eating patterns recommended for reducing the risk of chronic diseases (DHHS and USDA, 2015). The Healthy Vegetarian Eating Pattern is a lacto-ovo vegetarian dietary pattern that is considered within the realm of options to help "achieve and maintain a healthy body weight" (DHHS and USDA, 2015). Assessment of plant-based dietary patterns, through either observational or intervention studies, demonstrates that individuals who follow these patterns ad libitum often have a lower average kilocalorie intake than those following a nonvegetarian or omnivore pattern (Farmer et al., 2011; Turner-McGrievy et al., 2015).

7.1.3 WHY A PLANT-BASED DIET MAY REDUCE THE PREVALENCE OF OVERWEIGHT OR OBESITY

Plant-based diets have often been found to be high in fiber (Key et al., 1999, 2006; Farmer et al., 2011), which may help to increase satiety, thereby decreasing kilocalorie intake. Additionally, individuals who follow plant-based diets, particularly vegan diets, often consume less kilocalories and fat, while consuming higher amounts of phytochemicals and nutrient-dense foods, including fruits, vegetables, whole grains, legumes, and nuts (Key et al., 1999; Farmer et al., 2011; do Rosario et al., 2016). Additionally, fruits and vegetables are good sources of inulin-like fructans, which can affect gut microbiota in ways that impact adiposity (Delzenne et al., 2011).

7.2 OBSERVATIONAL STUDIES EXAMINING THE RELATIONSHIP BETWEEN PLANT-BASED DIETARY PATTERNS AND MEASURES OF ADIPOSITY

Various cohorts, in a variety of countries, have been used to examine the differences in weight and adiposity measures across dietary patterns. More than 60 publications have reported weight differences by dietary patterns (including plant based) for the past five decades. Associations between plant-based dietary patterns and measures of adiposity may help to assert that there is a relationship between vegetarian diets and a reduced risk or prevalence of overweight or obesity. Relevant findings of these studies are reported in Table 7.1.

7.2.1 STUDIES ON SEVENTH-DAY ADVENTISTS

Seventh-day Adventists (SDAs) comprise a unique population that, due to religious-related health beliefs and dietary habits, has been studied quite consistently over several decades. A substantial proportion of church members follow a plant-based dietary pattern, which ranges from vegan to semivegetarian, and health benefits have been observed for those members who follow such patterns (Key et al., 1999; Le and Sabate, 2014).

Early reports include several publications on Australian SDA members in the late 1970s to early 1980s. Several of these studies revealed that SDA vegetarians tend to weigh less than nonvegetarians (typically non-SDAs) (Armstrong et al., 1977, 1979; Simons et al., 1978). Assessment of weight without consideration of height is not very meaningful, but other studies have included measurements of relative weight, like BMI, which provide a better assessment of comparisons between groups. In 1981, Armstrong published results of a comparison of BMI between vegetarian and non-vegetarian postmenopausal women, but this comparison was not significantly different (Armstrong et al., 1981). Among male subjects in a 1983 comparison, BMI was significantly lower in lacto-ovo vegetarians (22.9 kg/m^2) than in SDA nonvegetarians (24.7 kg/m^2) and Mormon nonvegetarians (25.1 kg/m^2) (Rouse et al., 1983). Among the female subjects, BMI was significantly lower in SDA vegetarians (23.3 kg/m^2) than in Mormon nonvegetarians (26.3 kg/m^2) (Rouse et al., 1983).

TABLE 7.1
Observational Studies: Association between Dietary Patterns and Measures of Adiposity

Authors (Year), Country	Description of Subjects and Dietary Patterns	Study Findings
Chiu et al. (2015), Taiwan	Male/female; ≥20 years of age 1. Vegetarian ($n = 8,183$) 2. Nonvegetarian ($n = 40,915$)	BMI at baseline ($p < 0.0001$) - Vegetarians: 22.8 kg/m^2 - Nonvegetarians: 23.5 kg/m^2 Waist circumference ($p < 0.0001$) - Vegetarians: 75.5 cm - Nonvegetarians: 77.1 cm OR of waist circumference (90 cm for men or 80 cm for women) - Vegan: 0.69 (0.61, 0.78) - Lacto-vegetarian: 0.62 (0.55, 0.70) - LOV: 0.68 (0.62, 0.74) OR of BMI ≥27 kg/m^2 - Vegan: 0.68 (0.59, 0.78) - Lacto-vegetarian: 0.60 (0.52, 0.71) - LOV: 0.69 (0.62, 0.76) ORs adjusted for age, sex, education, leisure-time physical activity, alcohol, and study site
Fraser et al. (2015), United States and Canada	Adventist Health Study-2 subsample of black subjects Male/female; >30 years of age 1. Vegetarian (fish or meat) ($n = 146$) 2. Pesco-vegetarian (fish, no meat) ($n = 80$) 3. Nonvegetarian ($n = 366$)	After adjusting age, gender, education, substudy indicator, and physical activity, mean BMI and waist circumference were significantly higher in nonvegetarians than in vegetarians and vegans ($p < 0.05$) and significantly higher in nonvegetarians than in pesco-vegetarians ($p < 0.05$) BMI - Vegetarians: 27.3 kg/m^2 - Pesco-vegetarians: 27.6 kg/m^2 - Nonvegetarians: 30.7 kg/m^2 Waist circumference - Vegetarians: 91.6 cm - Pesco-vegetarians: 91.6 cm - Nonvegetarians: 99.2 cm Prevalence of overweight ($p < 0.0001$) - Vegetarians: 38% - Pesco-vegetarians: 46% - Nonvegetarians: 34% Prevalence of obesity ($p < 0.0001$) - Vegetarians: 27% - Pesco-vegetarians: 28% - Nonvegetarians: 47%

(Continued)

TABLE 7.1 (CONTINUED)
Observational Studies: Association between Dietary Patterns and Measures of Adiposity

Authors (Year), Country	Description of Subjects and Dietary Patterns	Study Findings
Jo et al. (2015), South Korea	Male/female (only in nonvegetarian group); average age: 43.4–49.3 years across dietary patterns 1. Vegetarian Buddhist priests ($n = 666$) 2. Nonvegetarian controls ($n = 17,817$)	BMI ($p = 0.021$) - Vegetarian: 24.3 kg/m^2 - Nonvegetarian: 23.4 kg/m^2
Tonstad et al. (2015), United States and Canada	Adventist Health Study-2 Male/female; >30 years of age 1. Vegan ($n = 5,389$) 2. LOV ($n = 18,390$) 3. Pesco-vegetarian ($n = 6,420$) 4. Semivegetarian ($n = 3,681$) 5. Nonvegetarian ($n = 32,101$)	BMI ($p < 0.0001$) - Vegan: 23.8 kg/m^2 - LOV: 25.6 kg/m^2 - Pesco-vegetarian: 25.9 kg/m^2 - Semivegetarian: 26.8 kg/m^2 - Nonvegetarian: 28.2 kg/m^2
Agrawal et al. (2014), India	Male/female; 20–49 years of age 1. Vegan (no animal products) ($n = 2,560$) 2. Lacto-vegetarian (no eggs, fish, chicken, or meat) ($n = 37,797$) 3. LOV (no fish, chicken, or meat) ($n = 5,002$) 4. Pesco-vegetarian (no chicken or meat) ($n = 3,446$) 5. Semivegetarian (no fish; daily/weekly/occasionally chicken and/or meat) ($n = 8,140$) 6. Nonvegetarian (animal products daily/weekly/ occasionally) ($n = 99,372$)	BMI (NS difference) - Vegans: 20.5 kg/m^2 - Lacto-vegetarians: 21.2 kg/m^2 - LOV: 21.0 kg/m^2 - Pesco-vegetarians: 20.3 kg/m^2 - Semivegetarians: 20.6 kg/m^2 - Nonvegetarians: 20.7 kg/m^2 Prevalence of overweight/obesity—BMI: ≥23 kg/m^2 (p for trend: <0.001) - Vegans: 21.5% - Lacto-vegetarians: 26.9% - LOV: 24.9% - Pesco-vegetarians: 19.5% - Semivegetarians: 21.8% - Nonvegetarians: 22.6% Prevalence of obesity—BMI: ≥25 kg/m^2 (p for trend: <0.001) - Vegans: 11.5% - Lacto-vegetarians: 16.2% - LOV: 14.9% - Pesco-vegetarians: 10.0% - Semivegetarians: 11.3% - Nonvegetarians: 12.7%

(Continued)

TABLE 7.1 (CONTINUED)

Observational Studies: Association between Dietary Patterns and Measures of Adiposity

Authors (Year), Country	Description of Subjects and Dietary Patterns	Study Findings
		BMI: ≥ 30 kg/m^2 (p for trend: <0.001)
		- Vegans: 2.3%
		- Lacto-vegetarians: 3.6%
		- LOV: 3.0%
		- Pesco-vegetarians: 1.7%
		- Semivegetarians: 1.6%
		- Nonvegetarians: 2.4%
Clarys et al. (2014), Belgium	Male/female; ≥ 20 years of age 1. Vegan (no animal products) ($n = 104$) 2. Vegetarian (no meat or fish) ($n = 573$) 3. Pesco-vegetarian (fish but no meat) ($n = 145$) 4. Semivegetarian (red meat, poultry, or fish ≤ 1/week) ($n = 498$) 5. Nonvegetarians (meat or fish almost every day) ($n = 155$)	Prevalence of overweight - Vegans: 10.6% - Vegetarians: 14.7% - Semivegetarians: 17.1% - Pesco-vegetarians: 15.9% - Nonvegetarians: 20.6% Prevalence of obesity - Vegans: 1.9% - Vegetarians: 3.5% - Semivegetarians: 2.4% - Pesco-vegetarians: 3.4% - Nonvegetarians: 8.4%
Gadgil et al. (2014), United States	Atherosclerosis in South Asians Living in America Study Male/female; 45–84 years of age 1. Vegetarian ($n = 59$) 2. Nonvegetarian ($n = 91$)	BMI ($p = 0.30$) - Vegetarian: 25.8 kg/m^2 - Nonvegetarian: 26.6 kg/m^2
Singh et al. (2014), United States	Adventist Health Study-2 subsample of Asian Indian subjects Male/female; >30 years of age 1. Vegan ($n = 9$) 2. LOV ($n = 44$) 3. Pesco-vegetarian ($n = 35$) 4. Semivegetarian ($n = 14$) 5. Nonvegetarian ($n = 119$)	Prevalence of overweight/obesity (BMI >23 kg/m^2) - Vegan: ~55% - LOV: ~50% - Pesco-vegetarian: ~58% - Semivegetarian: ≥ 80% - Nonvegetarian: ≥ 80%
Baig et al. (2013), Pakistan	Male/female; 20–80 years of age 1. Vegetarian ($n = 83$) 2. Nonvegetarian ($n = 93$)	BMI ($p = 0.027$) - Vegetarians: 20.43 kg/m^2 - Nonvegetarians: 21.24 kg/m^2

(Continued)

TABLE 7.1 (CONTINUED)
Observational Studies: Association between Dietary Patterns and Measures of Adiposity

Authors (Year), Country	Description of Subjects and Dietary Patterns	Study Findings
Orlich et al. (2013), Orlich and Fraser (2014), United States and Canada	Adventist Health Study-2 Male/female; average age: 57 years 1. Vegan ($n = 5,548$) 2. LOV ($n = 21,177$) 3. Pesco-vegetarian ($n = 7,194$) 4. Semivegetarian ($n = 4,031$) 5. Nonvegetarian ($n = 35,359$)	Age, sex, and race standardized average BMI - Vegans: 24.1 kg/m^2 - LOV: 26.1 kg/m^2 - Pesco-vegetarians: 26.0 kg/m^2 - Semivegetarians: 27.3 kg/m^2 - Nonvegetarians: 28.3 kg/m^2
Ho-Pham et al. (2012), Vietnam	Female; average age: ~60 years 1. Vegan nuns ($n = 88$) 2. Nonvegetarian regional residents ($n = 93$)	BMI (NS difference) - Vegans: 24 kg/m^2 - Nonvegetarians: 24 kg/m^2 NS difference in weight, lean mass, fat mass, and percent body mass between vegans and nonvegetarians
Timko et al. (2012), United States	Male/female; average age: 24.9 years 1. Vegan (no animal products) ($n = 35$) 2. Vegetarian ($n = 111$) 3. Semivegetarian (occasional consumption of fish and/or poultry) ($n = 75$) 4. Nonvegetarian (consumption of various animal foods) ($n = 265$)	BMI ($p < 0.01$) - Vegans: 21.29 kg/m^2 - Vegetarians: 23.79 kg/m^2 - Semivegetarians: 23.92 kg/m^2 - Nonvegetarians: 24.49 kg/m^2
Rizzo et al. (2011), United States and Canada	Adventist Health Study-2 substudy Male/female; average age: 60 years; $n = 773$ 1. Vegetarians (meat, poultry, or fish <1 time/month) 2. Semivegetarians (fish whenever but other meat <1 time/month or total meat ≥1/month and <1/week) 3. Nonvegetarians (meat or poultry ≥1 time/month and total meat ≥1 time/week)	BMI ($p < 0.001$) - Vegetarians: 25.7 kg/m^2 - Semivegetarians: 27.6 kg/m^2 - Nonvegetarians: 29.9 kg/m^2 Waist circumference was significantly lower in vegetarians and semivegetarians than in nonvegetarians ($p < 0.0001$; data n/a) Adjusted for age, gender, ethnicity, smoking, alcohol intake, physical activity, and kilocalorie intake

(Continued)

TABLE 7.1 (CONTINUED)
Observational Studies: Association between Dietary Patterns and Measures of Adiposity

Authors (Year), Country	Description of Subjects and Dietary Patterns	Study Findings
Karelis et al. (2010), Finland	Female; average age: 47.0–47.7 years across dietary patterns 1. Vegetarian ($n = 21$) 2. Age-matched nonvegetarian ($n = 41$)	BMI ($p < 0.05$) - Vegetarians: 21.7 kg/m² - Nonvegetarians: 23.8 kg/m²
Lee and Krawinkel (2009), South Korea	Female; average age: 30.4–31.4 years old across dietary patterns 1. Vegetarian Buddhist nuns ($n = 54$) 2. Nonvegetarian Catholic nuns ($n = 31$) (diets probably not that different)	BMI ($p = 0.010$) - Vegetarians: 22.6 kg/m² - Nonvegetarians: 20.7 kg/m² Weight, fat-free mass, and body fat were also significantly higher in vegetarians than in nonvegetarians ($p < 0.05$ for all comparisons) There was a higher prevalence of underweight in the nonvegetarian group
Baines et al. (2007), Australia	Australia Longitudinal Study on Women's Health; 22–27 years of age 1. Vegetarian (no red meat, fish, or poultry) ($n = 252$) 2. Semivegetarian (no red meat) $n = 827$ 3. Nonvegetarian $n = 8,034$	BMI - Vegetarians: 22.2 kg/m² (21.7–22.7) - Semivegetarians: 23.0 kg/m² (22.7–23.3) - Nonvegetarians: 23.7 kg/m² (23.6–23.8) Prevalence of overweight—BMI >25–30 kg/m² ($p < 0.001$) - Vegetarians: 12.4% - Semivegetarians: 15.4% - Nonvegetarians: 19.1% Prevalence of obesity—BMI >30 kg/m² ($p < 0.001$) - Vegetarians: 3.4% - Semivegetarians: 7.4% - Nonvegetarians: 10.3%
Fontana et al. (2007), United States	Male/female; average age: 53.1–53.2 years across dietary patterns 1. Low-kilocalorie, low-protein vegan ($n = 21$) 2. Age-, gender-, and height- matched Western diet ($n = 21$)	BMI ($p \leq 0.002$) - Vegans: 21.3 kg/m² - Western diet: 26.5 kg/m² Percent body fat—women ($p \leq 0.002$) - Vegans: 26.9% - Western diet: 42.3% Percent body fat—men ($p \leq 0.002$) - Vegans: 13.7% - Western diet: 21.0% NS difference in lean body mass

(Continued)

TABLE 7.1 (CONTINUED)

Observational Studies: Association between Dietary Patterns and Measures of Adiposity

Authors (Year), Country	Description of Subjects and Dietary Patterns	Study Findings

Rosell et al. (2006), United Kingdom	EPIC-Oxford
	Male/female; ≥20 years of age
	1. Vegan (no food of animal origin) ($n = 609$)
	2. Vegetarian (no meat or fish) ($n = 5,277$)
	3. Pesco-vegetarian (fish, no meat) ($n = 2,504$)
	4. Nonvegetarian ($n = 10,784$)
		Increase of BMI/year—women ($p = 0.017$)
		  - Vegans: 0.12 kg/m^2
		  - Vegetarians: 0.15 kg/m^2
		  - Pesco-vegetarians: 0.12 kg/m^2
		  - Nonvegetarians: 0.15 kg/m^2
		Increase of BMI/year—men (NS)
		  - Vegans: 0.10 kg/m^2
		  - Vegetarians: 0.12 kg/m^2
		  - Pesco-vegetarians: 0.12 kg/m^2
		  - Nonvegetarians: 0.12 kg/m^2

Alewaeters et al. (2005), Belgium	Male/female; ≥20 years of age
	1. Vegetarian ($n = 326$)
	2. Nonvegetarian ($n = 9,659$)
		BMI—women ($p < 0.001$)
		  - Vegetarians: 22.1 kg/m^2
		  - Nonvegetarians: 24.6 kg/m^2
		BMI—men ($p < 0.001$)
		  - Vegetarians: 22.6 kg/m^2
		  - Nonvegetarians: 25.7 kg/m^2

Bedford and Barr (2005), Canada	British Columbia Nutrition Survey
	Male/female; 19–84 years of age
	1. Vegetarian
	2. Nonvegetarian
		BMI—women ($p < 0.001$)
		  - Vegetarians: 23.1 kg/m^2
		  - Nonvegetarians: 25.7 kg/m^2
		BMI—men (NS difference)
		  - Vegetarians: 25.9 kg/m^2
		  - Nonvegetarians: 26.7 kg/m^2
		Prevalence of overweight in women ($p = 0.001$)
		  - Vegetarians: 12.7%
		  - Nonvegetarians: 21.2%
		Prevalence of overweight in men (NS)
		  - Vegetarians: 35.5%
		  - Nonvegetarians: 31.6%
		Prevalence of obesity in women ($p = 0.001$)
		  - Vegetarians: 4.2%
		  - Nonvegetarians: 18.1%
		Prevalence of obesity in men (NS)
		  - Vegetarians: 12.9%
		  - Nonvegetarians: 19.4%
		Vegetarian women had a significantly lower waist circumference than nonvegetarian women (79.8 cm vs. 75.0 cm)
		The comparison between men was NS
		Analyses were age-adjusted

(Continued)

TABLE 7.1 (CONTINUED)
Observational Studies: Association between Dietary Patterns and Measures of Adiposity

Authors (Year), Country	Description of Subjects and Dietary Patterns	Study Findings

Newby et al. (2005), Sweden	Swedish Mammography Cohort Female; average age: 51.1–54.8 years across categories of dietary patterns
	1. Vegan (no meat, poultry, fish, eggs, or dairy) ($n = 83$)
	2. Lacto-vegetarian (no meat, poultry, fish, or eggs) ($n = 159$)
	3. Semivegetarian (sometimes consume fish or eggs, but mainly LOV) ($n = 960$)
	4. Nonvegetarian ($n = 54,257$)
		BMI was also significantly higher in omnivores than in vegans, lacto-vegetarians, and semivegetarians ($p < 0.005$)
		  - Vegans: 23.3 kg/m^2
		  - Lacto-vegetarians: 23.4 kg/m^2
		  - Semivegetarians: 23.6 kg/m^2
		  - Nonvegetarians: 24.7 kg/m^2
		Prevalence of overweight ($p < 0.0001$)
		  - Vegans: 23%
		  - Lacto-vegetarians: 21%
		  - Semivegetarians: 24%
		  - Nonvegetarians: 30%
		Prevalence of obesity ($p < 0.0001$)
		  - Vegans: 6%
		  - Lacto-vegetarians: 4%
		  - Semivegetarians: 5%
		  - Nonvegetarians: 10%
		The average weight of omnivores was significantly higher than the weight of semivegetarians, lacto-vegetarians, and vegans ($p < 0.05$)

Rosell et al. (2005), United Kingdom	EPIC-Oxford
	Male/female; ≥20 years of age
	1. Lifelong vegetarian ($n = 379$)
	2. Became vegetarian 1–9 years old ($n = 328$)
	3. Became vegetarian 10–14 years old ($n = 1,160$)
	4. Became vegetarian 15–19 years old ($n = 2,764$)
	5. Became vegetarian ≥20 years old ($n = 10,891$)
	6. Nonvegetarian ($n = 29,250$)
		BMI—women ($p < 0.001$)
		  - Lifelong vegetarian: 23.7 kg/m^2
		  - Became vegetarian 1–9 years old: 23.9 kg/m^2
		  - Became vegetarian 10–14 years old: 23.8 kg/m^2
		  - Became vegetarian 15–19 years old: 23.6 kg/m^2
		  - Became vegetarian ≥20 years old: 23.5 kg/m^2
		  - Nonvegetarian: 23.2 kg/m^2
		BMI—men ($p < 0.001$)
		  - Lifelong vegetarian: 24.2 kg/m^2
		  - Became vegetarian 1–9 years old: 25.4 kg/m^2
		  - Became vegetarian 10–14 years old: 24.4 kg/m^2

(Continued)

TABLE 7.1 (CONTINUED)

Observational Studies: Association between Dietary Patterns and Measures of Adiposity

Authors (Year), Country	Description of Subjects and Dietary Patterns	Study Findings
		- Became vegetarian 15–19 years old: 24.2 kg/m^2
		- Became vegetarian ≥20 years old: 24.3 kg/m^2
		- Nonvegetarian: 25.2 kg/m^2
		Reference = became vegetarian ≥20 years of age
		Compared with reference nonvegetarians, differed $p < 0.0001$ for both sexes
		Those becoming vegetarian 1–9 years of age differed for men $p < 0.01$
		Those becoming vegetarian 10–14 years of age differed for women $p < 0.01$
Cade et al. (2004), United Kingdom	UK Women's Cohort Study; 35–69 years of age 1. Vegetarians (meat or fish <1 time/week) ($n = 6,478$) 2. Oily fish eaters (oily fish 2–4 times/week, meat <1 time/week) ($n = 870$) 3. Other fish eaters (fish ≥1 time/week, oily fish <2–4 times/week, meat <1/week) ($n = 6,478$) 4. Nonvegetarians (meat >1 time/week) ($n = 23,738$)	BMI - Vegetarians: 23.3 kg/m^2 - Oily fish eaters: 23.3 kg/m^2 - Other fish eaters: 23.2 kg/m^2 - Nonvegetarians: 25.0 kg/m^2
Brathwaite et al. (2003), Barbados	SDA Male/female; 18–74 years of age 1. Self-identified vegetarians 2. FFQ defined vegetarians 3. Self-identified nonvegetarians 4. FFQ-defined vegetarians	OR of being obese was greater for nonvegetarians: 1.70 (1.02, 2.83) NS difference is BMI, waist or hip circumference, or waist-to-hip ratio between groups Self-reported vegetarians >5 years had a significantly lower prevalence of overweight and obesity ($p < 0.05$)

(Continued)

TABLE 7.1 (CONTINUED)

Observational Studies: Association between Dietary Patterns and Measures of Adiposity

Authors (Year), Country	Description of Subjects and Dietary Patterns	Study Findings
Davey et al. (2003), United Kingdom	EPIC-Oxford Male/female; >20 years of age 1. Vegan (no food of animal origin) (n = 2,596) 2. Vegetarian (no meat or fish) (n = 18,840) 3. Pesco-vegetarian (fish, no meat) (10,110) 4. Nonvegetarian (n = 33,883)	BMI—women - Vegans: 21.9 kg/m^2 - Vegetarians: 22.7 kg/m^2 - Pesco-vegetarians: 22.9 kg/m^2 - Nonvegetarian: 24.3 kg/m^2 BMI—men - Vegans: 22.5 kg/m^2 - Vegetarians: 23.5 kg/m^2 - Pesco-vegetarians: 23.6 kg/m^2 - Nonvegetarians: 24.9 kg/m^2 Prevalence of obesity in women 20–65 years of age - Vegans: 2.5% - Vegetarians: 4.5% - Pesco-vegetarians: 4.4% - Nonvegetarians: 9.3% Prevalence of obesity in men 20–65 years of age - Vegans: 1.6% - Vegetarians: 3.5% - Pesco-vegetarians: 3.0% - Nonvegetarians: 7.1%
Spencer et al. (2003), United Kingdom	EPIC-Oxford Male/female; 20–97 years of age 1. Vegans (no meat, fish, eggs, or dairy) (n = 1,553) 2. Vegetarians (no meat or fish) (n = 12,307) 3. Pesco-vegetarians (fish, no meat) (n = 6,191) 4. Nonvegetarians (n = 17,824)	Age-, lifestyle-, and dietary factor–adjusted BMI (95% CI)—women - Vegans: 22.56 kg/m^2 (22.32, 22.79) - Vegetarians: 22.96 kg/m^2 (22.88, 23.04) - Pesco-vegetarians: 22.83 kg/m^2 (22.73, 22.92) - Nonvegetarians: 23.23 kg/m^2 (23.17, 23.31) Age-, lifestyle-, and dietary factor–adjusted BMI (95% CI)—men - Vegans: 23.12 kg/m^2 (22.83, 23.43) - Vegetarians: 23.67 kg/m^2 (23.54, 23.80) - Pesco-vegetarians: 23.45 kg/m^2 (23.27, 23.64) - Nonvegetarians: 24.09 kg/m^2 (23.97, 24.20)

(Continued)

TABLE 7.1 (CONTINUED)
Observational Studies: Association between Dietary Patterns and Measures of Adiposity

Authors (Year), Country	Description of Subjects and Dietary Patterns	Study Findings
Waldmann et al. (2003), Germany	German Vegan Study Male/female; average age: 42.4–44.9 years across dietary patterns 1. Strict vegan (no animal food products) ($n = 98$) 2. Moderate vegan (eggs and dairy <5% kcal/day)	BMI (NS) - Strict vegans: 21.2 kg/m^2 - Moderate vegans: 21.2 kg/m^2 Percent body fat was significantly lower in strict vegans (both sexes combined and females) than in moderate vegans ($p \leq 0.05$) Waist-to-hip ratio was significantly greater in strict vegans than in moderate vegans
Hoffmann et al. (2001), Germany	Giessen Wholesome Nutrition Study Female; 25–65 years of age 1. LOV ($n = 111$) 2. Low-meat eaters ($n = 131$) 3. Nonvegetarian controls ($n = 138$)	The difference in proportions of subjects within categories of BMI was significant when comparing LOV with controls and in comparing low-meat eaters with controls ($p \leq 0.05$) Prevalence of overweight - LOV: 18% - Low-meat eaters: 18% - Nonvegetarians: 39% Prevalence of obesity - LOV: 1% - Low-meat eaters: 2% - Nonvegetarians: 9%
Kennedy et al. (2001), United States	Continuing Survey of Food Intake by Individuals (CSFII 1994–1996) Male/female 1. Vegetarian (meat, poultry, or fish on day of recall) ($n = 643$) 2. Nonvegetarian ($n = 9,372$)	BMI—women ($p < 0.05$) - Vegetarians: 24.6 kg/m^2 - Nonvegetarians: 25.7 kg/m^2 BMI—men ($p < 0.05$) - Vegetarians: 25.2 kg/m^2 - Nonvegetarians: 26.4 kg/m^2
Lin et al. (2001), Taiwan	Male/female; ≥50 years of age 1. Vegetarian ($n = 20$) 2. Nonvegetarian ($n = 20$)	BMI (NS difference) - Vegetarians: 23.1 kg/m^2 - Nonvegetarians: 24.8 kg/m^2
Barr and Broughton (2000), Canada	Premenopausal women; 18–50 years of age 1. Vegetarians ($n = 90$) 2. Past vegetarians ($n = 35$) 3. Nonvegetarians ($n = 68$)	BMI (NS difference) - Vegetarians: 23.2 kg/m^2 - Past vegetarians: 25.3 kg/m^2 - Nonvegetarians: 23.5 kg/m^2 NS differences in weight or proportion within categories of BMI between vegetarians, nonvegetarians, and past vegetarians

(Continued)

TABLE 7.1 (CONTINUED)

Observational Studies: Association between Dietary Patterns and Measures of Adiposity

Authors (Year), Country	Description of Subjects and Dietary Patterns	Study Findings
Greenwood et al. (2000), United Kingdom	UK Women's Cohort Study; 35–69 years of age 1. High-diversity vegetarians (*n* = 4,379) 2. Low-diversity vegetarians (*n* = 5,190) 3. Conservative omnivores (*n* = 5,946) 4. Higher-diversity, traditional omnivores (*n* = 4,819) 5. Traditional meat, chips, and pudding eaters (*n* = 6,087) 6. Health-conscious omnivores (*n* = 2,131) 7. Monotonous low-quantity omnivores (*n* = 5,416)	BMI - Groups 1 and 2: 23 - Groups 3–5, and 7: 25 - Group 6: 24 Prevalence of obesity - Vegetarians: 5%–6% - Nonvegetarians: 9%–12% The mean waist-to-hip ratio ranged between 0.74 and 0.75 in all groups
Lu et al. (2000), Taiwan	Male/female; 31–45 years of age 1. Vegetarians 2. Age- and sex-matched nonvegetarians	BMI—women for two different regions ($p < 0.05$) - Vegetarians: 20.0 kg/m^2; 20.7 kg/m^2 - Nonvegetarians: 22.5 kg/m^2; 22.0 kg/m^2 BMI—men ($p < 0.05$) - Vegetarians: 20.8 kg/m^2 - Nonvegetarians: 22.9 kg/m^2 Average weight was significantly lower in vegetarians than in omnivores ($p < 0.05$)
Fraser (1999), United States and Canada	Adventist Health Study-1; ≥25 years of age 1. Vegetarian (no fish, poultry, or meat) (*n* = 17,488) 2. Semivegetarian (fish and poultry <1 time/week) (*n* = 12,525) 3. Nonvegetarian (*n* = 29,068)	BMI in women 45–64 years of age ($p = 0.0001$) - Vegetarians: 23.73 kg/m^2 - Semivegetarians: 24.83 kg/m^2 - Nonvegetarians: 25.88 kg/m^2 BMI in men 45–64 years of age ($p = 0.0001$) - Vegetarians: 24.26 kg/m^2 - Semivegetarians: 25.18 kg/m^2 - Nonvegetarians: 26.24 kg/m^2
Haddad et al. (1999), United States	Male/female; 20–60 years of age 1. Vegan (*n* = 25) 2. Nonvegetarian (*n* = 20)	BMI ($p < 0.001$) - Vegans: 20.5 kg/m^2 - Nonvegetarians: 25.5 kg/m^2

(Continued)

TABLE 7.1 (CONTINUED)
Observational Studies: Association between Dietary Patterns and Measures of Adiposity

Authors (Year), Country	Description of Subjects and Dietary Patterns	Study Findings
Hebbelinck et al. (1999), Belgium	Male/female; 16–30 years of age 1. LOV ($n = 44$) (compared with population reference value—data not shown)	BMI (NS difference from reference values) - Male: 22.1 kg/m² - Female: 21.8 kg/m² NS difference from reference population in terms of weight and skinfold measurements (triceps, suprailiac, calf)
Li et al. (1999), Australia	Male; age 20–50 years of age 1. Vegan (meat, eggs, or dairy <6 times/year) ($n = 18$) 2. LOV (dairy and eggs; meat <6 times/year) ($n = 43$) 3. Moderate-meat eaters (<285 g/day raw weight of meat) ($n = 60$) 4. High-meat eaters (≥285 g/day raw weight of meat) ($n = 18$)	LOVs' average BMI was significantly lower than high-meat and moderate-meat consumers ($p < 0.001$); similarly, the BMI in the vegan group was significantly lower than that for the moderate- and high-meat consumers ($p < 0.001$) - Vegans: 23.3 kg/m² - LOV: 23.6 kg/m² - Moderate-meat eaters: 26.4 kg/m² - High-meat eaters: 27.0 kg/m² Moderate-meat eaters had a significantly higher waist-to-hip ratio (0.88) than LOV (0.86) and vegans (0.85)
Appleby et al. (1998), United Kingdom	Oxford Vegetarian Study Male/female; 20–89 years of age 1. Vegetarian (including pesco-vegetarians) ($n = 2,847$) 2. Nonvegetarians ($n = 2,445$)	Age-adjusted BMI—women ($p < 0.0001$) - Vegetarians: 21.32 kg/m² - Nonvegetarians: 22.32 kg/m² Age-adjusted BMI—men ($p < 0.0001$) - Vegetarians: 22.05 kg/m² - Nonvegetarians: 23.18 kg/m² Prevalence of overweight or obesity in women ($p < 0.00001$) - Vegetarians: 8% - Nonvegetarians: 13% Prevalence of overweight or obesity in men ($p < 0.00001$) - Vegetarians: 10% - Nonvegetarians: 21%

(Continued)

TABLE 7.1 (CONTINUED)
Observational Studies: Association between Dietary Patterns and Measures of Adiposity

Authors (Year), Country	Description of Subjects and Dietary Patterns	Study Findings
Famodu et al. (1998), Nigeria	SDA Average age: 47–49 years across categories of dietary patterns 1. Vegan (no animal food products; dairy less than once per month) ($n = 40$) 2. Semivegetarian (meat less than once per month; dairy ≥2 times/week) ($n = 28$) 3. Nonvegetarian (meat ≥2 times/week) ($n = 8$)	BMI (NS difference) - Vegans: 26.9 kg/m^2 - Semivegetarians: 28.9 kg/m^2 - Nonvegetarians: 29.1 kg/m^2 Vegans weighed significantly less than nonvegetarians ($p < 0.05$) Triceps skinfold thickness was not significantly different between the groups
Toohey et al. (1998), United States	Black SDA members Male/female; average age: 45.6–52.1 years across dietary patterns 1. Vegans ($n = 45$) 2. LOV ($n = 143$)	BMI—women ($p = 0.03$) - Vegans: 25.3 kg/m^2 - LOV: 26.7 kg/m^2 BMI—men ($p = 0.03$) - Vegans: 23.6 kg/m^2 - LOV: 26.1 kg/m^2 NS difference in waist circumference between dietary patterns Waist-to-hip ratio was significantly ($p = 0.04$) lower in vegans than in LOV subjects
Janelle and Barr (1995), Canada	Female; age: 20–50 years 1. Vegan ($n = 8$) 2. Lacto-vegetarian ($n = 15$) 3. Nonvegetarian ($n = 22$)	BMI was significantly ($p < 0.05$) lower for vegans and vegetarians than for nonvegetarians - Vegans: 20.7 kg/m^2 - Lacto-vegetarians: 21.2 kg/m^2 - Nonvegetarians 22.7 kg/m^2 NS difference in lead body mass and percent body fat
Krajcovicova-Kudlackova et al. (1995), Slovakia	Male/female; 34–60 years of age 1. Vegetarian ($n = 67$) 2. Nonvegetarian (Melby et al., 1993) controls ($n = 75$)	BMI—women ($p < 0.001$) - Vegetarian: 22.7 kg/m^2 - Nonvegetarian: 25.4 kg/m^2 BMI—men ($p < 0.001$) - Vegetarian: 22.6 kg/m^2 - Nonvegetarian: 25.6 kg/m^2

(Continued)

TABLE 7.1 (CONTINUED)
Observational Studies: Association between Dietary Patterns and Measures of Adiposity

Authors (Year), Country	Description of Subjects and Dietary Patterns	Study Findings
Knutsen (1994), United States	Adventist Health Study-1 Male/female; ≥25 years of age 1. Vegetarian (meat, poultry, or fish <1 time/week) (n = 15,228) 2. Nonvegetarian (n = 12,538)	BMI—women ($p \leq 0.001$) - Vegetarians: 23.6 kg/m² - Nonvegetarians: 25.2 kg/m² BMI—men ($p \leq 0.001$) - Vegetarians: 24.2 kg/m² - Nonvegetarians: 25.7 kg/m²
Toth and Poehlman (1994), United States	1. Vegetarians (n = 17; 19–36 years of age) 2. Nonvegetarians (n = 40; 18–34 years of age)	NS differences in weight, fat mass, percent body fat, fat-free mass, sum of skinfold measurements (abdomen, axilla, biceps, calf, chest, subscapular, suprailiac, thigh, triceps), and waist-to-hip ratio
Melby et al. (1994), United States	Black SDA Male/female; average age 46–49 years across groups of dietary patterns 1. Vegetarian (no meat, fish, or poultry) (n = 66) 2. Semivegetarian (meat, fish, poultry 1–3 times/week) (n = 56) 3. Nonvegetarian (meat, fish, poultry daily) (n = 45)	BMI (NS difference) - Vegetarians: 26.8 kg/m² - Semivegetarians: 29.2 kg/m² - Nonvegetarians: 28.6 kg/m² Waist circumference ($p < 0.05$) for vegetarians compared with semi- and nonvegetarians - Vegetarians: 83.4 cm - Semivegetarians: 90.4 cm - Nonvegetarians: 89.4 cm Vegetarians weighed significantly less than semivegetarians ($p < 0.05$), but not when compared with nonvegetarians
Chang-Claude and Frentzel-Beyme (1993), Germany	Male/female; age ≥10 years (most are adults) 1. Strict vegetarian (no meat/fish) (n = 1,163) 2. Moderate vegetarian (occasionally consume meat/fish) (n = 741)	A lower proportion of strict vegetarians were in the upper third of BMI categories (>22.4 kg/m² in men; >21.6 kg/m² in women)

(Continued)

TABLE 7.1 (CONTINUED)
Observational Studies: Association between Dietary Patterns and Measures of Adiposity

Authors (Year), Country	Description of Subjects and Dietary Patterns	Study Findings
Melby et al. (1993), United States	SDA Male/female; average age: 65.2–69.3 years across dietary patterns and race 1. Vegetarian ($n = 112$) 2. Nonvegetarian ($n = 91$)	BMI—white subjects ($p < 0.05$) - Vegetarians: 25.0 kg/m^2 - Nonvegetarians: 27.6 kg/m^2 BMI—black subjects ($p < 0.05$) - Vegetarians: 27.0 kg/m^2 - Nonvegetarians: 31.7 kg/m^2 NS difference in waist-to-hip ratio and triceps skinfold thickness between vegetarians and nonvegetarians (black nonvegetarians had a higher waist circumference than white vegetarians)
Slattery et al. (1991), United States	CARDIA study Male/female; 18–30 years of age 1. Meat <1 time/week ($n = 79$) 2. Meat 1–3 times/week ($n = 211$) 3. Meat >3 times/week ($n = 4,821$)	BMI ($p \leq 0.05$; consumers of meat <1 time/week compared with those who consumed meat >3 times/week; those who consumed meat 1–3 times/week compared with those who consumed meat >3 times/week) - Meat <1 time/week: 22.7 kg/m^2 - Meat 1–3 times/week: 23.4 kg/m^2 - Meat >3 times/week: 24.6 kg/m^2
Millet et al. (1989), France	Male/female; average age 35.4–49.3 years across groups 1. Vegetarians (no meat, fish, or poultry >1 time/month) ($n = 37$) 2. Nonvegetarian controls ($n = 69$)	BMI—women ($p < 0.001$) - Vegetarian: 20.0 kg/m^2 - Nonvegetarian: 23.3 kg/m^2 BMI—men ($p < 0.001$) - Vegetarian: 21.2 kg/m^2 - Nonvegetarian: 24.7 kg/m^2 Weights were significantly lower in vegetarians than in nonvegetarians ($p < 0.001$ for men; $p < 0.05$ for women)
Faber et al. (1986), South Africa	Male/female; 18–40 years of age 1. LOV (SDA; no meat, fish, or poultry) ($n = 33$) 2. Nonvegetarian controls ($n = 22$)	BMI—women (NS difference) - LOV: 21.5 kg/m^2 - Nonvegetarians: 21.1 kg/m^2 BMI—men (NS difference) - LOV: 23.9 kg/m^2 - Nonvegetarians: 24.6 kg/m^2 Percent body fat in women (NS difference) - LOV: 26.6% - Nonvegetarians: 25.4% Percent body fat in men (NS difference) - LOV: 18.5% - Nonvegetarians: 15.4%

(Continued)

TABLE 7.1 (CONTINUED)
Observational Studies: Association between Dietary Patterns and Measures of Adiposity

Authors (Year), Country	Description of Subjects and Dietary Patterns	Study Findings
Melby et al. (1985), United States	SDA Male/female; average age: 51 years 1. Vegetarians (meat <1 time/month) ($n = 150$) 2. Nonvegetarians ($n = 65$)	BMI—women ($p = 0.0001$) - Vegetarians: 23.9 kg/m² - Nonvegetarians: 28.1 kg/m² BMI—men (NS difference) - Vegetarians: 23.9 kg/m² - Nonvegetarians: 28.1 kg/m²
Rouse et al. (1983), Australia	Male/female; 25–44 years of age 1. SDA LOV (rarely or never eat meat, fish, or poultry) ($n = 98$) 2. SDA nonvegetarians (meat, poultry, or fish ≥1 time/month) ($n = 82$) 3. Mormon nonvegetarians (meat, poultry, or fish >1 time/day on average) ($n = 113$)	BMI—women ($p < 0.01$ for difference between SDA LOV and Mormon nonvegetarians) - SDA LOV: 23.3 kg/m² - SDA nonvegetarian: 24.4 kg/m² - Mormon nonvegetarian: 26.3 kg/m² BMI—men ($p < 0.05$ for SDA LOV compared with SDA nonvegetarians; $p < 0.01$ for LOV compared with Mormon nonvegetarians) - SDA LOV: 22.9 kg/m² - SDA nonvegetarian: 24.7 kg/m² - Mormon nonvegetarian: 25.1 kg/m² Among the male subjects, omnivores (both SDA and Mormon) weighed significantly more than SDA LOV ($p < 0.05$ and $p < 0.01$, respectively) Among the female subjects, the differences were noted between SDA vegetarians and Mormon omnivores: weight, mid-upper arm circumference, and triceps skinfold thickness were significantly lower in SDA vegetarians than in Mormon omnivores ($p < 0.01$)
Shultz and Leklem (1983), United States	Male/female 1. SDA vegetarians ($n = 51$; 20–83 years old) 2. SDA nonvegetarians ($n = 16$; 24–38 years old) 3. Non-SDA nonvegetarians ($n = 53$; 19–78 years old)	BMI—women (NS difference) - SDA vegetarians: 24 kg/m² - SDA nonvegetarians: 25 kg/m² - Non-SDA nonvegetarians: 24 kg/m² BMI—men (NS difference) - SDA vegetarians: 23 kg/m² - SDA nonvegetarians: 22 kg/m² - Non-SDA nonvegetarians: 24 kg/m² NS difference in weight between the vegetarian and nonvegetarian groups

(Continued)

TABLE 7.1 (CONTINUED)
Observational Studies: Association between Dietary Patterns and Measures of Adiposity

Authors (Year), Country	Description of Subjects and Dietary Patterns	Study Findings
Knuiman and West (1982), Belgium and Netherlands	Male; 30–39 years of age 1. Macrobiotic (mainly whole grains, beans, vegetables, seaweed, fermented soy foods; very limited to no animal products) ($n = 33$) 2. LOV (very limited to no meat or fish) ($n = 56$) 3. Semi-lacto-vegetarians (meat or fish ≤1/week) ($n = 43$) 4. Nonvegetarian ($n = 52$)	The BMIs of macrobiotic, lacto-vegetarian, and semi-lacto-vegetarian men were significantly lower than those of the nonvegetarian group ($p < 0.01$ for each comparison) - Macrobiotics: 20.9 kg/m^2 - Lacto-vegetarians: 21.4 kg/m^2 - Semi-lacto-vegetarians: 22.2 kg/m^2 - Nonvegetarians: 24.4 kg/m^2
Armstrong et al. (1981), Australia	Postmenopausal women; 50–79 years of age 1. Vegetarian (SDA) ($n = 46$) 2. Nonvegetarian (matched regional residents) ($n = 47$)	BMI (NS difference) - Vegetarians: 23.1 kg/m^2 - Nonvegetarians: 24.0 kg/m^2 NS differences in weight, arm circumference, and triceps skinfold thickness between the vegetarian and nonvegetarian groups
Burr et al. (1981), United Kingdom	Male/female; 28–80 years of age 1. Vegetarian (meat and fish <1 time/month) ($n = 85$) 2. Nonvegetarian ($n = 215$)	BMI difference for women <60 years of age (NS) - Vegetarians: 22.4 kg/m^2 - Nonvegetarians: 23.2 kg/m^2 BMI difference for women ≥60 years of age ($p < 0.01$) - Vegetarians: 22.2 kg/m^2 - Nonvegetarians: 24.9 kg/m^2 BMI difference for men <60 years of age ($p < 0.001$) - Vegetarians: 20.5 kg/m^2 - Nonvegetarians: 24.5 kg/m^2 BMI difference for men ≥60 years of age ($p < 0.05$) - Vegetarians: 22.7 kg/m^2 - Nonvegetarians: 24.9 kg/m^2
Taber and Cook (1980), United States	Male/female; average age: 25.5–27.9 years across dietary patterns and genders 1. Vegetarian ($n = 28$) 2. Pesco-vegetarian ($n = 20$) 3. Nonvegetarians ($n = 49$)	NS difference between groups for weight, arm circumference, triceps skinfold, arm muscle area, and arm fat area

(Continued)

TABLE 7.1 (CONTINUED)
Observational Studies: Association between Dietary Patterns and Measures of Adiposity

Authors (Year), Country	Description of Subjects and Dietary Patterns	Study Findings
Armstrong et al. (1979), Australia	Male/female; matched pairs; 17–79 years of age 1. Vegetarians (including some SDAs; mostly no meat, fish, or poultry) ($n = 106$) 2. Nonvegetarians (meat, fish, or poultry ≥1 time/day) ($n = 106$)	BMI (NS difference) - Vegetarians: 22.9 kg/m^2 - Nonvegetarians: 23.9 kg/m^2 Average weight was lower in vegetarians than nonvegetarians ($p = 0.03$) NS difference was noted for triceps skinfold thickness between the groups
Sanders et al. (1978), United Kingdom	Male/female; 21–66 years of age 1. Vegans (no foods of animal origin for at least 1 year) 2. Nonvegetarian matched controls	Vegans had a significantly lower average standard weight for height than nonvegetarians ($p < 0.05$); they also had a significantly lower sum of skinfold measurements (biceps, triceps, subscapular, and suprailiac) than nonvegetarians ($p < 0.01$)
Simons et al. (1978), Australia	Male/female 1. Vegetarians (SDA) ($n = 20$; average age 39) 2. Nonvegetarians (SDA) ($n = 17$; average age 37) 3. Nonvegetarians 9regional residents) ($n = 38$; average age 46)	Proportion of subjects >10% overweight[a] - Vegetarians: 20% - Nonvegetarians: 47% Vegetarians weighed significantly less than nonvegetarians, but this analysis included both men and women, and there was a higher proportion of women in the vegetarian group than in the nonvegetarian group
Armstrong et al. (1977), Australia	Male/female; 30–79 years of age 1. Vegetarians (SDA; meat, fish, poultry <1/month) ($n = 418$) 2. Nonvegetarians (regional residents) ($n = 290$)	The nonvegetarians weighed significantly more than the vegetarians ($p < 0.005$ for differences by gender between vegetarians and nonvegetarians)
Sacks et al. (1975), United States	Male/female; 16–62 years of age 1. Macrobiotic/vegetarian (residing in commune) ($n = 115$) 2. Age- and gender-matched nonvegetarian controls (Framingham cohort offspring) ($n = 115$)	Vegetarians weighed significantly less than nonvegetarian controls ($p < 0.001$) Subscapular skinfold thickness was also significantly lower in vegetarians than in nonvegetarians ($p < 0.001$) Results for other skinfold measurements (triceps, abdomen) were not shown

Note: CARDIA = Coronary Artery Risk Development in Young Adults; FFQ = Food Frequency Questionaire; LOV = lacto-ovo vegetarian; NS = not significant or nonsignificant; n/a = not available.

[a] Not defined.

Cohorts in North America include the Adventist Health Study-1 (AHS-1) and Adventist Health Study-2 (AHS-2). Dietary patterns defined in the AHS-1 study (n = 59,081) include vegetarian (no fish, poultry, or meat), semivegetarian (fish and/or poultry <1 time/week), and nonvegetarian (Fraser, 1999). BMI differences between vegetarians (inclusive of semivegetarians) and nonvegetarians were significant for men (24.2 and 25.7 kg/m^2, respectively) and women (23.6 and 25.2 kg/m^2, respectively) (Knutsen, 1994). Among women 45–64 years of age, there was a significant difference in BMI by dietary patterns: vegetarians, 23.7 kg/m^2; semivegetarians, 24.8 kg/m^2; and nonvegetarians, 25.9 kg/m^2 (Fraser, 1999). BMI values among men of the same age group were also significantly different: 24.26, 25.18, and 26.24 kg/m^2 for vegetarians, semivegetarians, and nonvegetarians, respectively (Fraser, 1999).

In the AHS-2 cohort (>30 years of age; $n \geq$ 73,000), the defined dietary patterns include vegan (~7.7%), lacto-ovo vegetarian (~29.2%), pesco-vegetarian (~9.9%), semivegetarian (~5.4%), and nonvegetarian (~47.7%) (Orlich et al., 2013; Orlich and Fraser, 2014). The average age-, sex-, and race-adjusted BMI values of AHS-2 cohort members are 24.1 kg/m^2 (vegans), 26.1 kg/m^2 (lacto-ovo vegetarians), 26.0 kg/m^2 (pesco-vegetarians), 27.3 kg/m^2 (semivegetarians), and 28.3 kg/m^2 (nonvegetarians) (Orlich et al., 2013; Orlich and Fraser, 2014). Other publications on the AHS-2 cohort confirm that BMI differs significantly across categories of these dietary patterns (Tonstad et al., 2009, 2013, 2015).

In a subgroup study of 592 black subjects from AHS-2, vegetarians (vegans and lacto-ovo vegetarians) (27.3 kg/m^2) and pesco-vegetarians (27.6 kg/m^2) had a significantly lower average BMI than nonvegetarians (30.7 kg/m^2) (Fraser et al., 2015). The odds of being obese (OR 0.43 [0.28, 0.67]) were lower for vegetarians than for nonvegetarians (reference), and they were also lower for pesco-vegetarians (OR 0.47 [0.27, 0.81]) than for nonvegetarians (Fraser et al., 2015). The analyses on BMI were adjusted for several covariates, including age, gender, and physical activity (Fraser et al., 2015). The prevalence of overweight and obesity was also reported and significantly differed across dietary pattern groups: 27%, 28%, and 47% for vegetarians, pesco-vegetarians, and nonvegetarians, respectively (Fraser et al., 2015). Vegetarians had the highest prevalence of normal weight (35%) compared with pesco-vegetarians (26%) and nonvegetarians (19%) (Fraser et al., 2015). In subgroup analyses of Asian Indian subjects from AHS-2 (n = 211), the prevalence of overweight or obesity (BMI >23 kg/m^2) differed significantly between groups: ~55% for vegans, ~50% for lacto-ovo vegetarians, ~58% for pesco-vegetarians, and ~>80% for semivegetarians and nonvegetarians (Singh et al., 2014).

Smaller SDA cohorts have also been studied. Findings more or less support those found in AHS-1 and AHS-2 (Melby et al., 1985, 1993, 1994; Brathwaite et al., 2003) (Table 7.1). Even though the findings from most studies on SDAs have been positive, there are some studies where BMI differences between vegetarians and nonvegetarians were not significant (Shultz and Leklem, 1983; Faber et al., 1986; Famodu et al., 1998, 1999). It is possible that null findings may be partly related to the populations selected for comparisons and/or the number of subjects included in the studies.

7.2.2 STUDIES ON NORTH AMERICAN POPULATIONS

Aside from the North American studies in SDAs noted previously, there are several studies that have been published from other North American cohorts. Early studies focused on differences in weight (Sacks et al., 1975; Toth and Poehlman, 1994).

In the Coronary Artery Risk Development in Young Adults (CARDIA) study, investigators examined the BMI of subjects (18–30 years of age) according to their meat intake (Slattery et al., 1991). The groups that consumed meat <1 time/week (22.7 kg/m^2) and 1–3 times/week (23.4 kg/m^2) had a significantly lower BMI than those who consumed meat >3 times/week (24.6 kg/m^2) (Slattery et al., 1991).

Utilizing data from the Continuing Survey of Food Intake by Individuals (CSFII) 1994–1996, Kennedy et al. (2001) allocated subjects into vegetarian versus non-vegetarian patterns based on whether they consumed meat, poultry, or fish (based on one 24-hour dietary recall). In this particular study, the BMI of vegetarians (25.25 kg/m^2 for men, 24.65 kg/m^2 for women) was significantly lower than the BMI of nonvegetarians (26.65 kg/m^2 for men, 25.75 kg/m^2 for women). A higher proportion of vegetarians' BMI was <25 kg/m^2 compared with that of nonvegetarians, but these differences for men and women were not significant (Kennedy et al., 2001).

For the most part, other North American studies support lower BMI values in vegetarians than in nonvegetarians (Janelle and Barr, 1995; Haddad et al., 1999; Barr and Broughton, 2000; Bedford and Barr, 2005; Fontana et al., 2007; Timko et al., 2012).

7.2.3 STUDIES ON EUROPEAN POPULATIONS

There are various cohorts in the United Kingdom and Europe that have been used to examine the relationship between dietary patterns and anthropometric data. An early UK study by Burr and colleagues (1981) documented that the BMIs of vegetarian men <60 years of age (20.5 kg/m^2) and ≥60 years of age (22.7 kg/m^2) were significantly lower than those of nonvegetarian men of the same age ranges (24.5 and 24.9 kg/m^2, respectively). Similar results were noted for vegetarian women ≥60 years of age (22.2 kg/m^2 vs. 24.9 kg/m^2 in nonvegetarians), but the comparison for women <60 years of age was not significant (Burr et al., 1981).

In the Oxford Vegetarian Study, a significantly higher proportion of nonvegetarians (21% of men, 13% of women) are overweight or obese than vegetarians (10% of men, 8% of women) (Appleby et al., 1998). In this same group, the average age-adjusted BMI values are significantly higher in nonvegetarians (23.18 kg/m^2 in men, 22.32 kg/m^2 in women) than in vegetarians (22.05 kg/m^2 in men, 21.32 kg/m^2 in women) (Appleby et al., 1998). These differences continued to be significant even after adjustment for various lifestyle factors, including dietary fiber and exercise. There is also evidence of a possible trend in long-term vegetarians (>5 years) having a lower BMI than short-term vegetarians (≤5 years). It should be noted that only 1% of this cohort have a BMI ≥30 kg/m^2 (Appleby et al., 1998).

From the UK Women's Cohort Study, researchers reported a BMI of 23 kg/m^2 for low- and high-diversity vegetarians, whereas most of the nonvegetarian groups' average BMIs were ~25 kg/m^2 (no statistical test of differences noted) (Greenwood et al., 2000). The prevalence of obesity ranged from 5% to 6% for vegetarians and 9% to 12% for nonvegetarians (Greenwood et al., 2000). In this same cohort, vegetarians' and fish eaters' (similar to pesco-vegetarians) BMIs were lower than those of nonvegetarians (no statistical test of differences noted) (Cade et al., 2004).

A number of studies have been published on the UK European Prospective Investigation into Cancer and Nutrition (EPIC)–Oxford cohort (Davey et al., 2003; Spencer et al., 2003). The 2003 report based on the EPIC-Oxford cohort ($n = 65,429$) observed that the BMIs of vegan, vegetarian, pesco-vegetarian, and nonvegetarian women were 21.9, 22.7, 22.9, and 24.3 kg/m^2, respectively (no statistical test of differences noted), while the corresponding values for men were 22.5, 23.5, 23.6, and 24.6 kg/m^2, respectively (Davey et al., 2003). They also reported the prevalence of obesity in subjects 20–65 years of age. Among male subjects, the proportion of obesity was 1.6%, 3.5%, 3.9%, and 7.1% for vegans, vegetarians, pesco-vegetarians, and nonvegetarians, respectively (Davey et al., 2003), while the corresponding prevalence of obesity in women was 2.5%, 4.5%, 4.4%, and 9.3%, respectively (Davey et al., 2003). Spencer et al. (2003) also published findings on a sample ($n = 37,875$) from the EPIC-Oxford cohort. Age-, lifestyle-, and dietary factor–adjusted BMI (95% CI) values in women were 22.56 (22.23, 22.79) kg/m^2, 22.96 (22.88, 23.04) kg/m^2, 22.83 (22.73, 22.92) kg/m^2, and 23.23 (23.17, 23.31) kg/m^2 for the vegans, vegetarians, pesco-vegetarians, and nonvegetarians, respectively (Spencer et al., 2003). For men, the corresponding values were 23.12 (22.83, 23.43) kg/m^2, 23.67 (23.54, 23.80) kg/m^2, 23.45 (23.27, 23.64) kg/m^2, and 24.09 (23.97, 24.20) kg/m^2 (Spencer et al., 2003). The age-adjusted prevalence of obesity was lowest in vegans (1.9% for men, 1.8% for women) and highest in nonvegetarians (5% for men, 5.7% for women) (Spencer et al., 2003). Rosell et al. (2005) published differences related to when individuals commenced following a vegetarian diet (Rosell et al., 2005). Findings from longitudinal analyses ($n = 21,966$; median follow-up 5.3 years) determined a significant difference in the increases of BMI per year in women: 0.12 kg/m^2 for vegans, 0.15 kg/m^2 for vegetarians, 0.12 kg/m^2 for pesco-vegetarians, and 0.15 kg/m^2 for nonvegetarians (Rosell et al., 2006). These observations were not significant in men, with vegans gaining 0.10 kg/m^2 per year and all other groups 0.12 kg/m^2 per year. In terms of weight gain, vegan men gained significantly less weight than nonvegetarians. Those who converted their diet to a more plant-based pattern also gained less weight than nonvegetarians (Rosell et al., 2006). Vegan and pesco-vegetarian women gained significantly less weight per year than nonvegetarians, and those who converted to a more plant-based dietary pattern also gained significantly less over the years than nonvegetarians (Rosell et al., 2006).

Several studies have been done in other parts of Europe. Significant differences in BMI were noted across gradient patterns of meat intake in Belgian men (Knuiman and West, 1982; Alewaeters et al., 2005) and women (Alewaeters et al., 2005) and for combined analyses (Clarys et al., 2014). Among women in the Swedish Mammography Cohort ($n = 55,459$), the odds ratio for being overweight and/or obese (BMI ≥ 25 kg/m^2) (nonvegetarians as reference group) was 0.35 for vegans, 0.54 for lacto-vegetarians, 0.47 for vegans plus lacto-vegetarians, and 0.52 for semi-vegetarians. The logistic analyses were adjusted for various covariates, including age, energy intake, alcohol intake, smoking status, and parity (Newby et al., 2005).

The BMI of nonvegetarians (24.7 kg/m^2) was also significantly higher than that of vegans (23.3 kg/m^2), lacto-vegetarians (23.4), and semivegetarians (23.6 kg/m^2) (Newby et al., 2005).

Null findings have also been reported in European groups (Hebbelinck et al., 1999). Similarly, differences favoring vegans or vegetarians have been noted in France (Millet et al., 1989), Germany (Chang-Claude and Frentzel-Beyme, 1993; Hoffmann et al., 2001), Finland (Karelis et al., 2010), Sweden (Newby et al., 2005), and Slovakia (Krajcovicova-Kudlackova et al., 1995).

7.2.4 STUDIES ON OTHER POPULATIONS

Other cohorts, outside of North America and Europe, have also been evaluated. Findings have been mixed in Australian groups. In one study, the average BMI of lacto-ovo vegetarians (23.6 kg/m^2) and vegans (23.3 kg/m^2) was significantly lower than that of moderate-meat consumers (26.4 kg/m^2), and high-meat consumers (27 kg/m^2) (Li et al., 1999). In the Australian Longitudinal Study on Women's Health cohort (22–27 years of age), the prevalence of overweight and obesity was significantly lower in vegetarian (12.4% and 3.4%, respectively) than in semivegetarian (15.4% and 7.4%, respectively) and nonvegetarian (19.1% and 10.3%, respectively) women (Baines et al., 2007), while the average BMIs were not significantly different between the three groups (Baines et al., 2007).

In a large cohort study in India, there was a significant difference in prevalence of overweight (23.0–24.9 kg/m^2) and obesity (≥25.0 kg/m^2) for subjects following different dietary patterns. The prevalence of overweight and obesity, respectively, was 21.5% and 11.5% for vegans, 26.9% and 16.2% lacto-vegetarians, 24.9% and 14.9% for lacto-ovo vegetarians, 19.5% and 10.0% for pesco-vegetarians, 21.8% and 11.3% for semivegetarians, and 22.6% and 12.7% for nonvegetarians (Agrawal et al., 2014). BMI was also found to be lower among vegetarians in Taiwan (Lu et al., 2000; Chiu et al., 2015), South Korea (Jo et al., 2015), and Pakistan (Baig et al., 2013). Some studies in Asian populations reported no differences (Lin et al., 2001; Ho-Pham et al., 2012; Gadgil et al., 2014). Another study reported a higher BMI in vegetarians than in nonvegetarians (Lee and Krawinkel, 2009). These null findings may be partly related to particular characteristics of the groups selected for comparisons.

7.2.5 FINDINGS OF BODY COMPOSITION ANALYSES

There is evidence spanning at least five decades on differences in body composition, including abdominal obesity, between individuals following different dietary patterns. In a subgroup from the AHS-2 cohort, waist circumference was found to be significantly lower in vegetarians and semivegetarians than in nonvegetarians (analyses adjusted for age, gender, ethnicity, smoking, calorie intake, alcohol intake, and physical activity) (Rizzo et al., 2011). In a subgroup of black subjects from AHS-2, vegetarians and pesco-vegetarians had significantly smaller waist circumferences that nonvegetarians (Fraser et al., 2015). The waist circumference measurements for women and men, respectively, were 88.1 and 95.5 cm for vegetarians, 89.0 and

94.7 cm for pesco-vegetarians, and 95.6 and 103.5 cm for nonvegetarians (Fraser et al., 2015). The odds of abdominal obesity for men and women, respectively, were 0.48 and 0.55 for vegetarians and 0.43 and 0.53 for pesco-vegetarians, with non-vegetarians as the reference group. In another group of black SDA members, waist circumference was significantly lower in vegetarians (83.4 cm) than in semivegetarians (90.4 cm) and nonvegetarians (89.4 cm) (Melby et al., 1994). Waist-to-hip ratio was significantly lower in vegetarians (0.79) than in both semivegetarians (0.82) and nonvegetarians (0.82) (Melby et al., 1994).

Results from the British Columbia Nutrition Survey reveal that vegetarian women had a significantly lower age-adjusted waist circumference than nonvegetarian women (79.8 cm vs. 75.0 cm) (Bedford and Barr, 2005). The comparison was not significant in men. In a study from Taiwan, vegetarians had a significantly lower waist circumference than nonvegetarians (75.5 cm vs. 77.1 cm). (Chiu et al., 2015). A significantly greater proportion of nonvegetarians were abdominally obese (≥90 cm in men, ≥80 cm in women) than vegetarians (27.7% vs. 21.7%). After adjusting for covariates, the odds of a large waist circumference were significantly lower for lacto-ovo vegetarians only (OR 0.86) than for nonvegetarians (Chiu et al., 2015). Other researchers have reported that differences in waist circumference were not significant (Toohey et al., 1998; Brathwaite et al., 2003).

Most of the analyses on skinfold thickness measurements indicate that differences between vegetarians and nonvegetarians are not significant (Armstrong et al., 1979, 1981; Taber and Cook, 1980; Rouse et al., 1983; Melby et al., 1993, 1994; Toth and Poehlman, 1994; Famodu et al., 1998; Hebbelinck et al., 1999). However, a few studies do report differences. Vegans have been found to have significantly lower skinfold measurements (sum of biceps, triceps, subscapular, and suprailiac) than nonvegetarians (Sanders et al., 1978). Similarly, in a comparison among women of SDA vegetarians and Mormon nonvegetarians, triceps skinfold thickness measurements were significantly lower in the vegetarians (Rouse et al., 1983). In another study, subscapular skinfold thickness was significantly lower in vegetarians (including macrobiotic pattern) than in nonvegetarians (Sacks et al., 1975). In the CARDIA study, subjects who consumed meat less than once per week or 1–3 times/week had significantly lower skinfold thickness (sum of triceps, subscapular, and suprailiac) measurements than those who consumed meat >3 times/week (Slattery et al., 1991). It should be noted that interpretation of such measurements depends on the number of sites measured, use of formulas to estimate percent body fat, and/or availability of a good reference group to compare measurements to.

Reports on other measurements, such as arm circumference (Taber and Cook, 1980; Armstrong et al., 1981; Rouse et al., 1983), hip circumference (Brathwaite et al., 2003), and thigh circumference (Melby et al., 1994) have been varied.

Percent body fat was estimated or measured in only a few of the studies. Most reported no differences observed for percent body fat (Faber et al., 1986; Toth and Poehlman, 1994; Janelle and Barr, 1995; Ho-Pham et al., 2012). Fontana et al. (2007) found that vegans had significantly lower percent body fat than subjects on a Western dietary pattern (women 26.9% vs. 42.3%, men 13.7% vs. 21.0%). Vegan subjects, in the German Vegan Study, had significantly lower percent body fat than moderate vegans (Waldmann et al., 2003).

7.2.6 Conclusions

Most of the published studies examined here provide supporting evidence that plant-based dietary patterns are associated with lower excess adiposity, particularly when estimated by BMI. There are various caveats that should be noted, however. Most of the analyses in these studies were cross-sectional in nature and did not control for possible confounding variables, like age, gender, physical activity, and smoking status. Additionally, in some observational studies, the vegetarian group was selected from a different population than the nonvegetarian group. The definitions used for plant-based diets can be quite disparate, not allowing for complete comparisons between all studies. Also, vegans were not always included in analyses (at times excluded due to their small number). Anthropometric measurements were not always a main study outcome and were self-reported in some studies. It is possible that study design flaws and/or underpowered analyses contributed to mixed findings in some cases. These difficulties should be expected when examining a large number of studies published across several decades.

7.3 INTERVENTION STUDIES EXAMINING THE EFFECT OF PLANT-BASED DIETS ON MEASURES OF ADIPOSITY

One of the earliest intervention studies evaluating the effect of plant-based diets on anthropometric measurements was conducted by Ornish. In this study, 46 subjects with a history of ischemic heart disease were randomly assigned to receive either a vegetarian diet (minimal amount of nonfat yogurt allowed) or control diet for 24 days. Subjects in the intervention group experienced a significant amount of weight loss (5.6%) (Ornish et al., 1983). Later on, Ornish reported findings of a lifestyle program, which included a low-fat vegetarian diet as part of the intervention. The intervention group experienced 11% weight loss ($p < 0.0001$) following 1 year of treatment (Ornish et al., 1990). Five years later, Ornish followed up on this same group of subjects. The low-fat vegetarian diet group had sustained an overall average 5.8 kg (6.3%) of weight loss ($p = 0.001$), and the loss was significantly greater than what occurred for the control group (Ornish et al., 1998).

An Ornish-style vegetarian diet has been utilized as an intervention in a number of other studies. In one case, 160 subjects with a BMI of 27–42 kg/m^2 were randomly allocated to follow an Aktins, Zone, Weight Watchers, or Ornish diet for 1 year (Dansinger et al., 2005). The subjects in the Ornish group experienced significant reduction in weight (3.2%) and waist circumference (2.2 cm). These reductions were not significantly different from those in the other treatment groups. Similar results were noted in another randomized trial ($n = 311$) comparing Atkins, Zone, a lifestyle intervention (Lifestyle, Exercise, Attitudes, Relationships, Nutrition [LEARN]), and a high-carb Ornish diet for 2 months in overweight or obese individuals (Gardner et al., 2007). Weight loss was significant for all groups, with those on the Ornish diet losing 3%, although this reduction was not significantly different from that in the other groups. Changes in percent body fat and waist-to-hip ratio were not significant (Gardner et al., 2007).

In another study, a low-fat vegetarian diet was responsible for a 3.6% weight loss ($p < 0.05$) over the course of two menstrual cycles in a group of 35 premenopausal women. In this study, a trend was noted whereby the higher a subject's baseline BMI, the greater their weight loss (Barnard et al., 2000). Overweight or obese postmenopausal women on a low-fat vegan diet in another study experienced similar results. Compared with a group following the National Cholesterol Education Program (NCEP) diet, the women on the vegan diet lost significantly more weight (6.5%) after 14 weeks (Barnard et al., 2004, 2005; Turner-McGrievy et al., 2004). A similar study assessed adherence and weight loss 1 and 2 years after the initiation of a 14-week study comparing a low-fat vegan diet with the NCEP diet (Turner-McGrievy et al., 2007). The vegan group experienced significant weight loss over 1 and 2 years, and their loss was significantly greater than that of the NCEP group (Turner-McGrievy et al., 2007). Those in the vegan group who adhered to the diet for a year experienced more weight loss than nonadherers, but the difference was not significant (Turner-McGrievy et al., 2007).

In overweight or obese women ($n = 18$) previously diagnosed with polycystic ovary syndrome who were randomly assigned to either a vegan diet or low-calorie diet, significant weight loss (1.8%) was noted after 3 months for the vegan group. Weight loss was not significant after 6 months, with weight regain evident (Turner-McGrievy et al., 2014). The effects of a 2-month intervention were observed using different plant-based diets, including vegan, vegetarian, pesco-vegetarian, and semi-vegetarian diets, compared with a nonvegetarian diet in a group of 62 overweight or obese individuals. All groups experienced significant weight loss, but the loss in the vegan group was significantly greater than that in the nonvegetarian group (4.8% vs. 2.2%). After 6 months of follow-up, the loss in the vegan group (7.5%) was significantly more than that in the pesco-vegetarian (3.2%), semivegetarian (3.2%), and nonvegetarian (3.1%) groups (Turner-McGrievy et al., 2015).

The effect of an Eco-Atkins diet (low-carb vegan diet) was compared with that of a high-carb lacto-ovo vegetarian diet. After 1 month, no significant differences in weight were noted (Jenkins et al., 2009). Subjects included men and postmenopausal women with BMI >27 kg/m^2 (Jenkins et al., 2009). However, when the same subjects were followed for 6 months, the low-carb vegan diet resulted in greater weight loss than the high-carb lacto-ovo vegetarian diet (8.2% vs. 6.8%). Other measurements of adiposity, however, including percent body fat and waist circumference, did not differ between the groups (Jenkins et al., 2014).

Several other studies have reported significant weight losses due to vegan (Lindahl et al., 1984; Balliett and Burke, 2013) and lacto-ovo vegetarian diets (Mahon et al., 2007; Burke et al., 2008). Other studies have reported no significant changes (Margetts et al., 1986; Prescott et al., 1988; Delgado et al., 1996). Details of these studies are found in Table 7.2. Several studies have focused on the effect of short vegan fasts on health outcomes, but considering current expert weight loss recommendations, these studies are not included here (Bloomer et al., 2010; Trepanowski et al., 2012; McDougall et al., 2014).

7.3.1 Studies in Individuals with a History of Diabetes

Weight management is particularly beneficial for individuals diagnosed with type 2 diabetes, by improving insulin resistance and ultimately blood glucose control (Barnard et al., 2009c; Khazrai et al., 2014). Several studies have been published on the benefits of vegan or vegetarian diets for improving metabolic health for those with type 2 diabetes, including anthropometric data (Barnard et al., 2015). Details can be found in Table 7.3.

TABLE 7.2

Intervention Studies Examining the Effect of Plant-Based Diets on Measures of Adiposity

Authors (Year), Country	Study and Subject Descriptions	Interventions	Findings
Turner-McGrievy et al. (2015), United States	Randomized controlled trial Overweight/obese (BMI 25–49.9 kg/m^2) $n = 62$ Gender: Male, female Age: 18–65 years old	1. Vegan diet (n = 11) × 2 months 2. Vegetarian diet (n = 13) × 2 months 3. Pesco-vegetarian diet (n = 13) × 2 months 4. Semivegetarian diet (red meat limited to once per week and poultry to ≤5 times/week) (n = 13) × 2 months 5. Omnivorous diet (n = 12) × 2 months All: Limit fat and glycemic index; limit "fatty" plant foods Free-living	Weight loss was significant after 2 months ($p < 0.01$) - Vegan: 4.8% - Vegetarian: ~4.8% - Pesco-vegetarian: 4.3% - Semivegetarian: 3.7% - Omnivorous: 2.2% Weight loss in vegans was significantly different from that in the omnivore group after 2 months ($p < 0.01$) Weight loss was significant after 6 months ($p < 0.01$) - Vegan: 7.5% - Vegetarian: 6.3% - Pesco-vegetarian: 3.2% - Semivegetarian: 3.2% - Omnivorous: 3.1% Weight loss in the vegan group was significantly different from that in the pesco- and semivegetarian and omnivore groups after 6 months ($p < 0.03$ for each comparison)

(*Continued*)

TABLE 7.2 (CONTINUED)
Intervention Studies Examining the Effect of Plant-Based Diets on Measures of Adiposity

Authors (Year), Country	Study and Subject Descriptions	Interventions	Findings
Turner-McGrievy et al. (2014), United States	Randomized pilot study Overweight/obese (BMI 25–49.9 kg/m² with PCOS n = 18 Gender: Female Age: 18–35 years old	1. Vegan (n = 9) × 6 months 2. Low calorie (n = 9) × 6 months Free-living	Significant weight loss in vegan group at 3 months (−1.8%; p = 0.04) but NS at 6 months (−0.0%; p = 0.39)
Jenkins et al. (2014), Canada	Randomized controlled trial Healthy men and postmenopausal women with elevated LDL-C and BMI >27 kg/m² n = 47 Gender: Male, female Age: 21–70 years old	1. Low-carb vegan diet (26% carb kcal, 31% protein kcal, 43% fat kcal) × 1 month 2. Control: High-carb lacto-ovo vegetarian diet (58% carb kcal, 16% protein kcal, 25% fat kcal) × 1 month Continued self-selected (ad libitum) adherence to diet for 6 months with monthly visits with dietitian	The low carb vegan group experienced a significantly greater weight loss than the high carb lacto-ovo control group (−6.9 kg/8.2% vs. −5.8 kg/6.8%; difference of −1.1 kg; p = 0.047) The low-carb vegan group experienced a significantly greater reduction in BMI than the high-carb lacto-ovo control group (−2.4 vs. −1.9 kg/m²; −0.4 kg/m² difference between groups; p = 0.039) No significant differences between groups in terms of percent body fat, waist circumference, and satiety

(Continued)

TABLE 7.2 (CONTINUED)
Intervention Studies Examining the Effect of Plant-Based Diets on Measures of Adiposity

Authors (Year), Country	Study and Subject Descriptions	Interventions	Findings
Balliett and Burke (2013), United States	Uncontrolled study $n = 49$ Gender: Male, female Age: 20–60 years old	Low-calorie vegan diet × 21 days plus herbal supplements	Significant reduction in weight (–8.7 lb = 3.95 kg; ~5%), waist circumference (–1.5 in. = 3.81 cm), hip circumference (–1.2 in. = 3.05 cm), waist-to-hip ratio (–0.01), and waist-to-height ratio (–0.02); significant reduction in BMI (–1.4 kg/m²) Significant reduction in fat mass (–5.2 lb = 2.36 kg); decrease in fat-free mass but increase in percent at-free mass (–4.0 lb = 1.82 kg and +1.5%); NS change in percent fat mass (–1%) $p < 0.05$
Jenkins et al. (2009), Canada	Randomized controlled trial Healthy men and postmenopausal women with elevated LDL-C and BMI >27 kg/m² $n = 47$ Gender: Male, female Age: 21–70 years old	1. Low-carb vegan diet (26% carb kcal, 31% protein kcal, 43% fat kcal) × 1 month 2. Control: High-carb lacto-ovo vegetarian diet (58% carb kcal, 16% protein kcal, 25% fat kcal) × 1 month	NS weight change

(Continued)

TABLE 7.2 (CONTINUED)
Intervention Studies Examining the Effect of Plant-Based Diets on Measures of Adiposity

Authors (Year), Country	Study and Subject Descriptions	Interventions	Findings
Burke et al. (2008), United States	Randomized controlled trial BMI 27–43 kg/m² $n = 176$ Gender: Male, female Age: 18–55 years old	1. Self-selected lacto-ovo vegetarian (low-kilocalorie, low-fat) diet × 18 months 2. Self-selected standard low-kilocalorie, low-fat diet × 18 months 3. Assigned to lacto-ovo vegetarian (low-kilocalorie, low-fat) diet × 18 months 4. Assigned to standard low-kilocalorie, low-fat diet × 18 months (1–3 included gradual elimination of meat, poultry, and fish within the first 6 weeks)	Significant weight loss occurred in all groups after 6 months: 9.9% and 9.4%, respectively, in groups 1 and 3 ($p < 0.0001$) Weight loss after 18 months was 5.3% and 7.9% for groups 1 and 3, respectively ($p < 0.0001$) Those who self-selected the type of weight loss diet they would follow had significantly greater weight regain during months 6–18 than those who were assigned to their respective group ($p < 0.001$) There was also a significant reduction in BMI and waist circumference in all groups; the differences between groups were NS
Gardner et al. (2007), United States	Free-living Randomized trial BMI 25–50 kg/m² Premenopausal $n = 311$ Gender: Female Age: 25–50 years old	1. Atkins (low carb) × 2 months 2. Zone (low carb) × 2 months 3. LEARN × 2 months 4. Ornish (high carb) ($n = 76$) × 2 months	Significant reduction in BMI occurred in all groups but was greatest in the Atkins' group The Ornish (−0.77 kg/m²; $p < 0.01$) group was not significantly different from the Zone or LEARN groups in terms of reduction of BMI Weight loss was significant for all groups, with Ornish (−2.6 kg; 3.0%; $p < 0.001$) not being significantly different from the other three groups Changes in percent body fat and waist-to-hip ratio were NS

(Continued)

TABLE 7.2 (CONTINUED)
Intervention Studies Examining the Effect of Plant-Based Diets on Measures of Adiposity

Authors (Year), Country	Study and Subject Descriptions	Interventions	Findings
Mahon et al. (2007), United States	Randomized controlled trial Postmenopausal BMI 25–34 kg/m² $n = 54$ Gender: Female Age: 50–80 years old	1. Energy restricted Beef (1250 kcal; 20% beef kcal; 48% carb kcal, 26% protein kcal, 26% fat kcal) × 9 weeks 2. Energy restricted Chicken (1250 kcal; 20% chicken kcal; 48% carb kcal, 26% protein kcal, 26% fat kcal) × 9 weeks 3. Energy restricted Lacto-ovo carb (1250 kcal; 20% cookie and chocolate kcal—intentional to keep fiber intake the same between groups; 58% carb kcal, 16% protein kcal, 26% fat kcal) × 9 weeks 4. Isocaloric habitual diet control × 9 weeks Free-living	All the energy-restricted groups experienced a significant reduction in body mass, fat mass, percent body fat, and fat-free mass compared with the control group Group 3 had significantly larger reduction in BMI (-2.1 kg/m²) than the control (but significantly less than group 2); group 3's change in body mass (-5.6 kg) was significantly less than that of the chicken group but significantly greater than that of the control group Differences for changes in fat mass, percent body fat, and fat-free mass between groups 1, 2, and 3 were NS; for group 3, these changes were -3.9 kg, -2.1%, and -1.7 kg, respectively

(Continued)

TABLE 7.2 (CONTINUED)

Intervention Studies Examining the Effect of Plant-Based Diets on Measures of Adiposity

Authors (Year), Country	Study and Subject Descriptions	Interventions	Findings

Turner-McGrievy et al. (2007), United States	Randomized trial
	Postmenopausal overweight/obese
	$n = 62$
	Gender: Female
	Average age: 57.4 years old (vegan group), 55.7 years old (NCEP group)
		1. Low-fat vegan diet × 14 weeks
		  a. Social support vs.
		  b. None
		2. NCEP step II diet × 14 weeks
		  a. Social support vs.
		  b. None
		Free-living
			The vegan group experienced significant weight loss at 1 year (-4.9 kg; $p < 0.001$) and 2 years (-3.1 kg; $p < 0.01$); this was also significantly greater than the NCEP group's weight loss ($p < 0.05$)
			The vegan group subjects who received group support (1 year, -6.2 kg; 2 years, -5.3 kg; $p < 0.01$) lost significantly more weight than the unsupported (1 year, -2.1 kg; 2 years, -0.35 kg) ($p < 0.05$)
			The vegan group diet adherers experienced significant weight loss (1 year, -5.9; $p < 0.05$), but not significantly more than nonadherers (1 year, -3.6) after 1 year

Dansinger et al. (2005), United States	Randomized trial BMI 27–42 kg/m^2 plus 1 cardiometabolic risk factor $n = 160$ Gender: Male/female Average age: 49 years old	1. Atkins × 1 year 2. Zone × 1 year 3. Weight Watchers × 1 year 4. Ornish (vegetarian) × 1 year Free-living	The Ornish group had significant reductions in weight (-3.3 kg; 3.2%; $p < 0.01$), BMI (-1.4 kg/m^2; $p < 0.05$), and waist circumference (-2.2 cm; $p < 0.05$) after 1 year; these changes were not significantly different from those of other groups Among completers, these changes were of a larger magnitude for weight (-6.6 kg; $p < 0.01$), BMI (-2.3 kg/m^2; $p < 0.01$), and waist circumference (-4.3 cm)

(Continued)

TABLE 7.2 (CONTINUED)
Intervention Studies Examining the Effect of Plant-Based Diets on Measures of Adiposity

Authors (Year), Country	Study and Subject Descriptions	Interventions	Findings
Barnard et al. (2004, 2005), Turner-McGrievy et al. (2004), United States	Randomized controlled trial Overweight and obese (BMI 26–44 kg/m²) postmenopausal $n = 59$ Gender: Female Average age: 55.6–57.4 years old across treatment groups	1. Very-low fat vegan diet (75% carb kcal, 15% protein kcal, 10% fat kcal) × 14 weeks 2. NCEP diet (55% carb kcal, 15% protein kcal, ≤30% fat kcal; <200 mg cholesterol) × 14 weeks Free-living	The vegan group lost significantly more weight than the NCEP group (5.8 kg [6.5%] vs. 3.8 kg) $p < 0.05$ BMI was reduced significantly compared with that of the control group (−2.2 kg/m² vs. −1.4 kg/m²; $p = 0.012$), but this change was not significantly different over time Waist circumference was reduced significantly compared with that of the control group (−4.6 cm vs. −2.5 cm; $p = 0.023$), but this change was not significantly different over time Lean mass was reduced significantly (−0.7 kg; $p < 0.01$) in the intervention group, but this change was not significantly different from that in the control group NS changes were noted for percent body fat (−2.9% in the intervention group), hip circumference, and waist-to-hip ratio

(Continued)

TABLE 7.2 (CONTINUED)

Intervention Studies Examining the Effect of Plant-Based Diets on Measures of Adiposity

Authors (Year), Country	Study and Subject Descriptions	Interventions	Findings
Barnard et al. (2000), United States	Randomized crossover trial Premenopausal with abdominal pain $n = 35$ Gender: Female Age: >18 years old	1. Low-fat vegetarian diet (10% fat kcal) × 2 menstrual cycles 2. Placebo (typical diet) × 2 menstrual cycles Free-living	Significant reduction in weight (−2.5 kg; 3.6%; $p < 0.05$) and BMI (0.9 kg/m^2; $p < 0.01$) during the low-fat vegetarian intervention compared with baseline Total weight lost was different between these groups (NS between groups) - BMI <22 kg/m^2 = −1.4 kg - BMI 22–26.5 kg/m^2 = −3.3 kg - BMI >26.5 kg/m^2 = −2.9 kg
Ornish et al. (1998), United States	Randomized controlled trial Hx of atherosclerosis $n = 35$ Gender: Male, female (no female in intervention group) Average age: 57.4 years old (intervention), 61.8 years old (control)	1. Intensive lifestyle program × 5 years: Vegetarian diet (10% fat kcal), moderate aerobic exercise, stress management, smoking cessation, group psych support 2. Control: Personal physician's advice about lifestyle changes	Experimental group lost 10.9 kg (12%) by year 1 ($p = 0.001$) and sustained a 5.8 kg (6.3%) loss by year 5 ($p = 0.001$), which were significantly greater than changes in the control group
Delgado et al. (1996), Spain	Controlled trial Healthy physical education students or grads $n = 38$ Gender: Male, female Age: 20–25 years old	1. Lacto-ovo vegetarian diet × 2 months 2. Compared with nonvegetarian and vegetarian age-, weight-, dietary habit-, and physical activity–matched controls on habitual diet × 2 months Free-living	NS weight loss—weight actually stable in the experimental group (68.3–68.8 kg) after 2 months Similarly, NS change in percent body fat and lean body mass

(Continued)

TABLE 7.2 (CONTINUED)
Intervention Studies Examining the Effect of Plant-Based Diets on Measures of Adiposity

Authors (Year), Country	Study and Subject Descriptions	Interventions	Findings
Ornish et al. (1990), United States	Randomized controlled trial Hx of coronary heart disease $n = 41$ Gender: Male, female (only one female in experimental group) Age: 35–75 years old	1. Lifestyle program: Low-fat vegetarian diet (70%–75% carb kcal, 15%–20% protein kcal, 10% fat kcal), moderate aerobic exercise, stress management, smoking cessation, group support × 1 year 2. Control: Usual care ($n = 19$) × 1 year Prepared meals available if subjects chose to use them/free-living	Significant weight loss in experimental group: 10.1 kg (11%) ($p < 0.0001$)
Prescott et al. (1988), Australia	Randomized trial $n = 50$ Gender: Male, female Age: 18–60 years old	Abstain from consuming meat, fish, or poultry (2× weeks prior to a randomization and continuing for length of study) 1. Meat (protein) supplement (beef, chicken, lamb, sausage, pork: prawns) × 12 weeks 2. Nonmeat (protein) supplement (cereals, legumes, nuts, vegetables) × 12 weeks Some meals were provided (twice a day + weekends)	NS change in weight in either group

(Continued)

TABLE 7.2 (CONTINUED)
Intervention Studies Examining the Effect of Plant-Based Diets on Measures of Adiposity

Authors (Year), Country	Study and Subject Descriptions	Interventions	Findings
Margetts et al. (1986), Australia	Randomized crossover trial SBP 150–180 mmHg or DBP 90–110 mmHg and not on HTN medication n = 58 Gender: Male, female Age: 30–64 years old	1. Maintain habitual diet for duration of study 2. Lacto-ovo vegetarian diet × 6 weeks followed by habitual diet × 6 weeks 3. Habitual diet × 6 weeks followed by lacto-ovo vegetarian diet × 6 weeks	During lacto-ovo vegetarian period, group 2 gained ~2 kg and group 3 lost <2 kg (test of significance not noted)
Lindahl et al. (1984), Sweden	Uncontrolled study HTN n = 26 Gender: Male, female Age: 25–70 years old	Vegan foods provided (fruit juice only for first 7 days) × 1 year Free-living	Significant weight loss - At 4 months: 10.2 kg (13%) ($p < 0.001$) - At 1 year: 7.8 kg (10%) ($p < 0.001$)
Ornish et al. (1983), United States	Randomized controlled feeding trial Hx of ischemic heart disease n = 46 Gender: Male, female Age: 45–75 years old	1. Vegan diet (with minimal nonfat yogurt) × 24 days 2. Control Intervention included stress management training	Significant weight loss (−4.6 kg/5.6%) occurred in the intervention group ($p < 0.0001$)

Note: DBP = diastolic blood pressure; HTN = hypertension; Hx = history; LDL-C = low-density lipoprotein cholesterol; NS = not significant or nonsignificant; PCOS = polycystic ovary syndrome; SBP = systolic blood pressure.

TABLE 7.3

Intervention Studies Examining the Effect of Plant-Based Diets on Measures of Adiposity in Individuals with Diabetes

Authors (Year), Country	Study and Subject Descriptions	Interventions	Findings
Mishra et al. (2013), United States	Randomized, worksite pair-matched clusters, controlled trial Hx of type 2 DM and/or BMI ≥ 25 kg/m^2 $n = 10$ sites; 291 Gender: Male, Female Age: >18 years old	1. Low-fat vegan diet (75% carb kcal, 15% protein kcal, 10% fat kcal) × 18 weeks 2. Control × 18 weeks Free-living	Weight loss and BMI were significantly greater in the intervention group (-2.9 kg, 3%, $p < 0.0001$; -1.04 kg/m^2, $p < 0.0001$) than the control group (-0.06 kg and -0.01 kg/m^2) ($p < 0.001$ for both comparisons) even after adjusting for gender, cluster, and baseline value A greater proportion of the intervention group experienced $\geq 5\%$ weight loss (37%) compared with the control group (11%), $p < 0.001$ Weight loss and BMI were significantly reduced in the intervention group among program completers (-4.3 kg, 4.6%, $p < 0.001$; -1.5 kg/m^2, $p < 0.001$), whereas NS changes were noted in the control group (-0.08 kg; -0.02 kg/m^2); these changes differed significantly between groups ($p < 0.001$) even after adjusting for gender, cluster, and baseline value

(Continued)

TABLE 7.3 (CONTINUED)
Intervention Studies Examining the Effect of Plant-Based Diets on Measures of Adiposity in Individuals with Diabetes

Authors (Year), Country	Study and Subject Descriptions	Interventions	Findings
Kahleova et al. (2011), Czech Republic	Randomized controlled trial Hx of type 2 DM treated with oral hypoglycemics, HgbA1c 6%–11% BMI 25–53 kg/m^2 $n = 74$ Gender: Male, female Age: 30–70 years old	1. Isocaloric lacto-vegetarian diet (60% carb kcal, 15% protein kcal, 25% fat kcal) × 24 weeks 2. Control: Conventional diabetic diet (50% carb kcal, 20% protein kcal, <30% fat kcal) × 24 weeks Last 12 weeks included an exercise program Meals were provided	Significant weight loss in both groups, but it was greater in the vegetarian diet group (−6.2 kg; 6.1%; $p < 0.001$) than in the control (−3.2 kg; 3.2%; $p < 0.001$) ($p < 0.001$) Waist circumference decreased significantly in both groups but to a greater extent in the vegetarian diet group (−6.4 cm) than the control group (−5.3 cm) ($p < 0.001$); exercise helped to further decrease waist circumference in the vegetarian group (−1.9 cm; $p < 0.05$) but not the control group (+0.7 cm) Subcutaneous and visceral fat volumes decreased significantly in both groups, with exercise causing further reductions in the vegetarian diet group but not the control group

(Continued)

TABLE 7.3 (CONTINUED)
Intervention Studies Examining the Effect of Plant-Based Diets on Measures of Adiposity in Individuals with Diabetes

Authors (Year), Country	Study and Subject Descriptions	Interventions	Findings
Ferdowsian et al. (2010), Levin et al. (2010), United States	Site-specific designation of treatments GEICO employees with Hx of type 2 DM and/or BMI ≥25 kg/m^2 $n = 113$ Gender: Male, female Age: >18 years old	1. Low-fat vegan diet × 22 weeks 2. Control × 22 weeks Free-living	Subjects on the low-fat vegan diet significantly lost weight (-5.1 kg/5.2%; $p < 0.0001$), waist circumference (-4.7 cm; $p < 0.0001$), and hip circumference (-4.5 cm; $p < 0.0001$) These changes were also significantly greater than changes in the control group ($p < 0.0001$) The intervention group experienced a significant decrease in waist-to-hip circumference compared with the control group ($p = 0.0007$), but the change over time was NS

(*Continued*)

TABLE 7.3 (CONTINUED)
Intervention Studies Examining the Effect of Plant-Based Diets on Measures of Adiposity in Individuals with Diabetes

Authors (Year), Country	Study and Subject Descriptions	Interventions	Findings
Barnard et al. (2009a), United States	Randomized controlled trial Hx of type 2 DM $n = 99$ Gender: Male, female Average age: 56.7 years old (vegan group), 54.6 years old (ADA group)	1. Vegan diet (75% carb kcal, 15% protein kcal, ~10% fat kcal) × 74 weeks 2. 2003 ADA guidelines diet (60%–70% carb plus MUFAs kcal, 15%–20% protein kcal, <7% SAT fat kcal); if BMI >25 kg/m², then a 500–1000 kcal deficit was applied Free-living	Significant weight loss in both groups but not significantly different between groups - Vegan: 4.4 kg ($p < 0.0001$) - ADA: 3.0 kg ($p < 0.001$) Among adherent participants, those on the vegan treatment lost 6.8 kg, whereas those on the conventional treatment lost 4.9 kg (NS) Waist circumference was significantly reduced in both groups but not significantly different between groups - Vegan: 4.2 cm ($p < 0.001$) - Conventional: 1.8 cm ($p < 0.05$) Hip circumference was significantly reduced in both groups but not significantly between groups - Vegan: −3.4 cm ($p < 0.0001$) - Conventional: −2.3 cm ($p < 0.01$) NS changes in waist-to-hip ratio

(Continued)

TABLE 7.3 (CONTINUED)
Intervention Studies Examining the Effect of Plant-Based Diets on Measures of Adiposity in Individuals with Diabetes

Authors (Year), Country	Study and Subject Descriptions	Interventions	Findings
Barnard et al. (2006), United States	Randomized trial Hx of type 2 DM $n = 99$ Gender: Male, female Average age: 56.7 years old (vegan group), 54.6 years old (ADA group)	1. Low-fat vegan diet (75% carb kcal, 15% protein kcal, ~10% fat kcal) × 22 weeks 2. 2003 ADA guidelines diet (60%–70% carb plus MUFAs kcal, 15%–20% protein kcal, <7% SAT fat kcal, CHOL ≤200 mg/day) plus 500–1000 kcal restriction if BMI ≥25 × 22 weeks Free-living	Significant weight loss in both groups but NS between groups - Vegan: −5.8 kg/6% ($p < 0.0001$) - ADA: −4.3 kg/4.3% ($p < 0.0001$) Significant reduction in BMI (vegan: −2.1 kg/m^2) and hip circumference (vegan: −3.9 cm) in both groups but NS between groups Significant reduction in waist circumference (vegan: −5.3 cm) in both groups, but the reduction was significantly greater in vegans Significant reduction in waist-to-hip ratio (vegan: −0.02 cm) in the vegan group only
Nicholson et al. (1999), United States	Randomized controlled trial Hx of type 2 DM $n = 11$ Gender: Male, female Age: >25 years old	1. Low-fat vegan diet (restricted refined carbohydrates and sugars; 10%–15% protein kcal, <10% fat kcal) × 12 weeks 2. Control diet (encouraged reduction of red meat; poultry/fish encouraged instead; 55%–60% carb kcal, <30% fat kcal) × 12 weeks Most meals were provided—consumed off-site Free-living allowed	The low-fat vegan group experienced significantly greater weight loss (−7.2 kg/7.4% vs. −3.8 kg) than the control group ($p < 0.005$)

Note: CHOL = cholesterol; DM = diabetes mellitus; MUFA = monounsaturated fatty acid; SAT = saturated.

Several of these studies have been successful for weight management. A 12-week low-fat vegan diet resulted in significantly greater weight loss (7.4%) than the control diet (Nicholson et al., 1999). A 24-week lacto-vegetarian diet intervention resulted in a 6.1% weight loss, which was significantly greater than loss on a conventional diabetic diet (3.2%) (Kahleova et al., 2011). Additionally, waist circumference decreased significantly in both groups, but to a greater extent in the vegetarian group (6.4 cm vs. 5.3 cm) (Kahleova et al., 2011). The last 12 weeks of the intervention included an exercise program. Exercise was found to help further decrease waist circumference and subcutaneous and visceral fat in the vegetarian group but not the control group (Kahleova et al., 2011).

Barnard and colleagues (2006) compared a low-fat vegan diet to hypocaloric American Diabetes Association (ADA) guidelines for 22 weeks and later followed them for 74 weeks (Barnard et al., 2009a). After the initial 22-week intervention period, subjects in both groups experienced significant reductions in weight, BMI, and waist circumference, but the reductions were not significantly different between the groups. The vegan group also experienced a significant reduction in waist-to-hip ratio (0.02 cm) (Barnard et al., 2006). After 74 weeks, significant weight loss was noted for both the vegan (4.4 kg) and ADA (3.0 kg) groups (not significant between groups). Among those who remained adherent to the vegan diet, weight loss averaged 6.8 kg after 74 weeks (Barnard et al., 2009a). Waist circumference and hip circumference were significantly reduced for both groups, but the changes for average waist-to-hip ratio were not significant. The reduction in waist circumference in the vegan group was 4.2 cm at the end of 74 weeks.

A few worksite studies of GEICO employees have been conducted to evaluate the effect of a low-fat vegan diet on individuals with a history of type 2 diabetes and/or overweight and/or obesity (Ferdowsian et al., 2010; Levin et al., 2010; Mishra et al., 2013). In an initial study ($n = 113$), GEICO sites were designated for inclusion in either a low-fat vegan diet intervention or the control group (Ferdowsian et al., 2010; Levin et al., 2010). The low-fat vegan diet intervention resulted in a 5.2% weight loss ($p < 0.0001$), 4.7 cm reduction in waist circumference ($p < 0.0001$), and 4.5 cm reduction in hip circumference ($p < 0.0001$) after 22 weeks, and these reductions were significantly greater than changes in the control group (Ferdowsian et al., 2010; Levin et al., 2010). In an expanded GEICO worksite study ($n = 291$ subjects at 10 sites), sites were randomly allocated to a low-fat vegan diet or control diet for 18 weeks (Mishra et al., 2013). Weight loss (3%) and BMI (1.04 kg/m^2) were significantly reduced in the intervention group, and these changes were significantly greater than changes in the control group (Mishra et al., 2013). A greater proportion of the intervention group experienced ≥5% weight loss than the control group (37% vs. 11%; $p < 0.001$) (Mishra et al., 2013).

7.3.2 STUDIES IN INDIVIDUALS WITH A HISTORY OF RHEUMATOID ARTHRITIS

A few studies have been conducted to examine the effect of plant-based diets on relieving the symptoms of rheumatoid arthritis. Changes in weight were also measured in these studies. An uncontrolled study of a 4-week low-fat vegan diet intervention yielded a 4.4% weight loss ($p < 0.001$) (McDougall et al., 2002). A 4-month vegan intervention also resulted in significant weight loss (4.8 kg) (Skoldstam, 1986).

TABLE 7.4

Intervention Studies Examining the Effect of Plant-Based Diets on Measures of Adiposity in Individuals with Rheumatoid Arthritis

Authors (Year), Country	Study and Subject Descriptions	Interventions	Findings
McDougall et al. (2002), United States	Uncontrolled study Hx of rheumatoid arthritis $n = 24$ Gender: Male, female Average age: 56 years old	Low-fat vegan diet × 4 weeks Free-living	Body weight was significantly reduced (-3 kg/4.4%; $p < 0.001$)
Nenonen et al. (1998), Finland	Randomized controlled trial Hx of rheumatoid arthritis $n = 42$ Gender: Male, female Average age: 49.1 years old (vegan group), 55.6 years old (control group)	1. Raw vegan diet with fermented wheat drink (meals supplied) × 3 months 2. Control: Omnivore diet (free-living) × 3 months	The raw vegan group experienced significant weight loss (-9%; $p = 0.0001$) compared with the omnivore group ($+1\%$)
Kjeldsen-Kragh et al. (1991), Norway	Randomized controlled trial Hx of rheumatoid arthritis $n = 53$ Gender: Male, female Average age: 53 years old (vegetarian group), 56 years old (control group)	1. Vegetarian diet (7- to 10-day fast followed by elimination diet and abstaining from meat, fish, eggs, dairy, gluten, refined sugar, and citrus for 3.5 months; after 3.5 months, diary and gluten was reintroduced) × 1 year 2. Control diet × 1 year	Significant weight loss in the intervention group compared with the control group ($p < 0.02$) Most of the weight loss occurred in the first month, with some regained in the subsequent 12 months
Skoldstam (1986), Sweden	Pseudo-crossover study Hx of rheumatoid arthritis $n = 20$ Gender: Male, female Age: 35–68 years old	1. Vegan diet (no meat, fish, eggs, dairy, spices, preservatives, alcohol, tea, or coffee) intervention × 4 months compared with 2 Habitual diet period ($n = 20$) An inpatient dietary intervention lasted for 4 weeks, the first 7–10 days of which included a fast, then free-living for 3 months	Significant weight loss of 4.8 kg ($p < 0.001$) was documented

In a 3-month trial, subjects consuming a raw vegan diet experienced significantly greater weight loss (9%) than those in an omnivore group (gained 1%) (Nenonen et al., 1998). In another study, a vegetarian diet resulted in significant weight loss compared with the control group after 1 year (Kjeldsen-Kragh et al., 1991). See Table 7.4 for details.

7.4   CONCLUSION

A trend is apparent in that populations that include a variety of dietary patterns, those individuals on more of a plant-based pattern, including a spectrum of vegans to semivegetarians, will exhibit lower excess adiposity. In most intervention studies, subjects on the plant-based interventions have experienced significant weight loss, ranging from 1.8% to 13% for vegan interventions and 3.2% to 9.9% for vegetarians over a wide variety of intervention times. Even pesco- and semivegetarian dietary interventions are successful. The weight loss noted in most of these studies meets or exceeds AND recommendations for weight loss. Additionally, because adherence to a diet or dietary pattern is an important factor for maintaining weight loss, it is useful to consider the likelihood that individuals can adhere to a vegan or vegetarian diet long term. Good adherence has been demonstrated in a number of long-term studies, measured up to 5 years (Ornish et al., 1998; Turner-McGrievy et al., 2007; Burke et al., 2008; Barnard et al., 2009b; Moore et al., 2015). Even among subjects who do not fully adhere to study diets, they still exhibit a pattern closer to a vegetarian one and can still experience significant weight loss (Moore et al., 2015). Additionally, according to AND, when dietary patterns are used as weight loss interventions, they should "have either an explicit energy goal per day or provide an ad libitum approach without a formal energy goal that still produces a reduction in energy intake, usually by restriction or elimination of specific foods and/or food groups" (Raynor and Champagne, 2016, p. 134). The use of an ad libitum approach when recommending a plant-based pattern has successfully led to a reduction in calories in a number of intervention studies (Barnard et al., 2005; Dansinger et al., 2005; Gardner et al., 2007; Turner-McGrievy et al., 2015).

7.4.1   Mechanisms

There are possible mechanisms that help to explain why plant-based dietary patterns may be beneficial for weight management. These include differences in the nutrient, food group, and phytochemical profile between plant-based and omnivore patterns. These differences may have implications in gut microbiota profiles that can affect weight.

7.4.1.1   Nutrient Intake Trends in Plant-Based Patterns

Total kilocalorie intake, on average, tends to be lower in individuals on plant-based diets than in nonvegetarians. The reduction in energy intake is partly explained by a higher intake of fiber (Berkow and Barnard, 2006). Researchers report that for every 14 g/day increase of fiber, there is a concomitant reduction in kilocalorie intake of 10% (Berkow and Barnard, 2006).

Higher intakes of dietary fiber in vegans and vegetarians may help to explain the weight management benefits of such dietary patterns (Key et al., 2006). Individuals following plant-based diets tend to consume greater amounts of fiber-rich foods, like fruits, vegetables, and whole grains, than nonvegetarians (Newby et al., 2005; Farmer et al., 2011; Orlich et al., 2014). Fiber helps to increase satiety and reduce overall energy density of diets, both of which result in a lower kilocalorie intake (Berkow and Barnard, 2006; Barnard et al., 2009c). Viscous fiber may have an impact by slowing down digestion (Huang et al., 2016), which could theoretically reduce absorption. There is evidence to support an inverse relationship between fiber intake and weight (Berkow and Barnard, 2006; Huang et al., 2016).

Vegetarians and vegans typically tend to have higher intakes of carbohydrate, while having lower protein and fat intake than nonvegetarians (Berkow and Barnard, 2006; Farmer et al., 2011), and this pattern is evident in various cohorts (Appleby et al., 1999; Davey et al., 2003; Orlich and Fraser, 2014). This ratio of macronutrient intake is associated with a lower BMI (Berkow and Barnard, 2006). High intakes of carbohydrate may increase the thermic effect of food, thereby increasing energy expenditure (Berkow and Barnard, 2006). In terms of protein, it has been suggested that plant proteins may have less of an impact on insulin secretion and increases in glucagon secretion (Berkow and Barnard, 2006), which are catabolic actions.

7.4.1.2 Implications of Dietary Patterns on Gut Microbiota

Research on the effect of nutrients, nonnutritive compounds (like phytochemicals), foods, and dietary patterns on gut microbiota may help us to better elucidate the positive effects of plant-based dietary patterns. There is evidence that different dietary patterns result in variation of gut microbiota composition (Glick-Bauer and Yeh, 2014; Wong, 2014; Tomasello et al., 2016). Gut microbiota can be altered in such a way as to increase or decrease risk of weight gain (Delzenne et al., 2011). Microbiota can affect adiposity by impacting energy extraction during digestion, affecting metabolism of carbohydrate and fat, increasing inflammation, regulating enteroendocrine cells (which release glucagon-like peptides [GLPs]), and stimulating gut hormones (which affect appetite and weight) (Ley, 2010; Glick-Bauer and Yeh, 2014; Wong, 2014). Gut microbiota profiles that are related to increased obesity include reduced numbers of Bacteroidetes and *Bifidobacterium*, higher numbers of Firmicutes, and overall reduction in bacterial diversity (Ley, 2010; Delzenne et al., 2011; Wong, 2014). Gut microbiota interact with the endocannabinoid system to regulate the growth and reduction of adipose tissue (Delzenne et al., 2011).

There are a few dietary factors prevalent in plant-based patterns that can impact gut microbiota profiles positively. Carbohydrates, specifically resistant starches and dietary fiber, which are fermented in the colon, can alter gut microbiota (Delzenne et al., 2011; Wong, 2014; Tomasello et al., 2016). Dietary fiber, specifically inulin-type fructans, can increase *Bifidobacterium* and reduce *Bacteroides* numbers in the gut (Delzenne et al., 2011; Wong, 2014). Inulin-type fructans can impact the size of adipocytes by interacting with the endocannabinoid system and inhibiting the expression of G-protein-coupled receptor 43 (GPR43) (Delzenne et al., 2011). Fruits and vegetables are good sources of fructans (Delzenne et al., 2011).

Polyphenols have also been found to increase *Bifidobacterium* and reduce *Bacteroides* (do Rosario et al., 2016). Food sources of polyphenols include fruits, vegetables, legumes, chocolate, and coffee (Burkholder-Cooley et al., 2016). Among noncoffee consumers in the AHS-2 cohort, vegans have the highest mean consumption of polyphenols (Burkholder-Cooley et al., 2016).

A high intake of dietary fat can cause dysbiosis, leading to deleterious impacts on fat metabolism and inflammation (Ley, 2010; Tomasello et al., 2016). High-fat diets also decrease *Bifidobacterium* numbers (Ley, 2010). Additionally, omnivore patterns have been associated with lower gut microbiota diversity than plant-based patterns (Wong, 2014). Since healthy plant-based patterns, particularly vegan diets, tend to be low in fat and low or absent in animal food products, it can be hypothesized that they would not result in these deleterious effects.

Recent research indicates that individuals on plant-based diets have a greater number of Bacteroidetes, specifically *Prevotella*, and higher diversity of bacteria, but lower numbers of Firmicutes and *Bacteroides* in the gut (Liszt et al., 2009; Glick-Bauer and Yeh, 2014; Wong, 2014; do Rosario et al., 2016). Some studies have yielded contrary or null results, and some phyla include both harmful and protective species of bacteria (Tap et al., 2009; Glick-Bauer and Yeh, 2014; do Rosario et al., 2016). Clearly, much more research is needed to come to definitive conclusions.

7.4.1.3 Satiety

Inulin-type fructans can also increase GLP-1, which subsequently reduces appetite and increases satiety, leading to a reduction in kilocalorie intake (Delzenne et al., 2011). Additionally, GLP-1 has been found to reduce fat mass (Delzenne et al., 2011).

7.4.2 RESEARCH GAPS

Much more research is needed to fully elucidate the mechanisms that explain why plant-based diets are beneficial for weight loss. Additionally, although there have been studies that include various ethnic groups, there is not enough research in many groups in order to come to a consensus of the overall effectiveness of plant-based diets for weight management, especially the long-term maintenance of weight loss or a healthy weight. Long-term studies (beyond 5 years) are needed to evaluate the full impact of adherence with plant-based diets in terms of maintaining weight loss. Long-term studies may also help to assess whether changing dietary patterns can have a significant impact on altering gut microbiota.

REFERENCES

Agrawal S, Millett CJ, Dhillon PK, Subramanian SV, Ebrahim S. 2014. Type of vegetarian diet, obesity and diabetes in adult Indian population. *Nutr J* 13:89. doi: 10.1186/1475-2891-13-89.

Alewaeters K, Clarys P, Hebbelinck M, Deriemaeker P, Clarys JP. 2005. Cross-sectional analysis of BMI and some lifestyle variables in Flemish vegetarians compared with non-vegetarians. *Ergonomics* 48 (11–14):1433–44. doi: 10.1080/00140130500101031.

AND (Academy of Nutrition and Dietetics). 2014a. Adult weight management: Dietary approaches for caloric reduction 2014. http://www.andeal.org/ (accessed May 25, 2017).

AND (Academy of Nutrition and Dietetics). 2014b. Adult weight management: Realistic weight goal setting 2014. http://www.andeal.org/ (accessed May 25, 2017).

Appleby PN, Thorogood M, Mann JI, Key TJ. 1998. Low body mass index in non-meat eaters: The possible roles of animal fat, dietary fibre and alcohol. *Int J Obes Relat Metab Disord* 22 (5):454–60.

Appleby PN, Thorogood M, Mann JI, Key TJ. 1999. The Oxford Vegetarian Study: An overview. *Am J Clin Nutr* 70 (3 Suppl.):525S–31S.

Armstrong B, Clarke H, Martin C, Ward W, Norman N, Masarei J. 1979. Urinary sodium and blood pressure in vegetarians. *Am J Clin Nutr* 32 (12):2472–6.

Armstrong B, van Merwyk AJ, Coates H. 1977. Blood pressure in Seventh-day Adventist vegetarians. *Am J Epidemiol* 105 (5):444–9.

Armstrong BK, Brown JB, Clarke HT, Crooke DK, Hahnel R, Masarei JR, Ratajczak T. 1981. Diet and reproductive hormones: A study of vegetarian and nonvegetarian postmenopausal women. *J Natl Cancer Inst* 67 (4):761–7.

Baig JA, Sheikh SA, Islam I, Kumar M. 2013. Vitamin D status among vegetarians and non-vegetarians. *J Ayub Med Coll Abbottabad* 25 (1–2):152–5.

Baines S, Powers J, Brown WJ. 2007. How does the health and well-being of young Australian vegetarian and semi-vegetarian women compare with non-vegetarians? *Public Health Nutr* 10 (5):436–42. doi: 10.1017/S1368980007217938.

Balliett M, Burke JR. 2013. Changes in anthropometric measurements, body composition, blood pressure, lipid profile, and testosterone in patients participating in a low-energy dietary intervention. *J Chiropr Med* 12 (1):3–14. doi: 10.1016/j.jcm.2012.11.003.

Barnard ND, Cohen J, Jenkins DJ, Turner-McGrievy G, Gloede L, Green A, Ferdowsian H. 2009a. A low-fat vegan diet and a conventional diabetes diet in the treatment of type 2 diabetes: A randomized, controlled, 74-wk clinical trial. *Am J Clin Nutr* 89 (5):1588S–96S. doi: 10.3945/ajcn.2009.26736H.

Barnard ND, Cohen J, Jenkins DJ, Turner-McGrievy G, Gloede L, Jaster B, Seidl K, Green AA, Talpers S. 2006. A low-fat vegan diet improves glycemic control and cardiovascular risk factors in a randomized clinical trial in individuals with type 2 diabetes. *Diabetes Care* 29 (8):1777–83. doi: 10.2337/dc06-0606.

Barnard ND, Gloede L, Cohen J, Jenkins DJ, Turner-McGrievy G, Green AA, Ferdowsian H. 2009b. A low-fat vegan diet elicits greater macronutrient changes, but is comparable in adherence and acceptability, compared with a more conventional diabetes diet among individuals with type 2 diabetes. *J Am Diet Assoc* 109 (2):263–72. doi: 10.1016/j.jada.2008.10.049.

Barnard ND, Katcher HI, Jenkins DJ, Cohen J, Turner-McGrievy G. 2009c. Vegetarian and vegan diets in type 2 diabetes management. *Nutr Rev* 67 (5):255–63. doi: 10.1111/j.1753-4887.2009.00198.x.

Barnard ND, Levin SM, Yokoyama Y. 2015. A systematic review and meta-analysis of changes in body weight in clinical trials of vegetarian diets. *J Acad Nutr Diet* 115 (6):954–69. doi: 10.1016/j.jand.2014.11.016.

Barnard ND, Scialli AR, Bertron P, Hurlock D, Edmonds K, Talev L. 2000. Effectiveness of a low-fat vegetarian diet in altering serum lipids in healthy premenopausal women. *Am J Cardiol* 85 (8):969–72.

Barnard ND, Scialli AR, Turner-McGrievy G, Lanou AJ. 2004. Acceptability of a low-fat vegan diet compares favorably to a step II diet in a randomized, controlled trial. *J Cardiopulm Rehabil* 24 (4):229–35.

Barnard ND, Scialli AR, Turner-McGrievy G, Lanou AJ, Glass J. 2005. The effects of a low-fat, plant-based dietary intervention on body weight, metabolism, and insulin sensitivity. *Am J Med* 118 (9):991–7. doi: 10.1016/j.amjmed.2005.03.039.

Barr SI, Broughton TM. 2000. Relative weight, weight loss efforts and nutrient intakes among health-conscious vegetarian, past vegetarian and nonvegetarian women ages 18 to 50. *J Am Coll Nutr* 19 (6):781–8.

Bastien M, Poirier P, Lemieux I, Despres JP. 2014. Overview of epidemiology and contribution of obesity to cardiovascular disease. *Prog Cardiovasc Dis* 56 (4):369–81. doi: 10.1016/j.pcad.2013.10.016.

Bedford JL, Barr SI. 2005. Diets and selected lifestyle practices of self-defined adult vegetarians from a population-based sample suggest they are more 'health conscious'. *Int J Behav Nutr Phys Act* 2 (1):4. doi: 10.1186/1479-5868-2-4.

Berkow SE, Barnard N. 2006. Vegetarian diets and weight status. *Nutr Rev* 64 (4):175–88.

Bloomer RJ, Kabir MM, Canale RE, Trepanowski JF, Marshall KE, Farney TM, Hammond KG. 2010. Effect of a 21 day Daniel Fast on metabolic and cardiovascular disease risk factors in men and women. *Lipids Health Dis* 9:94. doi: 10.1186/1476-511X-9-94.

Brathwaite N, Fraser HS, Modeste N, Broome H, King R. 2003. Obesity, diabetes, hypertension, and vegetarian status among Seventh-day Adventists in Barbados: Preliminary results. *Ethn Dis* 13 (1):34–9.

Burke LE, Warziski M, Styn MA, Music E, Hudson AG, Sereika SM. 2008. A randomized clinical trial of a standard versus vegetarian diet for weight loss: The impact of treatment preference. *Int J Obes (Lond)* 32 (1):166–76. doi: 10.1038/sj.ijo.0803706.

Burkholder-Cooley N, Rajaram S, Haddad E, Fraser GE, Jaceldo-Siegl K. 2016. Comparison of polyphenol intakes according to distinct dietary patterns and food sources in the Adventist Health Study-2 cohort. *Br J Nutr* 115 (12):2162–9. doi: 10.1017/S0007114516001331.

Burr ML, Bates CJ, Fehily AM, St Leger AS. 1981. Plasma cholesterol and blood pressure in vegetarians. *J Hum Nutr* 35 (6):437–41.

Cade JE, Burley VJ, Greenwood DC, UK Women's Cohort Study Steering Group. 2004. The UK Women's Cohort Study: comparison of vegetarians, fish-eaters and meat-eaters. *Public Health Nutr* 7 (7):871–8.

CDC (Centers for Disease Control and Prevention). 2016a. Adult obesity facts. https://www.cdc.gov/obesity/data/adult.html (last modified September 1, 2016; accessed March 15, 2017).

CDC (Centers for Disease Control and Prevention). 2016b. Childhood obesity facts. https://www.cdc.gov/obesity/data/childhood.html (last modified December 22, 2016; accessed March 15, 2017).

CDC (Centers for Disease Control and Prevention). 2016c. Overweight and obesity. Adult obesity causes and consequences. https://www.cdc.gov/obesity/adult/causes.html (last modified August 15, 2016; accessed May 24, 2017).

CDC (Centers for Disease Control and Prevention). 2016d. Overweight and obesity. Defining adult overweight and obesity. https://www.cdc.gov/obesity/adult/defining.html (last modified June 16, 2016; accessed May 24, 2017).

CDC (Centers for Disease Control and Prevention). 2017. National Center for Health Statistics. Deaths and mortality. http://www.cdc.gov/nchs/fastats/deaths.htm (last modified March 17, 2017; accessed May 24, 2017).

Chang-Claude J, Frentzel-Beyme R. 1993. Dietary and lifestyle determinants of mortality among German vegetarians. *Int J Epidemiol* 22 (2):228–36.

Chiu YF, Hsu CC, Chiu TH, Lee CY, Liu TT, Tsao CK, Chuang SC, Hsiung CA. 2015. Cross-sectional and longitudinal comparisons of metabolic profiles between vegetarian and non-vegetarian subjects: A matched cohort study. *Br J Nutr* 114 (8):1313–20. doi: 10.1017/S0007114515002937.

Clarys P, Deliens T, Huybrechts I, Deriemaeker P, Vanaelst B, De Keyzer W, Hebbelinck M, Mullie P. 2014. Comparison of nutritional quality of the vegan, vegetarian, semi-vegetarian, pesco-vegetarian and omnivorous diet. *Nutrients* 6 (3):1318–32. doi: 10.3390/nu6031318.

Dansinger ML, Gleason JA, Griffith JL, Selker HP, Schaefer EJ. 2005. Comparison of the Atkins, Ornish, Weight Watchers, and Zone diets for weight loss and heart disease risk reduction: A randomized trial. *JAMA* 293 (1):43–53. doi: 10.1001/jama.293.1.43.

Davey GK, Spencer EA, Appleby PN, Allen NE, Knox KH, Key TJ. 2003. EPIC-Oxford: Lifestyle characteristics and nutrient intakes in a cohort of 33 883 meat-eaters and 31 546 non meat-eaters in the UK. *Public Health Nutr* 6 (3):259–69. doi: 10.1079/PHN2002430.

Delgado M, Gutierrez A, Cano MD, Castillo MJ. 1996. Elimination of meat, fish, and derived products from the Spanish-Mediterranean diet: Effect on the plasma lipid profile. *Ann Nutr Metab* 40 (4):202–11.

Delzenne NM, Neyrinck AM, Backhed F, Cani PD. 2011. Targeting gut microbiota in obesity: Effects of prebiotics and probiotics. *Nat Rev Endocrinol* 7 (11):639–46. doi: 10.1038/nrendo.2011.126.

DHHS (U.S. Department of Health and Human Services) and USDA (U.S. Department of Agriculture). 2015. *2015–2020 Dietary Guidelines for Americans.* Washington, DC: DHHS.

do Rosario VA, Fernandes R, Trindade EB. 2016. Vegetarian diets and gut microbiota: Important shifts in markers of metabolism and cardiovascular disease. *Nutr Rev* 74 (7):444–54. doi: 10.1093/nutrit/nuw012.

Faber M, Gouws E, Benade AJ, Labadarios D. 1986. Anthropometric measurements, dietary intake and biochemical data of South African lacto-ovovegetarians. *S Afr Med J* 69 (12):733–8.

Famodu AA, Osilesi O, Makinde YO, Osonuga OA. 1998. Blood pressure and blood lipid levels among vegetarian, semi-vegetarian, and non-vegetarian native Africans. *Clin Biochem* 31 (7):545–9.

Famodu AA, Osilesi O, Makinde YO, Osonuga OA, Fakoya TA, Ogunyemi EO, Egbenehkhuere IE. 1999. The influence of a vegetarian diet on haemostatic risk factors for cardiovascular disease in Africans. *Thromb Res* 95 (1):31–6.

Farmer B, Larson BT, Fulgoni VL 3rd, Rainville AJ, Liepa GU. 2011. A vegetarian dietary pattern as a nutrient-dense approach to weight management: An analysis of the National Health and Nutrition Examination Survey 1999–2004. *J Am Diet Assoc* 111 (6):819–27. doi: 10.1016/j.jada.2011.03.012.

Ferdowsian HR, Barnard ND, Hoover VJ, Katcher HI, Levin SM, Green AA, Cohen JL. 2010. A multicomponent intervention reduces body weight and cardiovascular risk at a GEICO corporate site. *Am J Health Promot* 24 (6):384–7. doi: 10.4278/ajhp.081027-QUAN-255.

Fontana L, Meyer TE, Klein S, Holloszy JO. 2007. Long-term low-calorie low-protein vegan diet and endurance exercise are associated with low cardiometabolic risk. *Rejuvenation Res* 10 (2):225–34. doi: 10.1089/rej.2006.0529.

Fraser G, Katuli S, Anousheh R, Knutsen S, Herring P, Fan J. 2015. Vegetarian diets and cardiovascular risk factors in black members of the Adventist Health Study-2. *Public Health Nutr* 18 (3):537–45. doi: 10.1017/S1368980014000263.

Fraser GE. 1999. Associations between diet and cancer, ischemic heart disease, and all-cause mortality in non-Hispanic white California Seventh-day Adventists. *Am J Clin Nutr* 70 (3 Suppl.):532S–8S.

Gadgil MD, Anderson CA, Kandula NR, Kanaya AM. 2014. Dietary patterns in Asian Indians in the United States: An analysis of the metabolic syndrome and atherosclerosis in South Asians Living in America study. *J Acad Nutr Diet* 114 (2):238–43. doi: 10.1016/j.jand.2013.09.021.

Gardner CD, Kiazand A, Alhassan S, Kim S, Stafford RS, Balise RR, Kraemer HC, King AC. 2007. Comparison of the Atkins, Zone, Ornish, and LEARN diets for change in weight and related risk factors among overweight premenopausal women: The A to Z Weight Loss Study: a randomized trial. *JAMA* 297 (9):969–77. doi: 10.1001/jama.297.9.969.

Glick-Bauer M, Yeh MC. 2014. The health advantage of a vegan diet: Exploring the gut microbiota connection. *Nutrients* 6 (11):4822–38. doi: 10.3390/nu6114822.

Global BMI Mortality Collaboration, Di Angelantonio E, Bhupathiraju Sh N, Wormser D, Gao P, Kaptoge S, Berrington de Gonzalez A et al. 2016. Body-mass index and all-cause mortality: Individual-participant-data meta-analysis of 239 prospective studies in four continents. *Lancet* 388 (10046):776–86. doi: 10.1016/S0140-6736(16)30175-1.

Greenwood DC, Cade JE, Draper A, Barrett JH, Calvert C, Greenhalgh A. 2000. Seven unique food consumption patterns identified among women in the UK Women's Cohort Study. *Eur J Clin Nutr* 54 (4):314–20.

Haddad EH, Berk LS, Kettering JD, Hubbard RW, Peters WR. 1999. Dietary intake and bio-chemical, hematologic, and immune status of vegans compared with nonvegetarians. *Am J Clin Nutr* 70 (3 Suppl.):586S–93S.

Hebbelinck M, Clarys P, De Malsche A. 1999. Growth, development, and physical fitness of Flemish vegetarian children, adolescents, and young adults. *Am J Clin Nutr* 70 (3 Suppl.):579S–85S.

Hoffmann I, Groeneveld MJ, Boeing H, Koebnick C, Golf S, Katz N, Leitzmann C. 2001. Giessen Wholesome Nutrition Study: Relation between a health-conscious diet and blood lipids. *Eur J Clin Nutr* 55 (10):887–95. doi: 10.1038/sj.ejcn.1601243.

Ho-Pham LT, Vu BQ, Lai TQ, Nguyen ND, Nguyen TV. 2012. Vegetarianism, bone loss, fracture and vitamin D: A longitudinal study in Asian vegans and non-vegans. *Eur J Clin Nutr* 66 (1):75–82. doi: 10.1038/ejcn.2011.131.

Huang RY, Huang CC, Hu FB, Chavarro JE. 2016. Vegetarian diets and weight reduction: A meta-analysis of randomized controlled trials. *J Gen Intern Med* 31 (1):109–16. doi: 10.1007/s11606-015-3390-7.

Janelle KC, Barr SI. 1995. Nutrient intakes and eating behavior scores of vegetarian and non-vegetarian women. *J Am Diet Assoc* 95 (2):180–6, 189, quiz 187–8.

Jenkins DJ, Wong JM, Kendall CW, Esfahani A, Ng VW, Leong TC, Faulkner DA, Vidgen E, Greaves KA, Paul G, Singer W. 2009. The effect of a plant-based low-carbohydrate ("Eco-Atkins") diet on body weight and blood lipid concentrations in hyperlipidemic subjects. *Arch Intern Med* 169 (11):1046–54. doi: 10.1001/archinternmed.2009.115.

Jenkins DJ, Wong JM, Kendall CW, Esfahani A, Ng VW, Leong TC, Faulkner DA et al. 2014. Effect of a 6-month vegan low-carbohydrate ('Eco-Atkins') diet on cardiovascular risk factors and body weight in hyperlipidaemic adults: A randomised controlled trial. *BMJ Open* 4 (2):e003505. doi: 10.1136/bmjopen-2013-003505.

Jensen MD, Ryan DH, Apovian CM, Ard JD, Comuzzie AG, Donato KA, Hu FB et al. 2014. 2013 AHA/ACC/TOS guideline for the management of overweight and obesity in adults: A report of the American College of Cardiology/American Heart Association Task Force on Practice Guidelines and The Obesity Society. *Circulation* 129 (25 Suppl. 2): S102–38. doi: 10.1161/01.cir.0000437739.71477.ee.

Jo HB, Lee JK, Choi MY, Han IW, Choi HS, Kang HW, Kim JH, Lim YJ, Koh MS, Lee JH. 2015. Is the prevalence of gallbladder polyp different between vegetarians and general population? *Korean J Gastroenterol* 66 (5):268–73. doi: 10.4166/kjg.2015.66.5.268.

Kahleova H, Matoulek M, Malinska H, Oliyarnik O, Kazdova L, Neskudla T, Skoch A, Hajek M, Hill M, Kahle M, Pelikanova T. 2011. Vegetarian diet improves insulin resistance and oxidative stress markers more than conventional diet in subjects with type 2 diabetes. *Diabet Med* 28 (5):549–59. doi: 10.1111/j.1464-5491.2010.03209.x.

Karelis AD, Fex A, Filion ME, Adlercreutz H, Aubertin-Leheudre M. 2010. Comparison of sex hormonal and metabolic profiles between omnivores and vegetarians in pre- and post-menopausal women. *Br J Nutr* 104 (2):222–6. doi: 10.1017/S0007114510000619.

Kennedy ET, Bowman SA, Spence JT, Freedman M, King J. 2001. Popular diets: Correlation to health, nutrition, and obesity. *J Am Diet Assoc* 101 (4):411–20. doi: 10.1016/S0002-8223(01)00108-0.

Key TJ, Appleby PN, Rosell MS. 2006. Health effects of vegetarian and vegan diets. *Proc Nutr Soc* 65 (1):35–41.

Key TJ, Davey GK, Appleby PN. 1999. Health benefits of a vegetarian diet. *Proc Nutr Soc* 58 (2):271–5.

Khazrai YM, Defeudis G, Pozzilli P. 2014. Effect of diet on type 2 diabetes mellitus: A review. *Diabetes Metab Res Rev* 30 (Suppl. 1):24–33. doi: 10.1002/dmrr.2515.

Kjeldsen-Kragh J, Haugen M, Borchgrevink CF, Laerum E, Eek M, Mowinkel P, Hovi K, Forre O. 1991. Controlled trial of fasting and one-year vegetarian diet in rheumatoid arthritis. *Lancet* 338 (8772):899–902.

Knuiman JT, West CE. 1982. The concentration of cholesterol in serum and in various serum lipoproteins in macrobiotic, vegetarian and non-vegetarian men and boys. *Atherosclerosis* 43 (1):71–82.

Knutsen SF. 1994. Lifestyle and the use of health services. *Am J Clin Nutr* 59 (5 Suppl.):1171S–5S.

Krajcovicova-Kudlackova M, Simoncic R, Bederova A, Babinska K, Ondreicka R. 1995. Selected prooxidative-antioxidative parameters in blood of adult vegetarians. *Oncol Rep* 2 (1):77–80.

Le LT, Sabate J. 2014. Beyond meatless, the health effects of vegan diets: Findings from the Adventist cohorts. *Nutrients* 6 (6):2131–47. doi: 10.3390/nu6062131.

Lee RD, Nieman DC. 2013. *Nutritional Assessment*. 6th ed. New York: McGraw-Hill.

Lee Y, Krawinkel M. 2009. Body composition and nutrient intake of Buddhist vegetarians. *Asia Pac J Clin Nutr* 18 (2):265–71.

Levin SM, Ferdowsian HR, Hoover VJ, Green AA, Barnard ND. 2010. A worksite programme significantly alters nutrient intakes. *Public Health Nutr* 13 (10):1629–35. doi: 10.1017/S136898000999303X.

Ley RE. 2010. Obesity and the human microbiome. *Curr Opin Gastroenterol* 26 (1):5–11. doi: 10.1097/MOG.0b013e328333d751.

Li D, Sinclair A, Mann N, Turner A, Ball M, Kelly F, Abedin L, Wilson A. 1999. The association of diet and thrombotic risk factors in healthy male vegetarians and meat-eaters. *Eur J Clin Nutr* 53 (8):612–9.

Lin CL, Fang TC, Gueng MK. 2001. Vascular dilatory functions of ovo-lactovegetarians compared with omnivores. *Atherosclerosis* 158 (1):247–51.

Lindahl O, Lindwall L, Spangberg A, Stenram A, Ockerman PA. 1984. A vegan regimen with reduced medication in the treatment of hypertension. *Br J Nutr* 52 (1):11–20.

Liszt K, Zwielehner J, Handschur M, Hippe B, Thaler R, Haslberger AG. 2009. Characterization of bacteria, clostridia and bacteroides in faeces of vegetarians using qPCR and PCR-DGGE fingerprinting. *Ann Nutr Metab* 54 (4):253–7. doi: 10.1159/000229505.

Lu SC, Wu WH, Lee CA, Chou HF, Lee HR, Huang PC. 2000. LDL of Taiwanese vegetarians are less oxidizable than those of omnivores. *J Nutr* 130 (6):1591–6.

Mahon AK, Flynn MG, Stewart LK, McFarlin BK, Iglay HB, Mattes RD, Lyle RM, Considine RV, Campbell WW. 2007. Protein intake during energy restriction: Effects on body composition and markers of metabolic and cardiovascular health in postmenopausal women. *J Am Coll Nutr* 26 (2):182–9.

Margetts BM, Beilin LJ, Vandongen R, Armstrong BK. 1986. Vegetarian diet in mild hypertension: A randomised controlled trial. *Br Med J (Clin Res Ed)* 293 (6560):1468–71.

McDougall J, Bruce B, Spiller G, Westerdahl J, McDougall M. 2002. Effects of a very low-fat, vegan diet in subjects with rheumatoid arthritis. *J Altern Complement Med* 8 (1): 71–5. doi: 10.1089/107555302753507195.

McDougall J, Thomas LE, McDougall C, Moloney G, Saul B, Finnell JS, Richardson K, Petersen KM. 2014. Effects of 7 days on an ad libitum low-fat vegan diet: The McDougall Program cohort. *Nutr J* 13:99. doi: 10.1186/1475-2891-13-99.

Melby CL, Goldflies DG, Toohey ML. 1993. Blood pressure differences in older black and white long-term vegetarians and nonvegetarians. *J Am Coll Nutr* 12 (3):262–9.

Melby CL, Hyner GC, Zoog B. 1985. Blood-pressure in vegetarians and nonvegetarians—A cross-sectional analysis. *Nutr Res* 5 (10):1077–82. doi: 10.1016/S0271-5317(85)80138-X.

Melby CL, Toohey ML, Cebrick J. 1994. Blood pressure and blood lipids among vegetarian, semivegetarian, and nonvegetarian African Americans. *Am J Clin Nutr* 59 (1):103–9.

Millet P, Guilland JC, Fuchs F, Klepping J. 1989. Nutrient intake and vitamin status of healthy French vegetarians and nonvegetarians. *Am J Clin Nutr* 50 (4):718–27.

Mishra S, Xu J, Agarwal U, Gonzales J, Levin S, Barnard ND. 2013. A multicenter randomized controlled trial of a plant-based nutrition program to reduce body weight and cardiovascular risk in the corporate setting: The GEICO study. *Eur J Clin Nutr* 67 (7):718–24. doi: 10.1038/ejcn.2013.92.

Moore WJ, McGrievy ME, Turner-McGrievy GM. 2015. Dietary adherence and acceptability of five different diets, including vegan and vegetarian diets, for weight loss: The New DIETs study. *Eat Behav* 19:33–8. doi: 10.1016/j.eatbeh.2015.06.011.

Nenonen MT, Helve TA, Rauma AL, Hanninen OO. 1998. Uncooked, lactobacilli-rich, vegan food and rheumatoid arthritis. *Br J Rheumatol* 37 (3):274–81.

Newby PK, Tucker KL, Wolk A. 2005. Risk of overweight and obesity among semivegetarian, lactovegetarian, and vegan women. *Am J Clin Nutr* 81 (6):1267–74.

Nicholson AS, Sklar M, Barnard ND, Gore S, Sullivan R, Browning S. 1999. Toward improved management of NIDDM: A randomized, controlled, pilot intervention using a lowfat, vegetarian diet. *Prev Med* 29 (2):87–91. doi: 10.1006/pmed.1999.0529.

Orlich MJ, Fraser GE. 2014. Vegetarian diets in the Adventist Health Study 2: A review of initial published findings. *Am J Clin Nutr* 100 (Suppl. 1):353S–8S. doi: 10.3945/ajcn.113.071233.

Orlich MJ, Jaceldo-Siegl K, Sabate J, Fan J, Singh PN, Fraser GE. 2014. Patterns of food consumption among vegetarians and non-vegetarians. *Br J Nutr* 112 (10):1644–53. doi: 10.1017/S000711451400261X.

Orlich MJ, Singh PN, Sabate J, Jaceldo-Siegl K, Fan J, Knutsen S, Beeson WL, Fraser GE. 2013. Vegetarian dietary patterns and mortality in Adventist Health Study 2. *JAMA Intern Med* 173 (13):1230–8. doi: 10.1001/jamainternmed.2013.6473.

Ornish D, Brown SE, Scherwitz LW, Billings JH, Armstrong WT, Ports TA, Mclanahan SM, Kirkeeide RL, Brand RJ, Gould KL. 1990. Can life-style changes reverse coronary heart-disease. *Lancet* 336 (8708):129–133. doi: 10.1016/0140-6736(90)91656-U.

Ornish D, Scherwitz LW, Billings JH, Brown SE, Gould KL, Merritt TA, Sparler S et al. 1998. Intensive lifestyle changes for reversal of coronary heart disease. *JAMA* 280 (23):2001–7.

Ornish D, Scherwitz LW, Doody RS, Kesten D, McLanahan SM, Brown SE, DePuey E et al. 1983. Effects of stress management training and dietary changes in treating ischemic heart disease. *JAMA* 249 (1):54–9.

Prescott SL, Jenner DA, Beilin LJ, Margetts BM, Vandongen R. 1988. A randomized controlled trial of the effect on blood pressure of dietary non-meat protein versus meat protein in normotensive omnivores. *Clin Sci (Lond)* 74 (6):665–72.

Raynor HA, Champagne CM. 2016. Position of the Academy of Nutrition and Dietetics: Interventions for the treatment of overweight and obesity in adults. *J Acad Nutr Diet* 116 (1):129–47. doi: 10.1016/j.jand.2015.10.031.

Rizzo NS, Sabate J, Jaceldo-Siegl K, Fraser GE. 2011. Vegetarian dietary patterns are associated with a lower risk of metabolic syndrome: The Adventist Health Study-2. *Diabetes Care* 34 (5):1225–7. doi: 10.2337/dc10-1221.

Rosell M, Appleby P, Key T. 2005. Height, age at menarche, body weight and body mass index in life-long vegetarians. *Public Health Nutr* 8 (7):870–5.

Rosell M, Appleby P, Spencer E, Key T. 2006. Weight gain over 5 years in 21,966 meat-eating, fish-eating, vegetarian, and vegan men and women in EPIC-Oxford. *Int J Obes (Lond)* 30 (9):1389–96. doi: 10.1038/sj.ijo.0803305.

Rouse IL, Armstrong BK, Beilin LJ. 1983. The relationship of blood pressure to diet and lifestyle in two religious populations. *J Hypertens* 1 (1):65–71.

Sacks FM, Castelli WP, Donner A, Kass EH. 1975. Plasma lipids and lipoproteins in vegetarians and controls. *N Engl J Med* 292 (22):1148–51. doi: 10.1056/NEJM197505292922203.

Sanders TA, Ellis FR, Dickerson JW. 1978. Haematological studies on vegans. *Br J Nutr* 40 (1):9–15.

Shultz TD, Leklem JE. 1983. Dietary status of Seventh-day Adventists and nonvegetarians. *J Am Diet Assoc* 83 (1):27–33.

Simons LA, Gibson JC, Paino C, Hosking M, Bullock J, Trim J. 1978. The influence of a wide range of absorbed cholesterol on plasma cholesterol levels in man. *Am J Clin Nutr* 31 (8):1334–9.

Singh PN, Arthur KN, Orlich MJ, James W, Purty A, Job JS, Rajaram S, Sabate J. 2014. Global epidemiology of obesity, vegetarian dietary patterns, and noncommunicable disease in Asian Indians. *Am J Clin Nutr* 100 (Suppl. 1):359S–64S. doi: 10.3945/ajcn.113.071571.

Skoldstam L. 1986. Fasting and vegan diet in rheumatoid arthritis. *Scand J Rheumatol* 15 (2):219–21.

Slattery ML, Jacobs Jr. DR, Hilner JE, Caan BJ, Van Horn L, Bragg C, Manolio TA, Kushi LH, Liu KA. 1991. Meat consumption and its associations with other diet and health factors in young adults: The CARDIA study. *Am J Clin Nutr* 54 (5):930–5.

Spencer EA, Appleby PN, Davey GK, Key TJ. 2003. Diet and body mass index in 38000 EPIC-Oxford meat-eaters, fish-eaters, vegetarians and vegans. *Int J Obes Relat Metab Disord* 27 (6):728–34. doi: 10.1038/sj.ijo.0802300.

Taber LA, Cook RA. 1980. Dietary and anthropometric assessment of adult omnivores, fish-eaters, and lacto-ovo-vegetarians. *J Am Diet Assoc* 76 (1):21–9.

Tap J, Mondot S, Levenez F, Pelletier E, Caron C, Furet JP, Ugarte E et al. 2009. Towards the human intestinal microbiota phylogenetic core. *Environ Microbiol* 11 (10):2574–84. doi: 10.1111/j.1462-2920.2009.01982.x.

Timko CA, Hormes JM, Chubski J. 2012. Will the real vegetarian please stand up? An investigation of dietary restraint and eating disorder symptoms in vegetarians versus non-vegetarians. *Appetite* 58 (3):982–90. doi: 10.1016/j.appet.2012.02.005.

Tomasello G, Mazzola M, Leone A, Sinagra E, Zummo G, Farina F, Damiani P et al. 2016. Nutrition, oxidative stress and intestinal dysbiosis: Influence of diet on gut microbiota in inflammatory bowel diseases. *Biomed Pap Med Fac Univ Palacky Olomouc Czech Repub* 160 (4):461–6. doi: 10.5507/bp.2016.052.

Tonstad S, Butler T, Yan R, Fraser GE. 2009. Type of vegetarian diet, body weight, and prevalence of type 2 diabetes. *Diabetes Care* 32 (5):791–6. doi: 10.2337/dc08-1886.

Tonstad S, Nathan E, Oda K, Fraser GE. 2015. Prevalence of hyperthyroidism according to type of vegetarian diet. *Public Health Nutr* 18 (8):1482–7. doi: 10.1017/S1368980014002183.

Tonstad S, Stewart K, Oda K, Batech M, Herring RP, Fraser GE. 2013. Vegetarian diets and incidence of diabetes in the Adventist Health Study-2. *Nutr Metab Cardiovasc Dis* 23 (4):292–9. doi: 10.1016/j.numecd.2011.07.004.

Toohey ML, Harris MA, DeWitt W, Foster G, Schmidt WD, Melby CL. 1998. Cardiovascular disease risk factors are lower in African-American vegans compared to lacto-ovo-vegetarians. *J Am Coll Nutr* 17 (5):425–34.

Toth MJ, Poehlman ET. 1994. Sympathetic nervous system activity and resting metabolic rate in vegetarians. *Metabolism* 43 (5):621–5.

Trepanowski JF, Kabir MM, Alleman Jr. RJ, Bloomer RJ. 2012. A 21-day Daniel fast with or without krill oil supplementation improves anthropometric parameters and the cardiometabolic profile in men and women. *Nutr Metab (Lond)* 9 (1):82. doi: 10.1186/1743-7075-9-82.

Turner-McGrievy GM, Barnard ND, Scialli AR. 2007. A two-year randomized weight loss trial comparing a vegan diet to a more moderate low-fat diet. *Obesity (Silver Spring)* 15 (9):2276–81. doi: 10.1038/oby.2007.270.

Turner-McGrievy GM, Barnard ND, Scialli AR, and Lanou AJ. 2004. Effects of a low-fat vegan diet and a Step II diet on macro- and micronutrient intakes in overweight post-menopausal women. *Nutrition* 20 (9):738–46. doi: 10.1016/j.nut.2004.05.005.

Turner-McGrievy GM, Davidson CR, Wingard EE, Billings DL. 2014. Low glycemic index vegan or low-calorie weight loss diets for women with polycystic ovary syndrome: A randomized controlled feasibility study. *Nutr Res* 34 (6):552–8. doi: 10.1016/j .nutres.2014.04.011.

Turner-McGrievy GM, Davidson CR, Wingard EE, Wilcox S, Frongillo EA. 2015. Comparative effectiveness of plant-based diets for weight loss: A randomized controlled trial of five different diets. *Nutrition* 31 (2):350–8. doi: 10.1016/j.nut.2014.09.002.

Waldmann A, Koschizke JW, Leitzmann C, Hahn A. 2003. Dietary intakes and lifestyle factors of a vegan population in Germany: Results from the German Vegan Study. *Eur J Clin Nutr* 57 (8):947–55. doi: 10.1038/sj.ejcn.1601629.

WHO (World Health Organization). 2016. Obesity and overweight. Fact sheet. http://www .who.int/mediacentre/factsheets/fs311/en/ (last modified June 2016; accessed March 15, 2017).

Wong JM. 2014. Gut microbiota and cardiometabolic outcomes: Influence of dietary patterns and their associated components. *Am J Clin Nutr* 100 (Suppl. 1):369S–77S. doi: 10.3945/ajcn.113.071639.

Section III

Plant Proteins

8 Soy and Human Health
Benefits and Controversies

Alison M. Duncan

CONTENTS

SUMMARY

Historically, observational studies have set the foundation for a relationship between plant-based dietary patterns and healthy weight status. Vegetarians, especially vegans, tend to weigh less than nonvegetarians and have a lower prevalence of overweight or obesity. Multiple studies, utilizing vegan and vegetarian dietary interventions, have demonstrated that plant-based diets may be successfully utilized in weight management treatment of overweight or obese individuals. Reduced energy, fat, and animal protein intake, and increased carbohydrate, fiber, whole grain, fruit, vegetable, and phytochemical intake, help to explain some of the weight management benefits of these patterns.

8.1   INTRODUCTION

Soybeans have been studied for their role in numerous health areas, in part due to the potential for their constituent isoflavones to provide a dietary alternative to hormone replacement therapy (HRT). This has prompted research into menopause-related health concerns, including breast cancer, menopausal symptoms, and bone health. Other health areas, also with an estrogen-related etiology but more relevant to men, such as prostate cancer, have been studied. However, there has also been concern about the safety of phytoestrogenic isoflavones in health areas such as breast cancer, thyroid health, and male fertility. This chapter provides background on soy isoflavones and examines the current state of the literature in these health and safety-related areas.

8.2   SOY ISOFLAVONE BACKGROUND

Soy is the most important source of isoflavones (Murphy and Hendrich, 2002), which are a type of phytoestrogen (Setchell, 1998). The structural similarity of isoflavones to endogenous estrogen allows them to bind to estrogen receptor (Shutt and Cox, 1972). The isoflavone content of soybeans ranges from 3 to 5 mg/g soy protein (Murphy et al., 1999) and depends on variables such as food processing, geographic location of cultivation, harvest year, and soybean variety (Wang and Murphy, 1994). A database of the isoflavone quantity of foods was developed by the U.S. Department of Agriculture and Iowa State University to inform research studies (USDA, 1999) and is publicly available. Isoflavones can occur in four different chemical forms, including an aglycone or conjugated to a glycoside unit (β-glycoside, malonlyl-β-glycoside, or acetyl-β-glycoside) (Murphy and Hendrich, 2002).

When soy foods are consumed, intestinal bacterial enzymes and/or mucosal β-glucosidases will cleave the isoflavone's glycosidic conjugate to produce an aglycone form of the isoflavone (Setchell, 1998; Setchell and Cassidy, 1999). At this point, the aglycone isoflavone can be absorbed or may further interact with intestinal bacteria to produce isoflavone metabolites, such as equol (from daidzein), O-desmethylangolensin (ODMA) (from daidzein), or p-ethylphenol (from genistein), all of which can also be absorbed (Setchell, 1998; Setchell and Cassidy, 1999). After absorption, isoflavones undergo extensive first-pass metabolism (Larkin et al., 2008) and are then conjugated to glucuronic acid or sulfate by hepatic phase II enzymes, after which they undergo an enterohepatic circulation (Setchell, 1998; Setchell and Cassidy, 1999). Isoflavone absorption and metabolism is influenced by many factors, the most important of which is the individual. As reviewed by Nielsen and Williamson (2007), isoflavone bioavailability can be influenced by chemical form, dose, source, frequency of consumption, sex, age, gut microflora, gastrointestinal transit time, food matrix, and background. There is particular interest in the large interindividual variation found in urinary excretion of the isoflavone metabolite equol (Kelly et al., 1993, 1995; Lampe et al., 1998; Rowland et al., 2000). Equol is produced by the gut microflora bacteria from daidzein and has numerous unique qualities among the isoflavone and isoflavone metabolites, the most obvious of which is the consistent observation that it is produced by approximately 30%–40% of the population (Kelly et al., 1993, 1995; Lampe et al., 1998; Rowland et al., 2000). Equol is also one of the most potent isoflavones; with a higher affinity for the estrogen receptor than its precursor daidzein (Shutt and Cox, 1972), it is able to exert a more estrogenic response than daidzein in cell culture (Markiewicz et al., 1993; Breinholt and Larsen, 1998), and it has a longer half-life than both genistein and daidzein (Kelly et al., 1995), suggesting that the ability to produce equol may increase soy isoflavone exposure. The clinical relevance of equol has been reviewed (Setchell et al., 2002; Lampe, 2009) and continues to be an active area of research with the working hypothesis that the equol production status of study participants is a major confounding variable to clarifying the health effects of soy isoflavone consumption.

8.3   BREAST CANCER PREVENTION

Breast cancer is one of the most frequently studied areas of health in relation to soy. Initial interest in soy and breast cancer prevention came from observations of lower breast cancer incidence in Asian countries (where soy intake is high) relative to Western countries (where soy intake is low) (Rose et al., 1986; Parkin, 1989). The totality of studies relating soy isoflavones to breast cancer has been documented in numerous meta-analyses. For example, Qin et al. (2006) pooled 14 case-control and 7 cohort studies to conclude an overall inverse association of breast cancer risk with intake of soy foods (RR 0.75; 95% CI 0.59–0.95) and soy isoflavones (RR 0.81; 95% CI 0.67–0.99). In the same year, Trock et al. (2006) published the results of their meta-analysis that included 12 case-control and 6 cohort studies that also found an inverse association of breast cancer risk with soy intake (RR 0.86; 95% CI 0.75–0.99). In another meta-analysis, the authors separated their analysis into studies of high-soy-consuming Asians and low-soy-consuming Western individuals and found a 14% risk reduction (RR 0.86; 95% CI 0.75–0.99) for an isoflavone intake of 10 mg/day and a 29% risk reduction (RR 0.71; 95% CI 0.60–0.85) for an isoflavone intake ≥20 mg/day, both compared with the lowest isoflavone intake of 5 mg/day (Wu et al., 2008). In another meta-analysis of 35 studies, a significant inverse association was found between soy isoflavone intake and breast cancer risk for pre- (OR 0.59) and post- (OR 0.59) menopausal Asian but not Western women (Chen et al., 2014). Overall, although these meta-analyses do provide support for a role of soy isoflavones in breast cancer prevention, there has been note of heterogeneity among studies (Trock et al., 2006) and there remains inconsistent results, with some studies having found no significant relationship between soy and breast cancer risk in Asian (Yuan et al., 1995; Key et al., 1999) and Western (Horn-Ross et al., 2001; Keinan-Boker et al., 2004) populations.

In possibly addressing the reason for inconsistent study results, a logical hypothesis has emerged that focuses on the age of exposure (Tomar and Shiao, 2008; Messina and Hilakivi-Clarke, 2009), from the idea that an intervention would have the maximal effect during the period of most active change, as would be the case for the developing breast during adolescence (Messina and Hilakivi-Clarke, 2009). Lamartiniere (2002) has studied the idea of timing of exposure and mammary cancer risk using a rat model and demonstrated relevant results, including significantly reduced mammary carcinogenesis with neonatal genistein exposure (Lamartiniere et al., 1995) and a lack of effect on mammary carcinogenesis with adult genistein exposure alone, but enhancement of an observed protective effect when combined with neonatal and prepubertal genistein exposure (Lamartiniere et al., 2002). The idea has been strengthened by human studies that have related adult breast cancer risk to soy and soy isoflavone exposure during adolescence or even childhood (5–11 years old) (Korde et al., 2009) and consistently shown a reduction in adult breast cancer risk in Chinese (Shu et al., 2001), Asian American (Wu et al., 2002; Korde et al., 2009), and Canadian (Thanos et al., 2006) women. The timing of exposure hypothesis is well supported and has added an informative dimension to the current understanding of the relationship between soy isoflavones and breast cancer prevention.

8.4 MENOPAUSAL SYMPTOMS

A dietary alternative to HRT for addressing menopausal symptoms has rationalized an examination of soy isoflavones. An early study by Messina and Hughes (2003) found that data from 13 soy intervention studies (34–100 mg of isoflavones/day) suggested that those with frequent hot flashes consider trying soy isoflavones for relief. This conclusion was confirmed by Howes et al. (2006) in their meta-analysis of 17 isoflavone (48–160 mg/day) intervention studies that found a significant reduction in hot flashes, the magnitude of which depended on the number of baseline hot flashes. Isoflavone composition was considered in another review of 11 studies, finding that hot flashes were significantly decreased with ≥15 mg genistein/day (5 studies, $n = 177$) but not <15 mg genistein/day (6 studies, $n = 201$) (Williamson-Hughes et al., 2006). This was corroborated by the most recent meta-analysis of 17 studies that found that isoflavones significantly reduced hot flash severity, and the effect was stronger when genistein was >18.8 mg/day (Taku, 2012). The idea that hot flash reduction is dependent on genistein but not total isoflavone dose introduces uncertainty into studies that have found no significant effects (Lethaby et al., 2007; Jacobs et al., 2009) and may not have considered isoflavone composition.

8.5 BONE HEALTH

Bone health is another health area in which soy isoflavones have been studied, primarily for potential as an alternative to HRT for postmenopausal women. Support for this comes from evidence showing that Asian women (who consume more soy) have a relatively lower incidence of fractures than Western women (Ross et al., 1991; Lauderdale et al., 1997). Also supportive are studies showing associations between increasing isoflavone intake and reduced bone resorption (Kritz-Silverstein and Goodman-Gruen, 2002), improved bone mineral density (BMD) (Mei et al., 2001; Kritz-Silverstein and Goodman-Gruen, 2002), and reduced risk of fracture (Zhang et al., 2005; Koh et al., 2009). Finally, ipriflavone, a synthetic isoflavone, has been shown to reduce bone loss and prevent osteoporosis in postmenopausal women (Zhang et al., 2009).

Randomized controlled trials that have examined the effect of soy isoflavones on bone health were summarized in two meta-analyses. One of the meta-analyses focused on markers of bone turnover by selecting nine studies that examined the effect of soy products or isoflavones (37.3–118 mg/day), for at least 4 weeks (range 4–48 weeks), in a total of 432 healthy females (Ma et al., 2008a). Results summarized significant favorable effects of isoflavone consumption on bone turnover, including a decrease in the bone resorption marker urinary deoxypyridinoline (DPD) and an increase in the bone formation marker bone alkaline phosphatase (BAP). The second meta-analysis focused on BMD by selecting 10 studies that intervened with soy products or isoflavones (range 4.4–150 mg/day), for at least 3 months (range 3–24 months), in a total of 608 females (Ma et al., 2008b). The results summarized a significant favorable increase in spine BMD due to isoflavone consumption. Unlike their bone turnover analysis results, which did not depend on dose or duration, the authors found greater effects on BMD with isoflavone intake >90 mg/day and treatment duration of at least 6 months. The 90 mg/day dose is consistent with a previous literature review (Branca, 2003) that emphasized the need for an isoflavone intake of at least 90 mg to realize bone health benefits. In contrast to the positive results from the two meta-analyses by Ma et al. described above, a 2009 meta-analysis of 10 randomized controlled trials including 896 women concluded that the average dose of 87 mg of soy isoflavones for at least 1 year did not significantly affect BMD (Liu et al., 2009). Finally, a 2016 meta-analysis of 23 studies that intervened for 7 weeks to 3 years in a total of 3494 participants with variable isoflavone treatments (including genistein alone or in combination with daidzein) reported significant beneficial effects on BMD and bone turnover biomarkers, although not in all studies (Abdi et al., 2016). Inconsistent results were also reported in an earlier meta-analysis of randomized controlled trials that included a total of 1240 menopausal women. It was concluded that soy isoflavone supplements (average dose, 82 mg of isoflavones) for 6–12 months significantly increased lumbar spine BMD but not femoral neck, hip total, or trochanter BMD (Taku et al., 2010). Overall, the study of soy isoflavones in relation to bone health has produced inconsistent results, with earlier studies summarizing favorable effects and more recent studies finding less consistent effects of isoflavones on bone health markers. These discrepancies will prompt continued investigation to further clarify the role of soy isoflavones in bone health.

8.6   PROSTATE CANCER

Evidence for a role for soy isoflavones in reducing prostate cancer risk comes from epidemiological observations of low prostate cancer rates in Asian countries (Pienta et al., 1996) and an increase in these rates when Asians migrate to the United States (Shimizu et al., 1991; Cook et al., 1999). Also relevant is that Japanese men, who have a lower risk of prostate cancer, have higher isoflavone concentrations in their blood (Adlercreutz et al., 1993), urine (Morton et al., 1997), and prostatic fluid (Morton et al., 1997) relative to their Western counterparts. Epidemiological studies that have focused on relating soy isoflavone intake to risk of prostate cancer have been summarized in three meta-analyses (Yan and Spitznagel, 2005, 2009; Hwang et al., 2009). The first one included two cohort and six case-control studies and found that soy consumption was associated with a 30% reduction in prostate cancer risk (RR 0.70; 95% CI 0.59–0.83). Four years later, an updated meta-analysis was published that included epidemiological studies that related prostate cancer to consumption of soy (15 studies) or isoflavones (9 studies). Results revealed combined RR/ORs of 0.74 (95% CI 0.63–0.89) for soy intake and 0.88 (95% CI 0.76–1.02) for isoflavone intake. Another meta-analysis was also published in 2009 that combined five cohort and eight case-control studies and reported results based on type of soy foods (Hwang et al., 2009). Consumption of both total soy foods (OR 0.69; 95% CI 0.57–0.84) and nonfermented soy foods (OR 0.75; 95% CI 0.62–0.89) was significantly associated with reduced prostate cancer risk, and among individual soy foods assessed (tofu, soybean milk, miso, and natto), tofu was the only specific food that signifi-cantly related to a reduced prostate cancer risk (0.73; 95% CI 0.57–0.92).

Other studies have related prostate cancer risk to circulating and urinary isofla-vones to overcome the limitations of dietary assessment and to consider the ability to produce equol, a metabolite of daidzein. This was the focus in two case-control stud-ies by Akaza and colleagues, the first of which showed that the proportion of those able to metabolize daidzein (to equol) was significantly higher in a group of 112 con-trols than in 141 men with prostate cancer (Akaza et al., 2002). The second case-control study showed that not only were there more equol producers among Japanese and Korean than American men, but within the Japanese and Korean men, the pro-portion of equol producers was significantly higher in the control (46% and 59%, respectively) than the prostate cancer (29% and 30%, respectively) groups (Akaza et al., 2004). The relation of equol production to prostate cancer risk was also identi-fied in a nested case-control study within the Japan Public Health Center–based pro-spective study that involved 14,203 men aged 40–69 years who had provided blood samples and were followed for an average of 12.8 years (Kurahashi et al., 2008). Results showed that total prostate cancer risk tended to be inversely associated with plasma genistein and was not significantly associated with plasma daidzein, but was significantly inversely associated with plasma equol (OR 0.60; 95% CI 0.36–0.99). Plasma isoflavones were also related to prostate cancer in a case-control substudy of the European Prospective Investigation into Cancer and Nutrition that reported an inverse association between plasma genistein and prostate cancer risk (RR 0.71; 95% CI 0.53–0.96), although no significant associations were found for plasma daidzein or equol (Travis et al., 2009). Finally, urinary daidzein was inversely related to pros-tate cancer risk (RR 0.55; 95% CI 0.31–0.98) in a multiethnic cohort case-control study conducted in Hawaii and California in 249 prostate cancer cases and 404 con-trols (Park et al., 2009). Overall, the role of soy isoflavones in prostate cancer risk is well studied and includes examination of associations with dietary, circulating, and urinary isoflavones. The relevance of equol is particularly interesting and logical based on the uniqueness of equol among the isoflavone metabolites.

8.7   BREAST CANCER SAFETY

Breast cancer, although an area of preventive research, is also a major area of safety-related research for soy isoflavones. These concerns stem from the possibility that a compound with estrogenic properties could cause an increase in the growth of an estrogen-dependent tumor. Providing evidence for this concern, cell culture studies that have examined the effect of genistein on the growth of estrogen receptor–positive breast cancer cells have shown stimulation at physiologically relevant concentrations (<10 μmol/L) and have only been able to show inhibition at higher (>10 μmol/L), physiologically irrelevant concentrations (de Lemos, 2001). Concern has also been generated from a series of studies conducted in an athymic nude mouse model that was ovariectomized and implanted with estrogen-dependent MCF-7 breast cancer cells. When these animals were fed soy protein or soy isoflavones in various forms, their breast tumors grew, often in a dose-dependent manner and at concentrations physiologically relevant to humans (Allred et al., 2001a, 2001b, 2004; Ju et al., 2001).

In terms of human data, two earlier studies prompted concern with reports of breast stimulatory effects of soy consumption (Petrakis et al., 1996; Hargreaves et al., 1999). The first study found that soy protein isolate (80 mg of isoflavones) caused stimulation of the breast tissue (through increased hyperplastic epithelial cells in breast nipple aspirate fluid and breast cell hyperplasia) in a 5-month study of healthy premenopausal (but not postmenopausal) women that did not contain a control group (Petrakis et al., 1996). The second study demonstrated estrogenic effects (increased levels of the estrogenic protein pS2) of 2 weeks' consumption of texturized vegetable protein (45 mg of isoflavones) on the tissue of the normal breast in premenopausal women who were undergoing breast biopsy or diagnostic surgery for breast cancer (Hargreaves et al., 1999).

In response to these safety concerns, human soy intervention studies have included functional markers of breast health, including mammographic density and breast biopsy samples to evaluate cell proliferation and estrogenic markers. Mammographic density is considered a valid biomarker of breast cancer risk (Boyd et al., 2001) and has therefore been included in several soy food and soy isoflavone human studies. In particular, Maskarinec and colleagues have completed multiple studies in this area and demonstrated that mammographic density was not significantly affected by interventions of either soy foods (50 mg of isoflavones/day) for 2 years (Maskarinec et al., 2004) or a soy isoflavone supplement (100 mg of isoflavones/day) for 1 year (Maskarinec et al., 2003) in premenopausal women or by an intervention of an 80 or 120 mg soy isoflavone supplement for 2 years in postmenopausal women (Maskarinec et al., 2009). In addition, Verheus et al. (2008) found that although mammographic density decreased over their 1-year intervention in healthy postmenopausal women consuming either soy (99 mg of isoflavone dose/day) or milk protein, there were no significant differences between the groups, nor did equol production status influence the results. In contrast, an associational study that overall found no significant association between soy intake and mammographic density in a sample of 232 healthy women 48–82 years old did detect an interaction with equol production status such that mammographic density was lower among equol producers (not significant; $p = 0.08$) but higher among equol nonproducers ($p = 0.03$) (Fuhrman et al., 2008).

The safety of soy in relation to human breast cancer is arguably best assessed in women who have had breast cancer in order to evaluate recurrence and survival (Boon et al., 2007). The first longitudinal study to examine this included 1459 breast cancer survivors who were followed for 5.2 years, with analysis revealing that soy intake prior to their diagnosis was unrelated to their breast cancer survival (HR 0.99; 95% CI 0.73–1.33) and that this association did not vary according to several relevant variables, including estrogen or progesterone receptor status, tumor stage, age at diagnosis, menopausal status, or estrogen receptor-β–related polymorphisms (Boyapati et al., 2005). The second study, published in 2009, included 5033 breast cancer survivors who were followed for 3.9 years, with their analysis showing an inverse association between intake of soy protein and both breast cancer survival (HR 0.68; 95% CI 0.54–0.87) and recurrence (HR 0.71; 95% CI 0.54–0.92), with similar results observed for soy isoflavones (Shu et al., 2009). These inverse associations did not vary according to type (estrogen receptor positive or negative) of breast cancer or tamoxifen use. Another study observed a reduction in all-cause mortality of breast cancer survivors in association with isoflavone intake in 1210 American women in Long Island, New York, who were followed for 5–6 years (HR 0.52; 95% CI 0.33–0.82), with a similar trend (but not significant) observed for isoflavone intake and reduced breast cancer recurrence (Fink et al., 2007). Another cohort study by Guha and colleagues (2009) utilized data from their Life After Cancer Epidemiology (LACE) study to examine the relationship between breast cancer recurrence and isoflavone intake. A sample of 1954 female breast cancer survivors were followed for 6.31 years, and when their isoflavone intake was related to their breast cancer recurrence, the result was a 52% risk reduction for the highest compared with the lowest daidzein intake among postmenopausal women treated with tamoxifen (HR 0.48; 95% CI 0.21–0.79) (Guha et al., 2009). More recently, Nechuta et al. (2012) completed an in-depth analysis of U.S. and Chinese cohort studies of breast cancer survivors (n = 9514 followed for 7.4 years) that had examined soy isoflavones and breast cancer recurrence. Results showed that isoflavone intake (≥10 mg/day) was inversely associated with breast cancer recurrence (HR 0.75; 95% CI 0.61, 0.92), and the same relationship was observed among both U.S. and Chinese women, regardless of whether data were analyzed separately by country or combined. It is encouraging that none of these studies have demonstrated cause for concern regarding soy isoflavone intake in breast cancer survivors, and in fact, many have demonstrated possible beneficial effects (Fink et al., 2007; Guha et al., 2009; Shu et al., 2009; Nechuta et al., 2012). It should be noted, however, that all these studies are associational and therefore do not establish causality. It is therefore prudent to remain conservative with respect to breast cancer safety, thus justifying continued research in this area.

8.8   THYROID HEALTH

Thyroid function is another area that has attracted safety concerns due to the structural similarity of isoflavones to thyroid hormones (Food Standards Agency, 2003) and observations that isoflavones can inhibit thyroid peroxidase (an enzyme involved in the synthesis of thyroid hormones) in cell culture (Divi et al., 1997) and in animals (Chang and Doerge, 2000). In addition, concern has been generated from early animal studies that observed goiter in rats fed raw soybeans in their iodine-deficient diets (McCarrison, 1933; Sharpless et al., 1939; Wilgus et al., 1941; Halverson et al., 1949), although it was discovered that the goiter could be prevented by the addition of iodine to the diet (Sharpless et al., 1939; Wilgus et al., 1941; Halverson et al., 1949). Similarly, in the late 1950s and early 1960s case studies reported incidence of goiter in infants fed soy-based formula (Van Wyk et al., 1959; Hydovitz, 1960; Shepard et al., 1960) that were eliminated once iodine was included in soy-based infant formula (Food Standards Agency, 2003).

With regards to infants currently consuming soy-based formula who are hypothyroid, a 2004 review concluded that elevated thyroid-stimulating hormone (TSH) did not result in the need for any alteration in thyroid replacement dose, although extra monitoring of free thyroxine and TSH levels is warranted (Conrad et al., 2004). The relationship between serum soy isoflavones and thyroid function in children without overt thyroid disease was examined in children from a region of the Czech Republic (low soy consumption) (Milerova et al., 2006). The results showed that serum genistein, although low in concentration, was positively associated with free thyroxine and thyroglobulin antibodies and negatively associated with thyroid volume. The magnitudes of the associations were modest, but the authors noted that they could become important if iodine intake were insufficient (Milerova et al., 2006).

With regards to adult soy intake, there has been little evidence for concern in healthy iodine-sufficient individuals. A 1991 Japanese study (without a control group) that reported a significant increase in TSH and occurrence of goiter among 11 of the 37 adults who consumed soybeans pickled in rice vinegar for 1 or 3 months is the only documentation of antithyroid effects of soy in healthy adults (Ishizuki et al., 1991). In a 2006 review, insufficient evidence was seen to support concern for adverse effects of soy isoflavones on thyroid function in euthyroid, iodone-replete individuals (Messina and Redmond, 2006). In addition, soy isoflavone intervention studies published after the 2006 review have reported no significant effects on circulating thyroid hormones in healthy men (Dillingham et al., 2007) or postmenopausal women (Teas et al., 2007), including a recent 3-year intervention of an isoflavone supplement (54 mg of genistein) in osteopenic postmenopausal women (Bitto et al., 2010). However, as also summarized in a 2006 review (Messina and Redmond, 2006), there may be reason for careful monitoring of thyroid replacement dosage in hypothyroid patients due to a case report of a female consuming a soy supplement who required an elevation in dose of thyroid replacement (Bell and Ovalle, 2001). Overall, the concern over the potential for soy isoflavones to influence thyroid health comes primarily from cell culture and experimental studies and has not translated to humans, with multiple studies demonstrating no significant effects of soy interventions on circulating thyroid hormones (Messina and Redmond, 2006; Dillingham et al., 2007; Teas et al., 2007; Bitto et al., 2010) with the exception of one study (Ishizuki et al., 1991) that has been criticized for its methodological limitations (Messina and Redmond, 2006). On the other hand, there is rationale for concern for those who are on thyroid replacement therapy due to potential medication interactions (Bell and Ovalle, 2001).

8.9 MALE FERTILITY

The idea that the weakly estrogenic soy isoflavones could cause feminization or infertility in men has been another safety focus area (West et al., 2005) that has also generated public concern through the media (Thornton, 2009). In terms of feminization, most relevant a meta-analysis of 15 high-quality clinical studies designed to evaluate the effect of soy on reproductive hormones in men that concluded that soy isoflavones do not significantly affect circulating levels of total testosterone, free testosterone, sex hormone binding globulin, or the free androgen index (Hamilton-Reeves et al., 2009). Fertility-related adverse effects of isoflavones have been documented, and frequently referred to, in early reports of Australian (female) sheep that were having breeding challenges, with their infertility linked to their consumption of formononetin-rich red clover and subsequent daidzein and the high amounts of equol that they are able to produce (Bennetts et al., 1946; Lightfoot et al., 1967). Fertility-related effects of isoflavone exposure during the adult period of life have been investigated in rodent, rabbit, and primate animal models with mixed results, including adverse sex gland (Cline et al., 2004) and sperm (Sliwa and Macura, 2005) changes in rodents, no significant changes in sperm parameters in rodents (Faqi et al., 2004; Lee et al., 2004; Glover and Assinder, 2006), beneficial changes in sperm parameters in rabbits (Yousef et al., 2003, 2004), and no significant changes in sperm count or testicular weight or prostate weight in primates (Perry et al., 2007). The documented species differences in isofla-vone metabolism and, most importantly, the production of equol (Gu et al., 2006) par-ticularly highlights the need for human research to address this safety area, although studies are more limited. A highly publicized study that prompted substantial media attention by Chavarro et al. (2008) reported on a retrospective analysis of intake of 15 soy-based foods over a 3-month period in 99 male partners of subfertile couples. Their data showed that soy intake was significantly inversely associated with sperm concentration, but no associations were found with sperm motility or morphology. Results from three clinical studies (Mitchell et al., 2001; Casini et al., 2006; Beaton et al., 2010) refuted the conclusions of Chavarro et al. (2008). The first is a case study of one oligospermic man who consumed an isoflavone supplement for 6 months and experienced improvements in sperm count, sperm motility, and sperm morphology (Casini et al., 2006). The other two studies are human interventions that examined the effects of soy isoflavone consumption on fertility in healthy men. Mitchell et al. (2001) studied 14 healthy men (18–35 years old) who consumed a soy extract supple-ment (40 mg of isoflavones) for 2 months and experienced no significant changes in their ejaculate volume, sperm count, sperm motility, or sperm morphology as moni-tored 2 months before, 2 months during, and 2 months after supplementation. Another intervention by Beaton et al. (2010) studied 32 healthy men (20–40 years old) who were randomized to consume a milk protein isolate (MPI), low-isoflavone soy protein isolate (1.64 mg of isoflavones/day), and high-isoflavone soy protein isolate (61.7 mg of isoflavones/day) for 57 days, each separated by 28-day washout periods in a crossover design. Results from semen collection and analysis before and after each treatment period showed no significant differences in semen parameters, including semen vol-ume, sperm concentration, sperm count, sperm percent motility, total motile sperm count, and sperm morphology. In summary, the idea that soy may influence fertil-ity has its roots in animal studies (Bennetts et al., 1946; Lightfoot et al., 1967), but despite the media reports (Thornton, 2009), the available human evidence does not provide cause for concern with respect to male feminization (Hamilton-Reeves et al., 2009) or fertility (Mitchell et al., 2001; Beaton et al., 2010). This conclusion is also summarized in a recent examination of the clinical evidence in the area of soy and feminization by Messina (2010).

8.10 SUMMARY

In summary, the relationship between soy and health has been extensively studied, and this chapter has focused on conditions relevant to menopause (breast cancer, menopausal symptoms, and bone health) and to men (prostate cancer). The safety of soy isoflavones has also been extensively studied, with focus areas including breast cancer, thyroid health, and male fertility. Despite the large amount of research in the area of soy and human health, there remains justification for continued research in many different health areas. Future human soy isoflavone interventions can be ideally designed according to the informative proceedings from a National Institutes of Health scientific workshop entitled "Soy Protein/Isoflavone Research: Challenges in Designing and Evaluating Intervention Studies," which was held July 28–29, 2009, and published in *Journal of Nutrition* (Klein et al., 2010).

REFERENCES

Abdi F, Alimoradi Z, Haqi P, Mahdizad F. 2016. Effects of phytoestrogens on bone mineral density during the menopause transition: A systematic review of randomized, controlled trials. *Climacteric* 19:535–45.

Adlercreutz H, Markkanen H, Watanabe S. 1993. Plasma concentrations of phyto-oestrogens in Japanese men. *Lancet* 342:1209–10.

Akaza H, Miyanaga N, Takashima N, Naito S, Hirao Y, Tsukamoto T, Fujioka T, Mori M, Kim WJ, Song JM, Pantuck AJ. 2004. Comparisons of percent equol producers between prostate cancer patients and controls: Case-controlled studies of isoflavones in Japanese, Korean and American residents. *Jpn J Clin Oncol* 34:86–9.

Akaza H, Miyanaga N, Takashima N, Naito S, Hirao Y, Tsukamoto T, Mori M. 2002. Is daidzein non-metabolizer a high risk for prostate cancer? A case-controlled study of serum soybean isoflavone concentration. *Jpn J Clin Oncol* 32:296–300.

Allred CD, Allred KF, Ju YH, Goeppinger TS, Doerge DR, Helferich WG. 2004. Soy processing influences growth of estrogen-dependent breast cancer tumors. *Carcinogenesis* 25:1649–57.

Allred CD, Allred KF, Ju YH, Virant SM, Helferich WG. 2001a. Soy diets containing varying amounts of genistein stimulate growth of estrogen-dependent (MCF-7) tumors in a dose-dependent manner. *Cancer Res* 61:5045–50.

Allred CD, Ju YH, Allred KF, Chang J, Helferich WG. 2001b. Dietary genistin stimulates growth of estrogen-dependent breast cancer tumors similar to that observed with genistein. *Carcinogenesis* 22:1667–73.

Beaton LK, McVeigh BL, Dillingham BL, Lampe JW, Duncan AM. 2010. Soy protein isolates of varying isoflavone content do not adversely affect semen quality in healthy young men. *Fertil Steril* 95:1717–22.

Bell DS, Ovalle F. 2001. Use of soy protein supplement and resultant need for increased dose of levothyroxine. *Endocr Pract* 7:193–4.

Bennetts HW, Underwood EJ, Shier FL. 1946. A specific breeding problem of sheep on subterranean clover pastures in Western Australia. *Aust Vet J* 22:2–11.

Bitto A, Polito F, Atteritano M, Altavilla D, Mazzaferro S, Marini H, Adamo EB et al. 2010. Genistein aglycone does not affect thyroid function: Results from a three-year, randomized, double-blind, placebo-controlled trial. *J Clin Endocrinol Metab* 95:3067–72.

Boon HS, Olatunde F, Zick SM. 2007. Trends in complementary/alternative medicine use by breast cancer survivors: Comparing survey data from 1998 and 2005. *BMC Womens Health* 7:4.

Boyapati SM, Shu XO, Ruan ZX, Dai Q, Cai Q, Gao YT, Zheng W. 2005. Soyfood intake and breast cancer survival: A followup of the Shanghai Breast Cancer Study. *Breast Cancer Res Treat* 92:11–7.

Boyd NF, Martin LJ, Stone J, Greenberg C, Minkin S, Yaffe MJ. 2001. Mammographic densities as a marker of human breast cancer risk and their use in chemoprevention. *Curr Oncol Rep* 3:314–21.

Branca F. 2003. Dietary phyto-oestrogens and bone health. *Proc Nutr Soc* 62:877–87.

Breinholt V, Larsen JC. 1998. Detection of weak estrogenic flavonoids using a recombinant yeast strain and a modified MCF7 cell proliferation assay. *Chem Res Toxicol* 11:622–9.

Casini ML, Gerli S, Unfer V. 2006. An infertile couple suffering from oligospermia by partial sperm maturation arrest: Can phytoestrogens play a therapeutic role? A case report study. *Gynecol Endocrinol* 22:399–401.

Casini ML, Marelli G, Papaleo E, Ferrari A, D'Ambrosio F, Unfer V. 2006. Psychological assessment of the effects of treatment with phytoestrogens on postmenopausal women: A randomized, double-blind, crossover, placebo-controlled study. *Fertil Steril* 85:972–8.

Chang HC, Doerge DR. 2000. Dietary genistein inactivates rat thyroid peroxidase in vivo without an apparent hypothyroid effect. *Toxicol Appl Pharmacol* 168:244–52.

Chavarro JE, Toth TL, Sadio SM, Hauser R. 2008. Soy food and isoflavone intake in relation to semen quality parameters among men from an infertility clinic. *Hum Reprod (Oxford, England)* 23:2584–90.

Chen M, Rao Y, Zheng Y, Wei S, Li Y, Guo T, Yin P. 2014. Association between soy isoflavone intake and breast cancer risk for pre- and post-menopausal women: A meta-analysis of epidemiological studies. *PLoS One* 9:e89288.

Cline JM, Franke AA, Register TC, Golden DL, Adams MR. 2004. Effects of dietary isoflavone aglycones on the reproductive tract of male and female mice. *Toxicol Pathol* 32:91–9.

Conrad SC, Chiu H, Silverman BL. 2004. Soy formula complicates management of congenital hypothyroidism. *Arch Dis Child* 89:37–40.

Cook LS, Goldoft M, Schwartz SM, Weiss NS. 1999. Incidence of adenocarcinoma of the prostate in Asian immigrants to the United States and their descendants. *J Urol* 161:152–5.

de Lemos ML. 2001. Effects of soy phytoestrogens genistein and daidzein on breast cancer growth. *Ann Pharmacother* 35:1118–21.

Dillingham BL, McVeigh BL, Lampe JW, Duncan AM. 2007. Soy protein isolates of varied isoflavone content do not influence serum thyroid hormones in healthy young men. *Thyroid* 17:131–7.

Divi RL, Chang HC, Doerge DR. 1997. Anti-thyroid isoflavones from soybean: Isolation, characterization, and mechanisms of action. *Biochem Pharmacol* 54:1087–96.

Faqi AS, Johnson WD, Morrissey RL, McCormick DL. 2004. Reproductive toxicity assessment of chronic dietary exposure to soy isoflavones in male rats. *Reprod Toxicol* 18:605–11.

Fink BN, Steck SE, Wolff MS, Britton JA, Kabat GC, Gaudet MM, Abrahamson PE et al. 2007. Dietary flavonoid intake and breast cancer survival among women on Long Island. *Cancer Epidemiol Biomarkers Prev* 16:2285–92.

Food Standards Agency, United Kingdom. 2003. *Phytoestrogens and Health*. London: Committee on Toxicity of Chemicals in Food, Consumer Products and the Environment, 1–444.

Fuhrman BJ, Teter BE, Barba M, Byrne C, Cavalleri A, Grant BJ, Horvath PJ, Morelli D, Venturelli E, Muti PC. 2008. Equol status modifies the association of soy intake and mammographic density in a sample of postmenopausal women. *Cancer Epidemiol Biomarkers Prev* 17:33–42.

Glover A, Assinder SJ. 2006. Acute exposure of adult male rats to dietary phytoestrogens reduces fecundity and alters epididymal steroid hormone receptor expression. *J Endocrinol* 189:565–73.

Gu L, House SE, Prior RL, Fang N, Ronis MJ, Clarkson TB, Wilson ME, Badger TM. 2006. Metabolic phenotype of isoflavones differ among female rats, pigs, monkeys, and women. *J Nutr* 136:1215–21.

Guha N, Kwan ML, Quesenberry CP Jr, Weltzien EK, Castillo AL, Caan BJ. 2009. Soy isoflavones and risk of cancer recurrence in a cohort of breast cancer survivors: The Life After Cancer Epidemiology study. *Breast Cancer Res Treat* 118:395–405.

Halverson AW, Zepplin M, Hart EB. 1949. Relation of iodine to the goitrogenic properties of soybeans. *J Nutr* 38:115–28.

Hamilton-Reeves JM, Vazquez G, Duval SJ, Phipps WR, Kurzer MS, Messina MJ. 2009. Clinical studies show no effects of soy protein or isoflavones on reproductive hormones in men: Results of a meta-analysis. *Fertil Steril* 94:997–1007.

Hargreaves DF, Potten CS, Harding C, Shaw LE, Morton MS, Roberts SA, Howell A, Bundred NJ. 1999. Two-week dietary soy supplementation has an estrogenic effect on normal premenopausal breast. *J Clin Endocrinol Metab* 84:4017–24.

Horn-Ross PL, John EM, Lee M, Stewart SL, Koo J, Sakoda LC, Shiau AC, Goldstein J, Davis P, Perez-Stable EJ. 2001. Phytoestrogen consumption and breast cancer risk in a multiethnic population: The Bay Area Breast Cancer Study. *Am J Epidemiol* 154:434–41.

Hwang YW, Kim SY, Jee SH, Kim YN, Nam CM. 2009. Soy food consumption and risk of prostate cancer: A meta-analysis of observational studies. *Nutr Cancer* 61:598–606.

Hydovitz JD. 1960. Occurrence of goiter in an infant on a soy diet. *N Engl J Med* 262:351–3.

Ishizuki Y, Hirooka Y, Murata Y, Togashi K. 1991. [The effects on the thyroid gland of soybeans administered experimentally in healthy subjects]. *Nippon Naibunpi Gakkai Zasshi* 67:622–9.

Jacobs A, Wegewitz U, Sommerfeld C, Grossklaus R, Lampen A. 2009. Efficacy of isoflavones in relieving vasomotor menopausal symptoms—A systematic review. *Mol Nutr Food Res* 53:1084–97.

Ju YH, Allred CD, Allred KF, Karko KL, Doerge DR, Helferich WG. 2001. Physiological concentrations of dietary genistein dose-dependently stimulate growth of estrogen-dependent human breast cancer (MCF-7) tumors implanted in athymic nude mice. *J Nutr* 131:2957–62.

Keinan-Boker L, van Der Schouw YT, Grobbee DE, Peeters PH. 2004. Dietary phytoestrogens and breast cancer risk. *Am J Clin Nutr* 79:282–8.

Kelly GE, Joannou GE, Reeder AY, Nelson C, Waring MA. 1995. The variable metabolic response to dietary isoflavones in humans. *Proc Soc Exp Biol Med* 208:40–3.

Kelly GE, Nelson C, Waring MA, Joannou GE, Reeder AY. 1993. Metabolites of dietary (soya) isoflavones in human urine. *Clin Chim Acta* 223:9–22.

Key TJ, Sharp GB, Appleby PN, Beral V, Goodman MT, Soda M, Mabuchi K. 1999. Soya foods and breast cancer risk: A prospective study in Hiroshima and Nagasaki, Japan. *Br J Cancer* 81:1248–56.

Klein MA, Nahin RL, Messina MJ, Rader JI, Thompson LU, Badger TM, Dwyer JT, Kim YS, Pontzer CH, Starke-Reed PE, Weaver CM. 2010. Guidance from an NIH workshop on designing, implementing, and reporting clinical studies of soy interventions. *J Nutr* 140:1192S–204S.

Koh WP, Wu AH, Wang R, Ang LW, Heng D, Yuan JM, Yu MC. 2009. Gender-specific associations between soy and risk of hip fracture in the Singapore Chinese Health Study. *Am J Epidemiol* 170:901–9.

Korde LA, Wu AH, Fears T, Nomura AM, West DW, Kolonel LN, Pike MC, Hoover RN, Ziegler RG. 2009. Childhood soy intake and breast cancer risk in Asian American women. *Cancer Epidemiol Biomarkers Prev* 18:1050–9.

Kritz-Silverstein D, Goodman-Gruen DL. 2002. Usual dietary isoflavone intake, bone mineral density, and bone metabolism in postmenopausal women. *J Womens Health Gend Based Med* 11:69–78.

Kurahashi N, Iwasaki M, Inoue M, Sasazuki S, Tsugane S. 2008. Plasma isoflavones and subsequent risk of prostate cancer in a nested case-control study: The Japan Public Health Center. *J Clin Oncol* 26:5923–9.

Lamartiniere CA. 2002. Timing of exposure and mammary cancer risk. *J Mammary Gland Biol Neoplasia* 7:67–76.

Lamartiniere CA, Cotroneo MS, Fritz WA, Wang J, Mentor-Marcel R, Elgavish A. 2002. Genistein chemoprevention: Timing and mechanisms of action in murine mammary and prostate. *J Nutr* 132:552S–8S.

Lamartiniere CA, Moore JB, Brown NM, Thompson R, Hardin MJ, Barnes S. 1995. Genistein suppresses mammary cancer in rats. *Carcinogenesis* 16:2833–40.

Lampe JW. 2009. Is equol the key to the efficacy of soy foods? *Am J Clin Nutr* 89:1664S–7S.

Lampe JW, Karr SC, Hutchins AM, Slavin JL. 1998. Urinary equol excretion with a soy challenge: Influence of habitual diet. *Proc Soc Exp Biol Med* 217:335–9.

Larkin T, Price WE, Astheimer L. 2008. The key importance of soy isoflavone bioavailability to understanding health benefits. *Crit Rev Food Sci Nutr* 48:538–52.

Lauderdale DS, Jacobsen SJ, Furner SE, Levy PS, Brody JA, Goldberg J. 1997. Hip fracture incidence among elderly Asian-American populations. *Am J Epidemiol* 146:502–9.

Lee BJ, Kang JK, Jung EY, Yun YW, Baek IJ, Yon JM, Lee YB, Sohn HS, Lee JY, Kim KS, Nam SY. 2004. Exposure to genistein does not adversely affect the reproductive system in adult male mice adapted to a soy-based commercial diet. *J Vet Sci* 5:227–34.

Lethaby AE, Brown J, Marjoribanks J, Kronenberg F, Roberts H, Eden J. 2007. Phytoestrogens for vasomotor menopausal symptoms. *Cochrane Database Syst Rev* (4):CD001395.

Lightfoot RJ, Crocker KP, Neil HG. 1967. Failure of sperm transport in relation to ewe infertility following prolonged grazing on oestrogenic pastures. *Aust J Agric Res* 18:755–65.

Liu J, Ho SC, Su YX, Chen WQ, Zhang CX, Chen YM. 2009. Effect of long-term intervention of soy isoflavones on bone mineral density in women: A meta-analysis of randomized controlled trials. *Bone* 44:948–53.

Ma DF, Qin LQ, Wang PY, Katoh R. 2008a. Soy isoflavone intake increases bone mineral density in the spine of menopausal women: Meta-analysis of randomized controlled trials. *Clin Nutr* 27:57–64.

Ma DF, Qin LQ, Wang PY, Katoh R. 2008b. Soy isoflavone intake inhibits bone resorption and stimulates bone formation in menopausal women: Meta-analysis of randomized controlled trials. *Eur J Clin Nutr* 62:155–61.

Markiewicz L, Garey J, Adlercreutz H, Gurpide E. 1993. In vitro bioassays of non-steroidal phytoestrogens. *J Steroid Biochem Mol Biol* 45:399–405.

Maskarinec G, Takata Y, Franke AA, Williams AE, Murphy SP. 2004. A 2-year soy intervention in premenopausal women does not change mammographic densities. *J Nutr* 134:3089–94.

Maskarinec G, Verheus M, Steinberg FM, Amato P, Cramer MK, Lewis RD, Murray MJ, Young RL, Wong WW. 2009. Various doses of soy isoflavones do not modify mammographic density in postmenopausal women. *J Nutr* 139:981–6.

Maskarinec G, Williams AE, Carlin L. 2003. Mammographic densities in a one-year isoflavone intervention. *Eur J Cancer Prev* 12:165–9.

McCarrison R. 1933. Goitrogenic action of soya-bean and ground-nut. *Indian J Med Res* 21:179–81.

Mei J, Yeung SS, Kung AW. 2001. High dietary phytoestrogen intake is associated with higher bone mineral density in postmenopausal but not premenopausal women. *J Clin Endocrinol Metab* 86:5217–21.

Messina M. 2010. Soybean isoflavone exposure does not have feminizing effects on men: A critical examination of the clinical evidence. *Fertil Steril* 93:2095–104.

Messina M, Hilakivi-Clarke L. 2009. Early intake appears to be the key to the proposed protective effects of soy intake against breast cancer. *Nutr Cancer* 61:792–8.

Messina M, Hughes C. 2003. Efficacy of soyfoods and soybean isoflavone supplements for alleviating menopausal symptoms is positively related to initial hot flush frequency. *J Med Food* 6:1–11.

Messina M, Redmond G. 2006. Effects of soy protein and soybean isoflavones on thyroid function in healthy adults and hypothryoid patients: A review of the relevant literature. *Thyroid* 16:249–58.

Milerova J, Cerovska J, Zamrazil V, Bilek R, Lapcik O, Hampl R. 2006. Actual levels of soy phytoestrogens in children correlate with thyroid laboratory parameters. *Clin Chem Lab Med* 44:171–4.

Mitchell JH, Cawood E, Kinniburgh D, Provan A, Collins AR, Irvine DS. 2001. Effect of a phytoestrogen food supplement on reproductive health in normal males. *Clin Sci (Lond)* 100:613–8.

Morton MS, Chan PS, Cheng C, Blacklock N, Matos-Ferreira A, Abranches-Monteiro L, Correia R, Lloyd S, Griffiths K. 1997. Lignans and isoflavonoids in plasma and prostatic fluid in men: Samples from Portugal, Hong Kong, and the United Kingdom. *Prostate* 32:122–8.

Murphy PA, Hendrich S. 2002. Phytoestrogens in foods. *Adv Food Nutr Res* 44:195–246.

Murphy PA, Song T, Buseman G, Barua K, Beecher GR, Trainer D, Holden J. 1999. Isoflavones in retail and institutional soy foods. *J Agric Food Chem* 47:2697–704.

Nechuta SJ, Caan BJ, Chen WY, Lu W, Chen Z, Kwan ML, Flatt SW, Zheng Y, Zheng W, Pierce JP, Shu XO. 2012. Soy food intake after diagnosis of breast cancer and survival: An in-depth analysis of combined evidence from cohort studies of US and Chinese women. *Am J Clin Nutr* 96:123–32.

Nielsen IL, Williamson G. 2007. Review of the factors affecting bioavailability of soy isoflavones in humans. *Nutr Cancer* 57:1–10.

Park SY, Wilkens LR, Franke AA, Le Marchand L, Kakazu KK, Goodman MT, Murphy SP, Henderson BE, Kolonel LN. 2009. Urinary phytoestrogen excretion and prostate cancer risk: A nested case-control study in the Multiethnic Cohort. *Br J Cancer* 101:185–91.

Parkin DM. 1989. Cancers of the breast, endometrium and ovary: Geographic correlations. *Eur J Cancer Clin Oncol* 25:1917–25.

Perry DL, Spedick JM, McCoy TP, Adams MR, Franke AA, Cline JM. 2007. Dietary soy protein containing isoflavonoids does not adversely affect the reproductive tract of male cynomolgus macaques (*Macaca fascicularis*). *J Nutr* 137:1390–4.

Petrakis NL, Barnes S, King EB, Lowenstein J, Wiencke J, Lee MM, Miike R, Kirk M, Coward L. 1996. Stimulatory influence of soy protein isolate on breast secretion in pre- and postmenopausal women. *Cancer Epidemiol Biomarkers Prev* 5:785–94.

Pienta KJ, Goodson JA, Esper PS. 1996. Epidemiology of prostate cancer: Molecular and environmental clues. *Urology* 48:676–83.

Qin LQ, Xu JY, Wang PY, Hoshi K. 2006. Soyfood intake in the prevention of breast cancer risk in women: A meta-analysis of observational epidemiological studies. *J Nutr Sci Vitaminol (Tokyo)* 52:428–36.

Rose DP, Boyar AP, Wynder EL. 1986. International comparisons of mortality rates for cancer of the breast, ovary, prostate, and colon, and per capita food consumption. *Cancer* 58:2363–71.

Ross PD, Norimatsu H, Davis JW, Yano K, Wasnich RD, Fujiwara S, Hosoda Y, Melton LJ 3rd. 1991. A comparison of hip fracture incidence among native Japanese, Japanese Americans, and American Caucasians. *Am J Epidemiol* 133:801–9.

Rowland IR, Wiseman H, Sanders TA, Adlercreutz H, Bowey EA. 2000. Interindividual variation in metabolism of soy isoflavones and lignans: Influence of habitual diet on equol production by the gut microflora. *Nutr Cancer* 36:27–32.

Setchell KD. 1998. Phytoestrogens: The biochemistry, physiology, and implications for human health of soy isoflavones. *Am J Clin Nutr* 68:1333S–46S.

Setchell KD, Brown NM, Lydeking-Olsen E. 2002. The clinical importance of the metabolite equol—A clue to the effectiveness of soy and its isoflavones. *J Nutr* 132:3577–84.

Setchell KD, Cassidy A. 1999. Dietary isoflavones: Biological effects and relevance to human health. *J Nutr* 129:758S–67S.

Sharpless GR, Pearsons J, Prato GS. 1939. Production of goiter in rats with raw and treated soy bean flour. *J Nutr* 17:545–55.

Shepard TH, Gordon EP, Kirschvink JF, McLean CM. 1960. Soybean goiter. *New Engl J Med* 262:1099–103.

Shimizu H, Ross RK, Bernstein L, Yatani R, Henderson BE, Mack TM. 1991. Cancers of the prostate and breast among Japanese and white immigrants in Los Angeles County. *Br J Cancer* 63:963–6.

Shu XO, Jin F, Dai Q, Wen W, Potter JD, Kushi LH, Ruan Z, Gao YT, Zheng W. 2001. Soyfood intake during adolescence and subsequent risk of breast cancer among Chinese women. *Cancer Epidemiol Biomarkers Prev* 10:483–8.

Shu XO, Zheng Y, Cai H, Gu K, Chen Z, Zheng W, Lu W. 2009. Soy food intake and breast cancer survival. *JAMA* 302:2437–43.

Shutt DA, Cox RI. 1972. Steroid and phyto-oestrogen binding to sheep uterine receptors in vitro. *J Endocrinol* 52:299–310.

Sliwa L, Macura B. 2005. Evaluation of cell membrane integrity of spermatozoa by hypoosmotic swelling test—"Water test" in mice after intraperitoneal daidzein administration. *Arch Androl* 51:443–8.

Taku K, Melby MK, Kronenberg F, Kurzer MS, Messina M. 2012. Extracted or synthesized soybean isoflavones reduce menopausal hot flash frequency and severity: Systematic review and meta-analysis of randomized controlled trials. *Menopause.* 19:776–90.

Taku K, Melby MK, Takebayashi J, Mizuno S, Ishimi Y, Omori T, Watanabe S. 2010. Effect of soy isoflavone extract supplements on bone mineral density in menopausal women: Meta-analysis of randomized controlled trials. *Asia Pac J Clin Nutr* 19:33–42.

Teas J, Braverman LE, Kurzer MS, Pino S, Hurley TG, Hebert JR. 2007. Seaweed and soy: Companion foods in Asian cuisine and their effects on thyroid function in American women. *J Med Food* 10:90–100.

Thanos J, Cotterchio M, Boucher BA, Kreiger N, Thompson LU. 2006. Adolescent dietary phytoestrogen intake and breast cancer risk (Canada). *Cancer Causes Control* 17:1253–61.

Thornton J. 2009. Is this (soy) the most dangerous food for men? *Men's Health* 146–52.

Tomar RS, Shiao R. 2008. Early life and adult exposure to isoflavones and breast cancer risk. *J Environ Sci Health C Environ Carcinog Ecotoxicol Rev* 26:113–73.

Travis RC, Spencer EA, Allen NE, Appleby PN, Roddam AW, Overvad K, Johnsen NF et al. 2009. Plasma phyto-oestrogens and prostate cancer in the European Prospective Investigation into Cancer and Nutrition. *Br J Cancer* 100:1817–23.

Trock BJ, Hilakivi-Clarke L, Clarke R. 2006. Meta-analysis of soy intake and breast cancer risk. *J Natl Cancer Inst* 98:459–71.

USDA (U.S. Department of Agriculture). 1999. USDA-Iowa State University Database on the isoflavone content of foods. Release 1.1–1999. Beltsville, MD: Beltsville Human Nutrition Research Center.

Van Wyk JJ, Arnold MB, Wynn J, Pepper F. 1959. The effects of a soybean product on thyroid function in humans. *Pediatrics* 24:752–60.

Verheus M, van Gils CH, Kreijkamp-Kaspers S, Kok L, Peeters PH, Grobbee DE, van der Schouw YT. 2008. Soy protein containing isoflavones and mammographic density in a randomized controlled trial in postmenopausal women. *Cancer Epidemiol Biomarkers Prev* 17:2632–8.

Wang HJ, Murphy PA. 1994. Isoflavone composition of American and Japanese soybeans in Iowa: Effects of variety, crop year, and location. *J Agric Food Chem* 42:1674–7.

West MC, Anderson L, McClure N, Lewis SE. 2005. Dietary oestrogens and male fertility potential. *Human Fertil (Camb)* 8:197–207.

Wilgus HS, Gassner FX, Patton AR, Gustavson RG. 1941. The goitrogenicity of soybeans. *J Nutr* 22:43–52.

Williamson-Hughes PS, Flickinger BD, Messina MJ, Empie MW. 2006. Isoflavone supplements containing predominantly genistein reduce hot flash symptoms: A critical review of published studies. *Menopause (New York, N.Y.)* 13:831–9.

Wu AH, Wan P, Hankin J, Tseng CC, Yu MC, Pike MC. 2002. Adolescent and adult soy intake and risk of breast cancer in Asian-Americans. *Carcinogenesis* 23:1491–6.

Wu AH, Yu MC, Tseng CC, Pike MC. 2008. Epidemiology of soy exposures and breast cancer risk. *Br J Cancer* 98:9–14.

Yan L, Spitznagel EL. 2005. Meta-analysis of soy food and risk of prostate cancer in men. *Int J Cancer* 117:667–9.

Yan L, Spitznagel EL. 2009. Soy consumption and prostate cancer risk in men: A revisit of a meta-analysis. *Am J Clin Nutr* 89:1155–63.

Yousef MI, El-Demerdash FM, Al-Salhen KS. 2003. Protective role of isoflavones against the toxic effect of cypermethrin on semen quality and testosterone levels of rabbits. *J Environ Sci Health B* 38:463–78.

Yousef MI, Esmail AM, Baghdadi HH. 2004. Effect of isoflavones on reproductive performance, testosterone levels, lipid peroxidation, and seminal plasma biochemistry of male rabbits. *J Environ Sci Health B* 39:819–33.

Yuan JM, Wang QS, Ross RK, Henderson BE, Yu MC. 1995. Diet and breast cancer in Shanghai and Tianjin, China. *Br J Cancer* 71:1353–8.

Zhang X, Li SW, Wu JF, Dong CL, Zheng CX, Zhang YP, Du J. 2009. Effects of ipriflavone on postmenopausal syndrome and osteoporosis. *Gynecol Endocrinol* 26:76–80.

Zhang X, Shu XO, Li H, Yang G, Li Q, Gao YT, Zheng W. 2005. Prospective cohort study of soy food consumption and risk of bone fracture among postmenopausal women. *Arch Intern Med* 165:1890–5.

9 The Role of Legumes in Maintaining Health

Peter Pribis

CONTENTS

SUMMARY

Legumes are exceptionally nutritious foods. They are high in protein and fiber and low in fat. Beans are an excellent source of several B vitamins (thiamin, riboflavin, and niacin), minerals (iron and potassium), phytochemicals (phytate and polyphenols), resistant starch, and oligosaccharides. Because of their nutritional profile, beans have cholesterol-lowering, blood glucose–lowering, and anti-inflammatory effects. There is accumulating evidence that regular consumption of beans may be useful for the preventionand treatment of several chronic diseases, including metabolic syndrome, hypertension, cardiovascular disease, blood dyslipidemias, obesity, diabetes, and certain cancers. Regular bean consumption may be associated with increased longevity in the Hispanic population.

9.1 INTRODUCTION

Legumes represent a vast family of plants (Leguminosae) with more than 650 genera and 18,000 species (Duke, 1981). Botanically, legumes are either the whole plants or the plants' fruits or seeds enclosed in a pod. *Legumes* is a general term that embraces four subgroups: pulses (dry beans and lentils), fresh green peas and beans (used as vegetables), soybeans and peanuts (used for oil extraction), and legumes that are used for sowing purposes (e.g., clover and alfalfa). The Food and Agriculture Organization (FAO) defines pulses as annual leguminous crops yielding 1–12 grains of dry, edible seeds in a pod that are eaten by humans and animals (FAO, 1994).

The most commonly used pulses for human consumption are dry beans, including kidney, navy, pinto, garbanzo, lima, black, Great Northern, fava, and mung beans; chickpeas, split peas, cowpeas, and black-eyed peas; and red, yellow, and green lentils. Because legumes, pulses, and dry beans usually refer to the same group of foods, the words are sometimes used interchangeably. Humans have cultivated legumes for thousands of years. The Egyptians, Incas, Aztecs, Greeks, Persians, and Romans farmed legumes not only because they provide large seeds that are easy to gather and store, but also because they restore nitrogen in soil (known as "green manure") that has been depleted by other crops (Champ, 2002; Schuszter-Gajzágó, 2004). Western dietary patterns, particularly after World War II, have led to a steady decline in legume intake in many European and South American countries (Hellendoorn, 1976). However, bean consumption has been on the rise in the United States over the last few decades, partially attributed to the rising number of Hispanic immigrants and a greater interest in ethnic foods featuring cooked dry beans (Lucier et al., 2000).

9.2 NUTRITIONAL COMPOSITION OF LEGUMES

Legumes are exceptionally nutrient-dense foods. They are an excellent source of protein (constituting 21%–26% of calories) and typically contain about twice the amount of protein found in cereal grains. Legumes are also high in complex carbohydrates, starches (particularly resistant starch [RS]), and fiber (soluble and insoluble); thus, they have a low glycemic index (GI). They are low in fat and are a good source of many micronutrients (folate, iron, zinc, magnesium, potassium, calcium, and B vitamins, including thiamin, riboflavin, and niacin), oligosaccharides, and phytochemicals (saponins and polyphenols) (Table 9.1). Although the mineral content of beans is high, the bioavailability can be low (between 1% and 30% depending on the mineral) (Sandberg, 2002) because of the presence of antinutritional factors, including protease inhibitors, lectins, phytic acid (PA), and oxalic acid. However, it is now recognized that the effects of these individual components when studied in isolation may be very different than when consumed in food as a part of a meal or diet (Lajolo and Genovese, 2002; Liener, 2012).

Both PA and oxalic acids can negatively affect calcium absorption, while PA alone, which is not destroyed by heat, can also reduce zinc and iron absorption. Absorption, however, can be improved when these inhibitors are deactivated by consuming beans with other foods (e.g., lemon as a source of ascorbic acid) as well as through enzymatic degradation during food processing (soaking, cooking, baking, sprouting, or fermentation) (Sandberg, 2002). High, moist temperatures during cooking can inactivate most protein inhibitors and lectins present in beans (Liener, 1994; Pusztai and Grant, 1998). Additionally, it was discovered that PA can actually exert beneficial effects as an antioxidant (Empson et al., 1991) by reducing the risk of several cancers, preventing kidney stones, and decreasing the risk of heart disease (Jenab and Thompson, 2002).

TABLE 9.1
Nutrient Content of Selected Dry Beans (Serving Size: ½ Cup)

Bean	Energy kcal (kJ)	Protein g	Fat g	Fiber g	Folate μg	Calcium mg	Zinc mg	Iron mg	Thiamin mg	Riboflavin mg	Niacin mg
Black	132 (552)	7.62	0.46	7.50	128	23	0.96	1.81	0.21	0.05	0.43
Garbanzo	134 (561)	7.27	2.12	6.20	141	40	1.25	2.37	0.09	0.05	0.43
Kidney	112 (469)	7.67	0.44	5.70	115	31	0.89	1.96	0.14	0.05	0.51
Lentils	115 (481)	8.93	0.38	7.80	179	19	1.26	3.30	0.16	0.07	1.04
Lima	108 (452)	7.33	0.36	6.60	78	16	0.89	2.25	0.15	0.05	0.39
Navy	140 (586)	8.23	0.62	9.60	127	63	0.94	2.15	0.21	0.06	0.59
Pinto	122 (510)	7.70	0.56	7.70	147	39	0.84	1.79	0.16	0.05	0.27

Source: U.S. Department of Agriculture, National nutrient database for standard reference, U.S. Department of Agriculture, Washington, DC, 2016. https://ndb.nal.usda .gov/ndb/.

Note: Values are presented for boiled mature seeds without salt.

One serving of beans (approximately 90 g or ½ cup of cooked beans) provides between 7 and 8 g of protein. Though beans are recognized for their high protein content, the quality of bean protein is often undervalued. Many textbooks (Edelstein, 2013) still state that dry beans are not complete proteins. This terminology is misleading since all proteins, animal or plant, with the exception of gelatin, contain all indispensable amino acids (IAAs) (Mangels et al., 2011; Nosworthy et al., 2017). Proteins are considered complete if they supply all IAAs necessary to meet biologic requirements when consumed at the recommended level of intake. When lower-quality proteins are consumed, more of the given protein must be consumed to meet the amino acid requirements (Mangels et al., 2011).

The FAO (1990) and the Food and Drug Administration (FDA) (Henley and Kuster, 1994) use the protein digestibility–corrected amino acid score (PDCAAS) method to evaluate protein quality. The PDCAAS values for individual protein-containing foods are primarily determined by their limiting amino acids. PDCAAS values are made up of two components, the amino acid score and the true protein digestibility (Schaafsma, 2000). The PDCAAS values for selected legumes are presented in Table 9.2.

A combination of two or more plant proteins with complementary amino acid profiles can improve protein quality. For example, the limiting amino acids in legumes are the sulfur amino acids, methionine (MET), and cysteine, while the limiting amino acid in cereal grains (wheat and rice) is lysine. Combining beans with wheat or rice increases the overall PDCAAS values (Pulse Canada, 2017) (Table 9.3). Humans usually consume diets with proteins from many different sources, thus providing

TABLE 9.2
PDCAA Values for Selected Legumes

Legume	Amino Acid Score[a]	True Protein Digestibility (%)[b]	PDCAAS[c]
Navy beans	0.83	80.0	0.67
Pea (yellow, split)	0.73	87.9	0.64
Lentil (green, whole)	0.71	87.9	0.63
Pinto beans	0.77	76.2	0.59
Kidney beans	0.70	78.6	0.55
Lentil (red, whole)	0.59	90.6	0.54
Black beans	0.76	70.0	0.53
Chickpeas	0.61	85.0	0.52
Pea (green, split)	0.59	85.2	0.50
Casein[d]	1.04	96.6	1.00

Source: Nosworthy MG et al., *Food Sci Nutr* 5 (4), 896–903, 2017. doi: https://doi .org/10.1002/fsn3.473.

[a] The amino acid score limits the amino acid with the lowest ratio relative to the established amino acid requirement values for humans, aged 2–5 years old.

[b] AOAC international test method: 991.29–1991.

[c] PDCAAS = Amino acid score × % True protein digestibility.

[d] Reference.

TABLE 9.3
PDCAAs Values for Selected Legumes and Grains

Legume and Grain	Amino Acid Score[a]	True Protein Digestibility (%)[b]	PDCAAS[c]
Lentil–wheat (25:75) blend[c]	0.78	0.91	0.71
Lentil–rice (20:80) blend[c]	0.82	90.0	0.74
Black bean–rice (25:75) blend[c]	0.81	93.0	0.75
Pea–wheat (30:70) blend[c]	0.83	90.0	0.75
Casein[d]	1.04	96.6	1.00

Source: Pulse Canada, Protein quality of cooked pulses, Pulse Canada, Winnipeg, Mannitoba, 2017.

[a] The amino acid score limits the amino acid with the lowest ratio relative to the established amino acid requirement values for humans, aged 2–5 years old.

[b] AOAC international test method: 991.29–1991.

[c] PDCAAS = Amino acid score × % True protein digestibility. Calculated data obtained from the 1989 WHO/FAO Report on Protein Quality.

[d] Reference.

adequate amounts of all amino acids, including IAAs. Furthermore, populations who consume mostly plant-based diets tend to eat complementary proteins at the same meal, like rice and soy in Asia or beans and corn in Latin America (Mangels et al., 2011).

Beans are also excellent prebiotics because of their high content of fiber and RS. RS is not digested in the small intestine, but instead it passes through the gastrointestinal tract to the large intestine (Raigond et al., 2015). These nondigestible components enhance the growth and activity of selected intestinal bacterial strains and favorably affect the intestinal microflora (Combrinck and Schellack, 2015). Gut microflora (microbiota) can influence several physiological aspects inside and outside of the intestinal system, including vitamin B_{12} and K production, the immune system, tissue regeneration, carcinogenesis, bone homeostasis, metabolism, and behavior (Sommer and Bäckhed, 2013; Barrett and Wu, 2017).

9.3 LEGUMES, METHIONINE, CHRONIC DISEASES, AND LONGEVITY

Recently, studies have demonstrated that dietary methionine restriction (MET-R) increases the life span in rats and mice, achieving an effect very similar to that of general energy restriction (McCarty et al., 2009). In humans, plant-based diets that are naturally low in MET could partly explain the observed reduction in chronic disease and increased longevity in vegetarian and vegan populations (Fraser and Shavlik, 2001). Moreover, MET-R not only increases rodent longevity, but also slows cataract development and age-related changes in T-cells; lowers serum glucose, insulin, insulin-like growth factor 1 (IGF-1), and thyroid hormone levels (Miller et al., 2005); decreases visceral fat; prevents age-related increases in triglycerides and cholesterol (Malloy et al., 2006); stops the division of cancer cells (Pavillard et al., 2006); and inhibits colon carcinogenesis (Komninou et al., 2006).

MET can induce damage to body tissues. One possible mechanism is the increased susceptibility of MET residues of proteins to oxidation by reactive oxygen species (ROS). The sensitivity of proteins to oxidative stress increases as a function of the number of MET residues (Pamplona and Barja, 2006). Experimental studies based on energy restriction or protein restriction resulting in MET-R suggest that decreased levels of mitochondrial oxidative stress lead to a decreased rate of DNA damage, lower rates of DNA mutations, and ultimately slower rates of aging and an increase in longevity (López-Torres and Barja, 2008). MET-R, however, can also be achieved by simply substituting animal proteins with low-MET, high-quality plant protein sources, like beans or nuts. Animal proteins, including meat, fish, and dairy, are naturally high in MET (Table 9.4). Bean proteins are naturally low in MET, which has been classically considered their main disadvantage. However, the capacity of MET-R to decrease the rate of mitochondrial ROS generation in internal organs, to lower the markers of chronic disease, and to increase maximum longevity ironically converts such a "disadvantage" into a strong advantage (López-Torres and Barja, 2008) and validates the important role of legumes in a healthy diet.

The longitudinal Food Habit in Later Life study conducted on five cohorts (Japanese in Japan, Swedes in Sweden, Anglo-Celts in Australia, and Greeks in Greece and Australia) of adults aged 70+ years showed that higher legume intake is the most protective predictor of survival among the elderly, regardless of ethnicity, with an 8% reduction in risk of premature death for every 20 g increase in daily legume intake (Darmadi-Blackberry et al., 2004).

TABLE 9.4
Methionine Content of Selected Foods

Food	Methionine g/100 g	Methionine g/100 g Protein
Lentil, raw	0.220	0.853
Chickpeas, mature seeds, raw	0.253	1.311
Lima beans, large, mature seeds, raw	0.271	1.263
Kidney beans, all types, mature seeds, raw	0.355	1.506
Black beans, mature seeds, raw	0.325	1.504
Milk, whole, 3.25%, without added vitamins A and D	0.073	2.317
Egg, white, raw, fresh	0.399	3.661
Pork, fresh, loin, raw	0.570	2.752
Turkey, all classes, meat and skin, raw	0.574	2.811
Beef, short loin, all grades, raw	0.491	2.559
Fish, salmon, Atlantic, wild, raw	0.587	2.959

Source: U.S. Department of Agriculture, National nutrient database for standard reference, U.S. Department of Agriculture, Washington, DC, 2016. https://ndb.nal.usda.gov/ndb/.

9.4 HISPANIC PARADOX

Health statistics and several epidemiologic studies show that Hispanics live longer than non-Hispanic whites and non-Hispanic blacks (Figure 9.1), despite a higher prevalence of cardiovascular disease (CVD) risk factors and an average lower socioeconomic status with a lack of health insurance (Medina-Inojosa et al., 2014). Hispanics have lower rates of coronary heart disease (CHD) events, lower CVD, and lower total mortality than other races, for both males and females, even after adjusting for age, sex, and comorbidities (Willey et al., 2012). Additionally, mortality rates from chronic obstructive pulmonary disease (COPD) and lung cancer are lowest in Hispanics and highest in African Americans, with non-Hispanic whites and Asians in between (Centers for Disease Control and Prevention, 2014; American Cancer Society, 2017). Hispanic subjects, compared with non-Hispanic whites, have improved survival rates from lung cancer, colon cancer, and breast cancer (Howe et al., 2006). Several hypotheses, including genetic (acculturation), geographic (healthy migrant and "salmon bias" hypothesis), psychosocial (high level of family support and social network among Hispanics), and nutritional factors, may explain this unexpected finding (Franzini et al., 2001). For some of these hypotheses, the evidence is lacking (Drummond, 2011). However, there is one protective "cultural factor" shared by a majority of Hispanics, namely, their high consumption of beans (Young and Hopkins, 2014). Although Hispanics represent only 11% of the U.S. population, they account for 33% of all dry bean consumption (Lucier et al., 2000). Hispanics consume up to fivefold more beans per capita than white subjects, at an estimated 14.24 kg (31.4 lb) versus 2.51 kg (5.5 lb) per year, respectively (Mitchell et al., 2009).

Consumption of legumes is associated with a significant reduction in systemic inflammatory markers, including interleukin-6 (IL-6) and C-reactive protein (CRP)

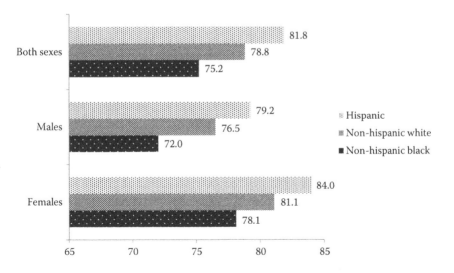

FIGURE 9.1   Life expectancy at birth by race in the United States, 2014. (From Centers for Disease Control and Prevention, National vital statistics report 2014, Centers for Disease Control and Prevention, Atlanta, GA, 2016. https://www.cdc.gov/nchs/fastats/life-expectancy.htm.)

(Esmaillzadeh et al., 2007; Hartman et al., 2010). A cross-sectional study of 489 females reported that participants in the highest tertile of legume consumption (≥237 g/week) experienced a 30%–50% reduction in IL-6 and CRP compared with the lowest tertile (<102 g/week). Additionally, individuals in the highest tertile of legume consumption had lower serum concentrations of adhesion molecules than those in the lowest tertile (Esmaillzadeh and Azadbakht, 2012). With an average bean intake of 1½ cups per week (273 g/week), Hispanics are well within that highest tertile (Esmaillzadeh and Azadbakht, 2012). There is substantial evidence that high legume consumption has anti-inflammatory effects that are likely mediated through the high fiber content (Ma et al., 2006, 2008). There is strong indirect evidence supporting the hypothesis that consumption of beans and bean-based products that are high in fiber can, in part, explain the lower mortality from CVD, COPD, and lung cancer and the lower total mortality observed in Hispanics compared with other ethnic groups (Young and Hopkins, 2014).

9.5   LEGUMES AND METABOLIC SYNDROME

Metabolic syndrome (MS) is characterized by the presence of at least three of the following five conditions: hypertension, hyperglycemia, hypertriglyceridemia, reduced high-density lipoprotein (HDL) cholesterol levels, and abdominal obesity (O'Neill and O'Driscoll, 2015). Studies have shown that MS doubles the risk of coronary artery disease and may also increase the risk of stroke, fatty liver disease, and cancer (Giovannucci, 2007). Subjects with MS suffer from chronic low-grade inflammation and increased oxidative stress (Brown et al., 2015). Recently, a systematic review of clinical trials on MS in animal models qualitatively summarized 41 studies including a wide variety of legumes (Martínez et al., 2016). The majority of the studies reported the beneficial effects of legume administration on the development and progression of MS and its related pathologies. Overall, legume administration positively affected glucose, lipid profiles, renal metabolism, and inflammation markers (Martínez et al., 2016).

Another meta-analysis of randomized controlled trials in humans found that 2–5 cups/week of beans for a period of 3–12 weeks produced favorable effects on MS risk factors (Sievenpiper et al., 2009). Consuming beans ad libitum (5 cups/week) was equally effective at reducing risk factors of MS as an energy-restricted diet. The bean and the energy-restricted diets both decreased energy intake, waist circumference, systolic blood pressure (BP), HbA1c, and insulin resistance. The bean diet increased HDL and fasting C-peptide (Mollard et al., 2012). Regular bean consumption may prevent or improve MS and should be recommended as a dietary treatment for MS.

9.6   LEGUMES AND HYPERTENSION

Elevated BP, also known as hypertension, represents a significant risk for stroke, CVD, renal failure, cognitive decline, and dementia (Mancia et al., 2007). A systematic review and meta-analysis of controlled feeding trials found that dietary pulses can significantly lower BP in people with and without hypertension (Jayalath et al., 2014). Eight isocaloric, randomized trials were included in the analysis with a pool of 544 participants, of which 215 were overweight or obese, 121 had diabetes, 119 had features of MS, and 103 were without disease at baseline. The average cooked bean consumption was 162 g/day (1 ⅔ servings/day; range 81–275 g/day) in the pooled analysis of the eight trials. Follow-up times ranged from 8 weeks to 1 year. Most trials incorporated whole beans, while three trials used dried and powdered beans. Consumption of beans significantly reduced systolic BP (mean difference –2.25 mmHg [95% confidence interval{95% CI} –4.22 to –0.28], $p = 0.03$) and mean arterial pressure (mean difference –0.75 mmHg [95% CI –1.44 to –0.06], $p = 0.03$). Diastolic BP was also reduced, though not statistically significant (mean difference –0.74 mmHg [95% CI –1.74 to 0.31], $p = 0.17$) (Jayalath et al., 2014).

Results from large observational studies also confirm the beneficial effect of bean consumption on BP (He and Whelton, 1999; Bazzano et al., 2001). A secondary analysis of National Health and Nutrition Examination Survey (NHANES) data found that bean consumers had higher intakes of dietary fiber, potassium, magnesium, iron, and copper than nonconsumers, while bean consumers had a lower body weight and a smaller waist size. In 20- to 40-year-old subjects who reported the consumption of beans, there was a 47% reduction in risk ($p = 0.037$) of elevated systolic BP and 1.7 mmHg lower systolic BP than in nonconsumers (Papanikolaou and Fulgoni, 2008). Dietary fiber, plant protein, and potassium, all of which are constituents of bean-based products, have BP-lowering effects (Lee et al., 2008). However, not all observational studies confirm these health effects.

Analyses of data from the Nurses' Health Study and the Health Professionals Follow-Up Study show that legume protein from dry beans, peas, soy, and tofu is associated with an increased risk of ischemic stroke (RR 1.45, 95% CI 1.06–2.00). The reason for these results is not clear (Bernstein et al., 2010). At the population level, a mean reduction of 2.25 mmHg in systolic BP could amend mortality from stroke, CVD, and other vascular diseases in a middle-aged population (Prospective Studies Collaboration, 2002). Use of canned cooked beans is convenient but can also add a significant amount of salt to the diet (Zanovec et al., 2011). It is recommended to purchase reduced-salt or no-salt-added varieties, rinse beans before cooking, or cook beans at home (Greger and Stone, 2015). Replacing animal protein with plant protein from beans (Altorf-van der Kuil et al., 2010) and increasing fiber intake from beans can be considered an evidence-based dietary strategy for the prevention and management of prehypertension and hypertension (McDougall, 2016).

9.7 LEGUMES AND CARDIOVASCULAR HEALTH

CVD is the leading cause of death worldwide in developed and developing countries (World Health Organization, 2007). Consumption of beans is associated with a reduction in the risk of CVD and improvement in blood lipid profiles (Padhi and Ramdath, 2017). A meta-analysis evaluated data from 10 randomized control trials (RCTs), of 3–8 weeks' duration, involving participants 18–78 years old who were not taking cholesterol-lowering drugs. Significant decreases were seen in both total cholesterol (–11.8 mg/dL, –0.305 mmol/L) and low-density lipoprotein (LDL) cholesterol (–11.8 mg/dL, –0.207 mmol/L) levels for those consuming beans compared with the controls (Bazzano et al., 2011). Most of the trials were matched for macronutrient and energy content with a wheat-based or canned vegetable substitute as a placebo. The intervention diets consisted of an addition of mixed legume dishes to the participants' current diet in the form of whole chickpeas, field beans grounded into flour, whole pinto beans, canned baked beans, whole peas, and whole navy beans.

More recently, a meta-analysis of 26 RCTs examined the impact of beans on CVD risk factors in 1037 adults, normolipidemic or hyperlipidemic, who were at moderate risk of coronary artery disease (Ha et al., 2014). A modest significant reduction in LDL of 5% from the baseline (–0.17 ml/L, 0.004 mmol/L) was reported for a median intake of 130 g of beans daily over a median follow-up of 6 weeks. No significant effects of bean intake on apolipoprotein B or non–HDL cholesterol were observed (Ha et al., 2014). Because most of the interventions included a heart-healthy diet, known to reduce LDL cholesterol by 5%–10%, the bean diet could further reduce LDL by 5% (Jenkins et al., 2011). Clinical studies have shown that regular consumption of beans can lower two major risk factors for CVD, total cholesterol and LDL cholesterol, while having little or no effect on HDL cholesterol levels (Mollard et al., 2012). Similar effects, reductions of total and LDL cholesterol without also lowering the HDL cholesterol, cannot presently be achieved with cholesterol-lowering drugs, including statins. Evidence suggests that regular nut consumption can have similar effects (Sabate and Wien, 2010).

Data from observational studies consistently demonstrate that consuming beans lowers CVD incidence and mortality. The mechanism underlying this cardioprotective effect appears to be related to the ability of beans to attenuate total cholesterol and LDL cholesterol levels (Padhi and Ramdath, 2017).

9.8 LEGUMES AND WEIGHT MANAGEMENT

The nutritional composition of beans, high in protein and fiber while low in fat, makes them a suitable food for weight management. Studies have demonstrated that consumption of foods high in fiber and protein promotes weight loss and maintenance (Slavin, 2005; Anderson et al., 2009). Recently, a meta-analysis of 21 randomized trials involving 940 overweight or obese middle-aged men and women was published (Kim et al., 2016). The median baseline BMI across the studies was 30.2. The median number of participants per trial was 27, with a median follow-up of 6 weeks. The median intake of cooked beans was 132 g/day (½–¾ cups) and included mixed beans, chickpeas, dried peas, or lentils. All the trials were isocaloric. In four trials, caloric intake was also restricted to a negative energy balance to promote weight loss. In the remaining 17, the design was to provide matched neutral energy balances between control and intervention groups to promote weight maintenance. The meta-analysis revealed a significant weight reduction of 0.34 kg ($p = 0.03$) in those consuming beans. The weight reduction in the weight loss trials was 1.74 kg ($p = 0.02$) and in the weight maintenance trials 0.29 kg ($p = 0.03$) (Kim et al., 2016).

A cross-sectional study using NHANES data reported that bean consumption was associated with lower weight and waist size. Individuals who consumed beans were 22% ($p = 0.03$) less likely to be obese than those who did not consume beans (Papanikolaou and Fulgoni, 2008).

There are several ways that bean consumption could support weight management. The high protein content of beans could influence satiety through the modulation of intestinal hormones, such as cholecystokinin (CCK) and glucagon-like peptide-1 (GLP-1) (McCrory et al., 2010; Murty et al., 2010), and through the stimulation of satiety receptors in the brain (Sufian et al., 2007). Beans contain 14–32 g of fiber per 100 g serving, of which 55%–88% is insoluble fiber. High-fiber foods contribute to satiety by increasing chewing time and slowing the transit of digested food in the upper gastrointestinal tract (Howarth et al., 2001). Soluble fiber has the ability to slow the absorption of nutrients, helping to regulate insulin release and promoting lower glucose concentrations following consumption (Jenkins et al., 2008). The high fiber content of beans can decrease fat and protein digestibility and significantly limit the absorption of energy-containing nutrients, including carbohydrates (Baer et al., 1997; Noah et al., 1998; Zou et al., 2007).

Strategies to increase bean consumption should be included in any short- or long-term weight management recommendations, particularly for overweight or obese individuals at risk or those diagnosed with prediabetes or diabetes.

9.9   LEGUMES AND DIABETES

With a low-fat, high-fiber content and low GI, legumes are suitable for people with diabetes (Sievenpiper et al., 2009). Consuming beans can help manage blood glucose levels since beans have a low GI, varying from 36 to 69 (Table 9.5). Additionally, beans are rich in RS, which slows digestion and absorption, thus reducing sudden, high rises in blood glucose.

Recently, a meta-analysis of two observational studies representing 2746 persons with diabetes reported an association between legumes and diabetic-related

TABLE 9.5
Glycemic Index (Bread = 100) of Selected Legumes

Legume	Index Value
Baked beans, canned	69
Black-eyed beans, boiled	59
Butter beans, boiled	44
Garbanzo beans, boiled	39
Kidney beans, boiled	39
Lentils, green, boiled	42
Lentils, red, boiled	36
Pinto beans, boiled	55

Source: Foster-Powell K et al., *Am J Clin Nutr* 76 (1):5–56, 2002.

morbidities (Afshin et al., 2014). The Iowa Women's Health Study followed 35,988 women for 6 years (Meyer et al., 2000), while the Shanghai Women's Health Study followed 64,227 women for 4.6 years (Villegas et al., 2008). The median consumption of legumes in the lowest category was 12 g/day, compared with 80 g/day in the highest category. Legume consumption was not significantly associated with incident diabetes (RR 0.78, 95% CI 0.05–1.24). However, the Shanghai Women's Health Study did observe an inverse association between quintiles of total legume intake and three mutually exclusive legume categories (peanuts, soybeans, and other legumes) and incidence of type 2 diabetes. The multivariate-adjusted relative risk of type 2 diabetes for the upper quintiles compared with the lower quintile of all legumes was 0.62 (p-trend = <0.0001) and 0.76 (p-trend = <0.0001) for other legumes (Villegas et al., 2008). The Iowa Women's Health Study did not find any significant protective effect of legumes or fiber from legumes on incident type 2 diabetes. However, there was an inverse association between whole-grain, dietary fiber, cereal fiber, and dietary magnesium intakes and incident type 2 diabetes (Meyer et al., 2000).

A meta-analysis of 41 trials reported that pulses alone (11 trials) lowered fasting blood glucose (standardized mean difference [SMD] = −0.82, 95% CI −1.36 to −0.27) and fasting insulin levels (SMD = −0.49, 95% CI −0.93 to −0.04). Pulses as part of low-GI diets (19 trials) significantly lowered glycosylated blood proteins, measured as HbA1c or fructosamine (SMD = −0.28, 95% CI −0.42 to −0.14). Finally, pulses in high-fiber diets (11 trials) significantly lowered fasting blood glucose (SMD = −0.32, 95% CI −0.49 to −0.15) and glycosylated blood proteins (SMD = −0.27, 95% CI −0.45 to −0.09) (Sievenpiper et al., 2009). There is emerging evidence that shows a beneficial effect of bean consumption against the development of diabetes as part of a high-fiber, low-GI diet.

9.10   LEGUMES AND CANCER

Cancer is a group of diseases that involve abnormal cell growth with the potential to invade or spread to other parts of the body (National Cancer Institute, 2015). Because of the complexities of cancer, there is no universal evidence for a protective effect of beans against all cancers. Some evidence suggests protective effects for some cancers (stomach, prostate, colon, and pancreatic) but lack of evidence for others (Greger and Stone, 2015). In a literature review by the World Cancer Research Fund/ American Institute for Cancer Research, a limited protective effect against stomach and prostate cancer was found, although most of the protection was attributed to soy foods (Marmot et al., 2007).

Data from the Adventist Health Study showed that those who consumed beans, lentils, and peas three times or more every week had a 57% reduction in risk of fatal pancreatic cancer (p-trend = 0.044) (Mills et al., 1988). Results from the same study also showed that the consumption of beans, lentils, or peas three times or more every week was associated with a 47% reduction (p-trend = 0.02) in the risk of colon cancer (Singh and Fraser, 1998).

Results from the Nurses' Health Study showed that women who consumed four or more servings of legumes per week had a 33% lower incidence of colorectal adenomas than women who reported consuming one serving per week or less (p-trend =

0.005) (Michels et al., 2006). The National Cancer Institute's Polyp Prevention Trial reported that participants who increased their bean consumption by less than ¼ cup per day decreased their odds of precancerous colorectal recurrence by 65% (Lanza et al., 2006). An ecological study in China reported that residents in low-risk areas for gastric cancer consumed kidney beans, raw vegetables, fruit, tomatoes, and soy products more frequently than those in high-risk areas (Takezaki et al., 1999). Hispanics, known for their high bean consumption, have lower lung cancer rates and better survival rates from lung, colon, and breast cancers (Howe et al., 2006; American Cancer Society, 2017).

There are many possible mechanisms explaining the impact of beans on cancer risk. Beans are rich in many potential protective components, including vitamins and the minerals folate, selenium, and zinc; RS; oligosaccharides; and bioactive compounds, like protease inhibitors, saponins, phytosterols, and phytates.

Phytate (inositol hexaphosphate) has demonstrated a remarkable anticancer effect in different experimental models (*in vitro*, in diet, intratumoral, and peritumoral) for leukemia, colon, liver, lung, breast, melanoma, pancreas, skin, and uterine cervix cancers (Vucenik and Shamsuddin, 2003). Phytate is capable of enhancing immunity, reducing inflammation, reducing cell proliferation, inducing differentiation of malignant cells, and contributing to tumor cell destruction (Vucenik and Shamsuddin, 2006). After the phytate from food is absorbed into the bloodstream, the tumors utilize the phytate so efficiently that phytate scans can be used to trace the spread of cancer in the body (Ogawa et al., 2010). Beans' high fiber content is able to dilute carcinogens, decrease overall transit time, and bind bile acids (Fleming et al., 1985), processes that may reduce the development and/or proliferation of cancer cells.

Beans contain RS and oligosaccharides that are digested in very limited amounts in the small intestine and reach the colon intact. In the colon, RS and oligosaccharides are fermented producing butyrate. There is substantial evidence that butyrate suppresses tumor growth and induces apoptosis (Cho et al., 2014), while also enhancing immunity (Frei et al., 2015). Beans are naturally low in MET and could potentially be used as supplemental nutrition therapy in MET-sensitive cancers (Cavuoto and Fenech, 2012).

Even though current evidence is inconclusive, beans have the potential to reduce the risk of cancer at several sites.

9.11 FLATULENCE

Fear of flatulence is a common reason people are reluctant to consume more beans. Participants in three studies testing the effect of beans on heart disease completed a weekly gastrointestinal discomfort questionnaire to assess flatulence. The test meals were ½ cup of either pinto beans, baked beans, or black-eyed peas, while controls consumed a ½ cup of canned carrots. During the first week, less than 50% of participants reported increased flatulence from eating pinto or baked beans, and only 19% reported increased flatulence with black-eyed peas. A small percentage of those on the control diet (3%–11%) reported increased flatulence during the first week. The authors concluded that people's concern about excessive flatulence might be exaggerated (Winham and Hutchins, 2011).

Undigested fibers in the large intestine are fermented, generating odorless and colorless gases such as carbon dioxide and methane. A small amount of odoriferous sulfur-containing gas, containing hydrogen sulfide, methanethiol, and dimethyl sulfide, may also be produced. Garlic and cauliflower are also sources of sulfur metabolites. However, the predominant source of sulfur in feces comes from animal proteins, which are high in sulfur-containing amino acids, MET, cysteine, and taurine (McDougall, 2017). Soaking, thorough cooking, sprouting, or adding enzymes that help partially break down some of the oligosaccharides responsible for gas production are methods suggested to decrease flatulence (McDougall, 2017). In the long term, most people on high-fiber, plant-based diets do not seem to have significant problems with gas (McEligot et al., 2002).

9.12   CONCLUSION

Legumes are a rich nutritional resource. There is growing evidence that regular consumption of beans can be recommended for the prevention or treatment of chronic diseases such as hypertension, CVD, obesity, diabetes, and cancer. The good nutritional profile of legumes is most likely the "nutritional reason" for the "paradoxical" longevity observed in Hispanics. Many governmental (U.S. Department of Agriculture) and health-promoting (Academy of Nutrition and Dietetics, American Heart Association, American Cancer Society, and FAO/World Health Organization [WHO]) organizations and Dietary Food Guides (such as 2015 Dietary Guidelines and My Plate) recommend daily consumption of at least ½ cup of cooked beans.

ACKNOWLEDGMENTS

I would like to express my gratitude to Kathryn Coakley, PhD, RD, LD, my colleague at the University of New Mexico, for her invaluable help in editing this chapter. I would also like to thank my daughters, Abigail and Aimee, for their technical assistance.

REFERENCES

Afshin A, Micha R, Khatibzadeh S, Mozaffarian D. 2014. Consumption of nuts and legumes and risk of incident ischemic heart disease, stroke, and diabetes: A systematic review and meta-analysis. *Am J Clin Nutr* 100 (1):278–88.

Altorf-van der Kuil W, Engberink MF, Brink EJ, van Baak MA, Bakker SJL, Navis G, van't Veer P, Geleijnse JM. 2010. Dietary protein and blood pressure: A systematic review. *PLoS One* 5 (8):e12102.

American Cancer Society. 2017. Cancer facts and statistics 2017. https://www.cancer.org /research/cancer-facts-statistics.html (accessed May 31, 2017).

Anderson JW, Baird P, Davis RH, Ferreri S, Knudtson M, Koraym A, Waters V, Williams CL. 2009. Health benefits of dietary fiber. *Nutr Rev* 67 (4):188–205.

Baer DJ, Rumpler WV, Miles CW, Fahey GC. 1997. Dietary fiber decreases the metabolizable energy content and nutrient digestibility of mixed diets fed to humans. *J Nutr* 127 (4):579–86.

Barrett KE, Wu GD. 2017. Influence of the microbiota on host physiology—Moving beyond the gut. *J Physiol* 595 (2):433–5.

Bazzano LA, He J, Ogden LG, Loria C, Vupputuri S, Myers L, Whelton PK. 2001. Legume consumption and risk of coronary heart disease in US men and women: NHANES I Epidemiologic Follow-Up Study. *Arch Intern Med* 161 (21):2573–8.

Bazzano LA, Thompson AM, Tees MT, Nguyen CH, Winham DM. 2011. Non-soy legume consumption lowers cholesterol levels: A meta-analysis of randomized controlled trials. *Nutr Metab Cardiovasc Dis* 21 (2):94–103.

Bernstein AM, Sun Q, Hu FB, Stampfer MJ, Manson JE, Willett WC. 2010. Major dietary protein sources and risk of coronary heart disease in women. *Circulation* 122 (9):876–83.

Brown L, Poudyal H, Panchal SK. 2015. Functional foods as potential therapeutic options for metabolic syndrome. *Obes Rev* 16 (11):914–41.

Cavuoto P, Fenech MF. 2012. A review of methionine dependency and the role of methionine restriction in cancer growth control and life-span extension. *Cancer Treat Rev* 38 (6):726–36.

Centers for Disease Control and Prevention. 2014. Chronic obstructive pulmonary disease. Atlanta, GA: Centers for Disease and Prevention. https://www.cdc.gov/copd/data.html (accessed May 31, 2017).

Champ MM. 2002. Foreword. *Br J Nutr* 88 (S3):237. doi: 10.1079/BJN/2002762.

Cho Y, Turner ND, Davidson LA, Chapkin RS, Carroll RJ, Lupton JR. 2014. Colon cancer cell apoptosis is induced by combined exposure to the n-3 fatty acid docosahexaenoic acid and butyrate through promoter methylation. *Exp Biol Med* 239 (3):302–10.

Combrinck Y, Schellack N. 2015. Probiotics and prebiotics: Review. *Prof Nurs Today* 19 (3):16–20.

Darmadi-Blackberry I, Wahlqvist ML, Kouris-Blazos A, Steen B, Lukito W, Horie Y, Horie K. 2004. Legumes: The most important dietary predictor of survival in older people of different ethnicities. *Asia Pac J Clin Nutr* 13 (2):217–20.

Drummond MB. 2011. The Hispanic paradox unraveled? *Am J Respir Crit Care Med* 184 (11):1222–3. doi: http://10.1164/rccm.201109-1684ED.

Duke JA. 1981. *Handbook of Legumes of World Economic Importance*. New York: Plenum Press: 302–6.

Edelstein S. 2013. *Food Science, an Ecological Approach*. Jones & Bartlett Publishers.

Empson KL, Labuza TP, Graf E. 1991. Phytic acid as a food antioxidant. *J Food Sci* 56 (2):560–3.

Esmaillzadeh A, Azadbakht L. 2012. Legume consumption is inversely associated with serum concentrations of adhesion molecules and inflammatory biomarkers among Iranian women. *J Nutr* 142 (2):334–9.

Esmaillzadeh A, Kimiagar M, Mehrabi Y, Azadbakht L, Hu FB, Willett WC. 2007. Dietary patterns and markers of systemic inflammation among Iranian women. *J Nutr* 137 (4):992–8.

Fleming SE, O'Donnell AU, Perman JA. 1985. Influence of frequent and long-term bean consumption on colonic function and fermentation. *Am J Clin Nutr* 41 (5):909–18.

FAO (Food and Agriculture Organization). 1990. Protein quality evaluation. FAO Food and Nutrition Paper 51. Rome: FAO.

FAO (Food and Agriculture Organization). 1994. Definition and classification of commodities. Rome: FAO. http://www.fao.org/es/faodef/fdef04e.htm (accessed May 18, 2017).

Franzini L, Ribble JC, Keddie AM. 2001. Understanding the Hispanic paradox. *Ethn Dis* 11:496–518.

Fraser GE, Shavlik DJ. 2001. Ten years of life: Is it a matter of choice? *Arch Intern Med* 161 (13):1645–52.

Frei R, Akdis M, O'Mahony L. 2015. Prebiotics, probiotics, synbiotics, and the immune system: Experimental data and clinical evidence. *Curr Opin Gastroenterol* 31 (2):153–8.

Giovannucci E. 2007. Metabolic syndrome, hyperinsulinemia, and colon cancer: A review. *Am J Clin Nutr* 86 (3):836S–42S.

Greger M, Stone G. 2015. *How Not to Die: Discover the Foods Scientifically Proven to Prevent and Reverse Disease.* New York: Flatiron Books.

Ha V, Sievenpiper JL, de Souza RJ, Jayalath VH, Mirrahimi A, Agarwal A, Chiavaroli L, Mejia SB, Sacks FM, Di Buono M. 2014. Effect of dietary pulse intake on established therapeutic lipid targets for cardiovascular risk reduction: A systematic review and meta-analysis of randomized controlled trials. *Can Med Assoc J* 186 (8):E252–62.

Hartman TJ, Albert PS, Zhang Z, Bagshaw D, Kris-Etherton PM, Ulbrecht J, Miller CK, Bobe G, Colburn NH, Lanza E. 2010. Consumption of a legume-enriched, low-glycemic index diet is associated with biomarkers of insulin resistance and inflammation among men at risk for colorectal cancer. *J Nutr* 140 (1):60–7.

He J, Whelton PK. 1999. Effect of dietary fiber and protein intake on blood pressure: A review of epidemiologic evidence. *Clin Exp Hypertens* 21 (5–6):785–96.

Hellendoorn EW. 1976. Beneficial physiologic action of beans. *J Am Diet Assoc* 69 (3):248–53.

Henley EC, Kuster JM. 1994. Protein quality evaluation by protein digestibility-corrected amino acid scoring. *Food Technol* 48 (4):74–7.

Howarth NC, Saltzman E, Roberts SB. 2001. Dietary fiber and weight regulation. *Nutr Rev* 59 (5):129–39.

Howe HL, Wu X, Ries LAG, Cokkinides V, Ahmed F, Jemal A, Miller B, Williams M, Ward E, Wingo PA. 2006. Annual report to the nation on the status of cancer, 1975–2003, featuring cancer among US Hispanic/Latino populations. *Cancer* 107 (8):1711–42.

Jayalath VH, de Souza RJ, Sievenpiper JL, Ha V, Chiavaroli L, Mirrahimi A, Di Buono M, Bernstein AM, Leiter LA, Kris-Etherton PM. 2014. Effect of dietary pulses on blood pressure: A systematic review and meta-analysis of controlled feeding trials. *Am J Hypertens* 27 (1):56–64.

Jenab M, Thompson LU. 2002. *Role of Phytic Acid in Cancer and other Diseases.* Boca Raton, FL: CRC Press.

Jenkins DJA, Jones PJH, Lamarche B, Kendall CWC, Faulkner D, Cermakova L, Gigleux I, Ramprasath V, de Souza R, Ireland C. 2011. Effect of a dietary portfolio of cholesterol-lowering foods given at 2 levels of intensity of dietary advice on serum lipids in hyperlipidemia: A randomized controlled trial. *JAMA* 306 (8):831–9.

Jenkins DJA, Kendall CWC, McKeown-Eyssen G, Josse RG, Silverberg J, Booth GL, Vidgen E, Josse AR, Nguyen TH, Corrigan S. 2008. Effect of a low–glycemic index or a high–cereal fiber diet on type 2 diabetes: A randomized trial. *JAMA* 300 (23):2742–53.

Kim SJ, de Souza RJ, Choo VL, Ha V, Cozma AI, Chiavaroli L, Mirrahimi A, Mejia SB, Di Buono M, Bernstein AM. 2016. Effects of dietary pulse consumption on body weight: A systematic review and meta-analysis of randomized controlled trials. *Am J Clin Nutr* 103 (5):1213–23.

Komninou D, Leutzinger Y, Reddy BS, Richie JP Jr. 2006. Methionine restriction inhibits colon carcinogenesis. *Nutr Cancer* 54 (2):202–8.

Lajolo FM, Genovese MI. 2002. Nutritional significance of lectins and enzyme inhibitors from legumes. *J Agric Food Chem* 50 (22):6592–8.

Lanza E, Hartman TJ, Albert PS, Shields R, Slattery M, Caan B, Paskett E, Iber F, Kikendall JW, Lance P. 2006. High dry bean intake and reduced risk of advanced colorectal adenoma recurrence among participants in the polyp prevention trial. *J Nutr* 136 (7):1896–1903.

Lee YP, Puddey IB, Hodgson JM. 2008. Protein, fibre and blood pressure: Potential benefit of legumes. *Clin Exp Pharmacol Physiol* 35 (4):473–6.

Liener IE. 1994. Implications of antinutritional components in soybean foods. *Crit Rev Food Sci Nutr* 34 (1):31–67.

Liener IE. 2012. *The Lectins: Properties, Functions, and Applications in Biology and Medicine.* Amsterdam: Elsevier.

López-Torres M, Barja G. 2008. Lowered methionine ingestion as responsible for the decrease in rodent mitochondrial oxidative stress in protein and dietary restriction: Possible implications for humans. *BBA Gen Subjects* 1780 (11):1337–47.

Lucier G, Lin B-H, Allshouse J, Kantor LS. 2000. Factors affecting dry bean consumption in the United States. agmrc.org/media/cms/DryBeanConEF5442C497B.pdf.

Ma Y, Griffith JA, Chasan-Taber L, Olendzki BC, Jackson E, Stanek EJ, Li W, Pagoto SL, Hafner AR, Ockene IS. 2006. Association between dietary fiber and serum C-reactive protein. *Am J Clin Nutr* 83 (4):760–6.

Ma Y, Hébert JR, Li W, Bertone-Johnson ER, Olendzki B, Pagoto SL, Tinker L, Rosal MC, Ockene IS, Ockene JK. 2008. Association between dietary fiber and markers of systemic inflammation in the Women's Health Initiative Observational Study. *Nutrition* 24 (10):941–9.

Malloy VL, Krajcik RA, Bailey SJ, Hristopoulos G, Plummer JD, Orentreich N. 2006. Methionine restriction decreases visceral fat mass and preserves insulin action in aging male Fischer 344 rats independent of energy restriction. *Aging Cell* 5 (4):305–14.

Mancia G, De Backer G, Dominiczak A, Cifkova R, Fagard R, Germano G, Grassi G, Heagerty AM, Kjeldsen SE, Laurent S. 2007. 2007 Guidelines for the management of arterial hypertension. *Eur Heart J* 28 (12):1462–536.

Mangels R, Messina V, Messina M. 2011. *The Dietitian's Guide to Vegetarian Diets.* Jones & Bartlett Publishers.

Marmot M, Atinmo T, Byers T, Chen J, Hirohata T, Jackson A, James W, Kolonel L, Kumanyika S, Leitzmann C. 2007. Food, nutrition, physical activity, and the prevention of cancer: A global perspective. Washington, DC: American Institute for Cancer Research.

Martínez R, López-Jurado M, Wanden-Berghe C, Sanz-Valero J, Porres JM, Kapravelou G. 2016. Beneficial effects of legumes on parameters of the metabolic syndrome: A systematic review of trials in animal models. *Br J Nutr* 116 (03):402–24.

McCarty MF, Barroso-Aranda J, Contreras F. 2009. The low-methionine content of vegan diets may make methionine restriction feasible as a life extension strategy. *Med Hypotheses* 72 (2):125–8.

McCrory MA, Hamaker BR, Lovejoy JC, Eichelsdoerfer PE. 2010. Pulse consumption, satiety, and weight management. *Adv Nutr Inter Rev J* 1 (1):17–30.

McDougall J. 2016. *The Healthiest Diet on the Planet: Why the Foods You Love—Pizza, Pancakes, Potatoes, Pasta, and More—Are the Solution to Preventing Disease and Looking and Feeling Your Best.* New York: HarperCollins.

McDougall J. 2017. Lectines: Plants' self-defense system circuitously kills people. *McDougall Newsletter*, May.

McEligot AJ, Gilpin EA, Rock CL, Newman V. 2002. High dietary fiber consumption is not associated with gastrointestinal discomfort in a diet intervention trial. *J Am Diet Assoc* 102 (4):549–51.

Medina-Inojosa J, Jean N, Cortes-Bergoderi M, Lopez-Jimenez F. 2014. The Hispanic paradox in cardiovascular disease and total mortality. *Prog Cardiovasc Dis* 57 (3):286–92.

Meyer KA, Kushi LH, Jacobs DR, Slavin J, Sellers TA, Folsom AR. 2000. Carbohydrates, dietary fiber, and incident type 2 diabetes in older women. *Am J Clin Nutr* 71 (4):921–30.

Michels KB, Giovannucci E, Chan AT, Singhania R, Fuchs CS, Willett WC. 2006. Fruit and vegetable consumption and colorectal adenomas in the Nurses' Health Study. *Cancer Res* 66 (7):3942–53.

Miller RA, Buehner G, Chang Y, Harper JM, Sigler R, Smith-Wheelock M. 2005. Methionine-deficient diet extends mouse lifespan, slows immune and lens aging, alters glucose, T4, IGF-I and insulin levels, and increases hepatocyte MIF levels and stress resistance. *Aging Cell* 4 (3):119–25.

Mills PK, Beeson WL, Abbey DE, Fraser GE, Phillips RL. 1988. Dietary habits and past medical history as related to fatal pancreas cancer risk among Adventists. *Cancer* 61 (12):2578–85.

Mitchell DC, Lawrence FR, Hartman TJ, Curran JM. 2009. Consumption of dry beans, peas, and lentils could improve diet quality in the US population. *J Am Diet Assoc* 109 (5):909–13.

Mollard RC, Luhovyy BL, Panahi S, Nunez M, Hanley A, Anderson GH. 2012. Regular consumption of pulses for 8 weeks reduces metabolic syndrome risk factors in overweight and obese adults. *Br J Nutr* 108 (S1):S111.

Murty CM, Pittaway JK, Ball MJ. 2010. Chickpea supplementation in an Australian diet affects food choice, satiety and bowel health. *Appetite* 54 (2):282–8.

National Cancer Institute. 2015. Defining cancer. Bethesda, MD: National Cancer Institute. https://www.cancer.gov/about-cancer/understanding/what-is-cancer (accessed June 4, 2017).

Noah L, Guillon F, Bouchet B, Buleon A, Molis C, Gratas M, Champ M. 1998. Digestion of carbohydrate from white beans (*Phaseolus vulgaris* L.) in healthy humans. *J Nutr* 128 (6):977–985.

Nosworthy MG, Neufeld J, Frolich P, Young G, Malcolmson L, House JD. 2017. Determination of protein quality of cooked Canadian pulses. *Food Sci Nutr* 5 (4):896–903. doi: https://doi.org/10.1002/fsn3.473.

Ogawa S, Kobayashi H, Amada S, Yahata H, Sonoda K, Abe K, Baba S, Sasaki M, Kaku T, Wake N. 2010. Sentinel node detection with 99mTc phytate alone is satisfactory for cervical cancer patients undergoing radical hysterectomy and pelvic lymphadenectomy. *Int J Clin Oncol* 15 (1):52–8.

O'Neill S, O'Driscoll L. 2015. Metabolic syndrome: A closer look at the growing epidemic and its associated pathologies. *Obes Rev* 16 (1):1–12.

Padhi EMT, Ramdath DD. 2017. A review of the relationship between pulse consumption and reduction of cardiovascular disease risk factors. *J Funct Foods*. doi: https://doi.org/10.1016/j.jff.2017.03.043.

Pamplona R, Barja G. 2006. Mitochondrial oxidative stress, aging and caloric restriction: The protein and methionine connection. *BBA Bioenergetics* 1757 (5):496–508.

Papanikolaou Y, Fulgoni VL III. 2008. Bean consumption is associated with greater nutrient intake, reduced systolic blood pressure, lower body weight, and a smaller waist circumference in adults: Results from the National Health and Nutrition Examination Survey 1999–2002. *J Am Coll Nutr* 27 (5):569–76.

Pavillard V, Nicolaou A, Double JA, Phillips RM. 2006. Methionine dependence of tumours: A biochemical strategy for optimizing paclitaxel chemosensitivity in vitro. *Biochem Pharmacol* 71 (6):772–8.

Prospective Studies Collaboration. 2002. Age-specific relevance of usual blood pressure to vascular mortality: A meta-analysis of individual data for one million adults in 61 prospective studies. *Lancet* 360 (9349):1903–13.

Pulse Canada. 2017. Protein quality of cooked pulses. Winnipeg, Mannitoba: Pulse Canada.

Pusztai A, Grant G. 1998. Assessment of lectin inactivation by heat and digestion. *Methods Mol Med* 9:505–14.

Raigond P, Ezekiel R, Raigond B. 2015. Resistant starch in food: A review. *J Sci Food Agric* 95 (10):1968–78.

Sabate J, Wien M. 2010. Nuts, blood lipids and cardiovascular disease. *Asia Pac J Clin Nutr* 19 (1):131–6.

Sandberg A. 2002. Bioavailability of minerals in legumes. *Br J Nutr* 88 (S3):281–5.

Schaafsma G. 2000. The protein digestibility–corrected amino acid score. *J Nutr* 130 (7):1865S–7S.

Schuszter-Gajzágó I. 2004. Nutritional aspects of legumes. In *Encyclopedia of Food and Agricultural Sciences, Engineering and Technology Resources*. Oxford: EOLSS Publishers.

Sievenpiper JL, Kendall CWC, Esfahani A, Wong JMW, Carleton AJ, Jiang HY, Bazinet RP, Vidgen E, Jenkins DJA. 2009. Effect of non-oil-seed pulses on glycaemic control: A systematic review and meta-analysis of randomised controlled experimental trials in people with and without diabetes. *Diabetologia* (52):1479–95. doi: http://dx.doi.org/10 .1007%2Fs00125-009-1395-7.

Singh PN, Fraser GE. 1998. Dietary risk factors for colon cancer in a low-risk population. *Am J Epidemiol* 148 (8):761–74.

Slavin JL. 2005. Dietary fiber and body weight. *Nutrition* 21 (3):411–8.

Sommer F, Bäckhed F. 2013. The gut microbiota—Masters of host development and physiology. *Nat Rev Microbiol* 11 (4):227–38.

Sufian MK, Hira T, Asano K, Hara H. 2007. Peptides derived from dolicholin, a phaseolin-like protein in country beans (*Dolichos lablab*), potently stimulate cholecystokinin secretion from enteroendocrine STC-1 cells. *J Agric Food Chem* 55 (22):8980–6.

Takezaki T, Gao C-M, Ding J-H, Liu T-K, Li M-S, Tajima K. 1999. Comparative study of lifestyles of residents in high and low risk areas for gastric cancer in Jiangsu Province, China; with special reference to allium vegetables. *J Epidemiol* 9 (5):297–305.

Villegas R, Gao Y-T, Yang G, Li H-L, Elasy TA, Zheng W, Shu XO. 2008. Legume and soy food intake and the incidence of type 2 diabetes in the Shanghai Women's Health Study. *Am J Clin Nutr* 87 (1):162–7.

Vucenik I, Shamsuddin AM. 2003. Cancer inhibition by inositol hexaphosphate (IP6) and inositol: From laboratory to clinic. *J Nutr* 133 (11):3778S–84S.

Vucenik I, Shamsuddin AM. 2006. Protection against cancer by dietary IP6 and inositol. *Nutr Cancer* 55 (2):109–25.

Willey JZ, Rodriguez CJ, Moon YP, Paik MC, Di Tullio MR, Homma S, Sacco RL, Elkind MSV. 2012. Coronary death and myocardial infarction among Hispanics in the Northern Manhattan Study: Exploring the Hispanic paradox. *Ann Epidemiol* 22 (5):303–9.

Winham DM, Hutchins AM. 2011. Perceptions of flatulence from bean consumption among adults in 3 feeding studies. *Nutr J* 10 (1):128. doi: 10.1186/1475-2891-10-128.

World Health Organization. 2007. Prevention of cardiovascular disease. Geneva: World Health Organization. www.who.org (accessed June 12, 2017).

Young RP, Hopkins RJ. 2014. A review of the Hispanic paradox: Time to spill the beans? *Eur Respir Rev* 23 (134):439–49.

Zanovec M, O'Neil CE, Nicklas TA. 2011. Comparison of nutrient density and nutrient-to-cost between cooked and canned beans. *Food Nutr Sci* 2 (02):66.

Zou ML, Moughan PJ, Awati A, Livesey G. 2007. Accuracy of the Atwater factors and related food energy conversion factors with low-fat, high-fiber diets when energy intake is reduced spontaneously. *Am J Clin Nutr* 86 (6):1649–56.

Section IV

Nutrient Profiles

10 Critical Nutrients in a Plant-Based Diet

Winston J. Craig and Angela V. Saunders

CONTENTS

SUMMARY

A well-planned vegetarian diet, rich in antioxidants and phytochemicals, can be health promoting, lower the risk of many chronic diseases, and meet nutritional needs of all age groups. Vegetarians may have a marginal intake of a few vitamins and minerals, or their bioavailability may be limited in a plant-based diet. Of major concern, especially for the vegan, are vitamins B12 and D, calcium, iron, and zinc. The more foods that are eliminated from the diet, the greater the risk of nutritional deficiency. Clearly, vegans who eliminate dairy and egg products, and who subsist totally on foods that are not fortified with certain vitamins and minerals, place themselves at most risk of falling short of the Dietary Reference Intake (DRI) for the critical nutrients. The use of appropriately fortified foods and some supplements safeguards the vegetarian from nutrient shortfall.

10.1 INTRODUCTION

A plant-based diet rich in dietary fiber, potassium, magnesium, folic acid, and a variety of phytochemicals and antioxidants, and low in saturated fat and cholesterol, is recognized for its health-promoting characteristics and its ability to lower the risk of many chronic diseases (Craig and Mangels, 2009). Vegetarian diets have been shown to be not only healthful but also nutritionally adequate across the life cycle (Craig and Mangels, 2009). Nevertheless, there are a few micronutrients of concern that necessitate attention

(Craig, 2010). These few vitamins and minerals may be in short supply in some plant-based diets, or their absorption may be hindered by dietary inhibitors. The situation is most problematic in vegans who follow a whole-food diet devoid of all fortified foods and can be exacerbated when supplements have no place in the diet.

10.2   IRON

Dietary iron is necessary for the formation of hemoglobin and myoglobin for oxygen delivery to the cells. Iron deficiency anemia affects about 25% of the world's population, or 2 billion people, mostly women and children (World Health Organization, 2001; De Benoist et al., 2008) who have restricted access to a varied diet. Also included are overweight females who follow poorly planned, restricted weight loss diets (O'Connor et al., 2011). A deficiency of iron has serious consequences, particularly during pregnancy, where it may result in premature delivery and higher risk of infant morbidity and mortality.

Vegetarians who eat a varied and well-balanced diet are not at any greater risk of iron deficiency anemia than nonvegetarians (Craig, 1994; Hunt, 2003). In fact, there is no significant difference in hemoglobin and hematocrit values between vegetarians and nonvegetarians (Craig, 1994; Obeid et al., 2002). Vegetarian diets generally contain as much or more iron than omnivore diets (Davey et al., 2003; Craig and Mangels, 2009). A diet that is rich in whole grains, legumes, nuts, seeds, dried fruits, iron-fortified cereal products, and green leafy vegetables provides an adequate iron intake. The DRI for iron assumes that a significant amount of iron comes from non-meat sources, as approximately 80%–90% of iron in the typical diet comes from plant sources, with the remainder being heme iron (Hallberg, 1981; Carpenter and Mahoney, 1992). Heme iron is absorbed easily and may contribute up to 50% of the total iron absorbed by an omnivore (Crichton, 2016). The body is very conservative of its iron, recycling the iron from its short-lived red blood cells (Samman, 2007a).

Iron absorption is carefully regulated by the gut. Absorption of nonheme iron, but not heme iron, is inversely related to the body's iron stores (Geissler et al., 2005). This situation has importance since we have only a limited ability to excrete excess stored iron (Hunt, 2003). Volume of menstrual flow is the most significant factor affecting iron status for women. Those who have the highest monthly losses tend to have the lowest ferritin stores (Harvey et al., 2005). The absorption of nonheme iron increases during the physiological demand of pregnancy (Hunt, 2003; Hurrell and Egli, 2010). During the third trimester of pregnancy, this may reach as high as 60% (Whittaker et al., 2001).

Excessive amounts of heme iron may be unhealthful, since it can act as a pro-oxidant. Different researchers have reported the association of heme iron intake with an increased risk of chronic diseases, such as heart disease, diabetes, metabolic syndrome, and colorectal cancer (Qi et al., 2007; Cross et al., 2010; Agarwal, 2013; White and Collinson, 2013). Hence, consuming nonheme iron from a plant-based diet may convey protective qualities so that an omnivore should be encouraged to consume more nonheme iron foods (Haider et al., 2016).

It has been suggested that iron absorption from a mixed diet (including meat) is about 18%, whereas it is 10% from a plant-based diet (Food and Nutrition Board, Institute of Medicine, 2001). Nonheme iron absorption is influenced by various inhibitors and enhancers (Hallberg and Hulthen, 2000). Nonheme iron absorption is enhanced significantly when vitamin C–rich fruits and vegetables are eaten at the same meal (Hallberg and Hulthen, 2000). Other organic acids in plant foods also enhance absorption (Garcia-Casal et al., 1998). Erythorbic acid, an antioxidant used in processed food, is a potent enhancer of nonheme-iron absorption acid, even more potent than ascorbic acid (Fidler et al., 2004). While phytates (found in legumes, nuts, and whole grains) can inhibit nonheme iron absorption, usual cooking methods can diminish their inhibitory effect (Davidsson, 2003). Polyphenols in beverages, like tea and coffee, may also inhibit nonheme iron absorption (Hurrell et al., 1999).

However, the overall long-term effect of enhancers and inhibitors of iron may be less important than once thought, particularly when eaten as part of a whole diet (Scientific Advisory Committee on Nutrition, 2011; Armah et al., 2013). Iron absorption from whole diets can vary from 1% to 23% depending on the body's iron stores *and* the presence of inhibitors and enhancers. Absorption was low (1.8%–3%) in people with good iron stores (serum ferritin levels of 100 µg/L), but higher (14%–23%) when serum ferritin levels were low (6 µg/L) (Collings et al., 2013). It is interesting to note that iron in soy and other legumes (plant ferritin) is a significant and easily absorbed source of dietary iron (Lonnerdal, 2009; Theil et al., 2012; Zielinska-Dawidziak, 2015). Plant ferritin is absorbed independently through a separate transport system, so it does not compete with other dietary sources of iron. Its absorption varies from 22% to 34%. Along with other plant sources of iron in a varied diet, plant ferritin can provide the nutritional needs of iron (Theil et al., 2012; Zielinska-Dawidziak, 2015).

Vegetarians typically have lower iron stores (as reflected in lower serum ferritin levels) even when their iron intake is adequate (Alexander et al., 1994; Ball and Bartlett, 1999; Wilson and Ball, 1999; Lim et al., 2013; Rizzo et al., 2013). It has been suggested that lower stores may not be a disadvantage (Haider et al., 2016), as higher ferritin levels may be associated with increased risk of chronic disease (Park et al., 2012) and lower serum ferritin may be associated with improved insulin sensitivity and reduced risk of type 2 diabetes mellitus. Lower iron stores will be associated with a greater absorption of the nonheme iron (Hunt, 2003; Collings et al., 2013). Another adaptive response for vegetarians is that they tend to excrete less iron (conserving losses) than meat eaters (Hunt and Roughead, 1999).

According to the current DRI (Food and Nutrition Board, Institute of Medicine, 2001), iron requirements for vegetarians have been set 1.8 times higher than those for nonvegetarians. This increased requirement is based on very limited research (Food and Nutrition Board, Institute of Medicine, 2001). Overall, research to date has been unable to accurately measure adaptive absorption rates of nonheme iron in vegetarians (Armah et al., 2013). Further research is needed to reassess the higher dietary iron requirements recommended by the Institute of Medicine for vegetarians (Saunders et al., 2013b).

10.3 VITAMIN B12

Vitamin B12 deficiency is an important issue not fully appreciated by all vegetarians. It manifests itself with both hematological and neurological changes. Megaloblastic anemia with diminished energy, fatigue, pallor of the skin, and neutropenia are common manifestations of B12 deficiency. Neurological effects commonly include tingling and numbness in the extremities, unsteadiness in walking, disorientation, memory loss, and dementia.

For the lacto-ovo vegetarian, dairy (milk, yogurt, and cheese) and eggs are considered good sources of vitamin B12. However, the absorption of vitamin B12 from cooked eggs is <10% (Doscherholmen et al., 1975) compared with an absorption of 50% for other animal foods. Losses of up to 50% can occur through food processing, such as cooking and pasteurization (Watanabe, 2007).

Vegans must obtain their vitamin B12 either from a regular use of vitamin B12–fortified foods, such as fortified soy, almond, coconut, and rice beverages; fortified breakfast cereals; meat analogs; and fortified nutritional yeast, or from a daily vitamin B12 supplement. Unfortified plant foods, such as fermented soy foods (such as tempeh), leafy vegetables, seaweeds (except nori), mushrooms (except Shiitake), and algae (including spirulina), do not contain significant amounts of active vitamin B12 to provide daily needs (Watanabe et al., 2014). Some of the foods claimed to have vitamin B12 may actually contain inactive corrinoids (Watanabe et al., 2013).

Typically, the mean intake of vitamin B12 of a vegan is well below the DRI, while that of lacto-ovo vegetarians may be marginal (Herrmann et al., 2001; Craig, 2010; Gilsing et al., 2010). Adequate vitamin B12 intake is especially important during pregnancy and breastfeeding. Infants born to long-term vegan mothers, and who are breastfed, are at measurable risk of B12 deficiency. Symptoms of B12 deficiency in breastfed infants and small children fed a vegan diet include developmental delay or regression, lethargy, apathy, anemia, and failure to thrive (Doyle et al., 1989). A B12 deficiency during infancy can increase the risk of neurological problems, which may not always be reversible after treatment.

Many vegans feel reluctant to use supplements or B12-fortified foods. They may even avoid using them altogether, viewing such products as unnatural, and that the danger of B12 deficiency is quite remote. However, research shows that the use of supplements or B12-fortified foods do prevent B12 deficiency (Rizzo et al., 2016). Omnivores who switched to a strict vegan diet and consumed only natural foods experienced falling serum B12 levels over a 5-year period, while those omnivores who switched to a vegan diet containing B12-fortified foods did not experience those changes in blood levels (Madry et al., 2012). A Swiss study revealed that despite having a negligible dietary intake of vitamin B12, the use of B12 supplements protected vegans against B12 deficiency (Schupbach et al., 2017).

If an individual's folic acid intake is high, hematological symptoms of vitamin B12 deficiency may be masked and go undetected until neurological symptoms are manifested (Herrmann et al., 2001). As a person ages, the level of pepsin and acid in the stomach decreases. With the loss of normal gastric function, and the chronic use of proton pump inhibitors, B12 is not removed very effectively from the food proteins, and B12 absorption is greatly diminished (Rizzo et al., 2016). It is recommended that individuals over 50 years of age consume B12-fortified foods or a regular supplement since these forms of B12 do not require digestion before absorption.

Absorption of B12 occurs by two processes, and there are no data to suggest that absorption depends on one's B12 status. About 50% of dietary B12 is normally absorbed via receptors in the ileum. The B12 is carried to the ileum by the intrinsic factor from the stomach. The ileal receptors become saturated with 1.5–2 µg of B12, limiting further absorption (Watanabe, 2007). Absorption can also occur by passive diffusion and does not involve the intrinsic factor, with fractional absorption of vitamin B12 being inversely related to the size of the dose ingested.

When ingesting large doses of supplemental B12, up to 1% of the dose can be absorbed by mass action (Food and Nutrition Board, Institute of Medicine, 1998). Consuming a 500–1000 µg vitamin B12 (cyanocobalamin) supplement three to four times a week or a 250 µg tablet daily can provide sufficient B12 for adult needs. Sublingual or chewable tablets are the most effective. In healthy adults, the absorption of vitamin B12 (either free or protein-bound cobalamin) does not appear to diminish with aging (Van Asselt et al., 1996). While methylcobalamin and adenosylcobalamin are active metabolic forms of vitamin B12 in the body, taking them in supplemental form does not appear to be more effective than using the cheaper and commonly available cyanocobalamin supplement (Obeid et al., 2015). In addition to oral supplementation, vitamin B12 (hydroxocobalamin) may also be administered by injection. Once absorbed, vitamin B12 circulates in the blood bound to three transcobalamins. Of these proteins, transcobalamin II is responsible for the receptor-mediated uptake of vitamin B12 into cells (Food and Nutrition Board, Institute of Medicine, 1998).

The body stores amount to about 2–4 mg on average, with most of that occurring as adenosylcobalamin in the liver. A deficiency of vitamin B12 may take years to develop due to the vitamin's long biological half-life. The enterohepatic circulation of B12 plays a major role in conserving vitamin B12 since most of the B12 secreted in the bile is reabsorbed. Losses of B12 amount to about 0.1%–0.2% of the body's B12 pool per day (Food and Nutrition Board, Institute of Medicine, 1998). With a deficient intake, clinical signs of a B12 deficiency will be manifest after the body stores run low.

Vitamin B12 is a vital coenzyme necessary for both the conversion of homocysteine to methionine and the conversion of L-methylmalonic coenzyme A (CoA) to succinyl CoA. Hence, a subclinical B12 deficiency results in elevated serum homocysteine and methylmalonic acid (MMA). Since other deficiencies produce elevated homocysteine levels, this indicator has poor specificity for determining B12 status (Food and Nutrition Board, Institute of Medicine, 1998). Laboratory tests to assess vitamin B12 status normally include measuring serum MMA levels or serum or plasma vitamin B12 levels (Food and Nutrition Board, Institute of Medicine, 1998). An elevated serum MMA level is a reliable indicator of B12 deficiency, while serum B12 levels are an insensitive indicator with poor predictive value. Serum B12 levels below 200 pg/mL (148 pmol/L) are considered deficient by most labs, while those between 200 and 300 pg/mL (148–221 pmol/L) suggest borderline deficiency (Chatthanawaree, 2011). However, a significant number of elderly subjects with unequivocal clinical evidence of B12 deficiency had serum cobalamin levels within the conventionally defined normal range (Lindenbaum et al., 1994). A person may have normal serum levels but low tissue concentrations (Beck, 1991) and manifest neuropsychiatric problems and memory loss. Every individual over the age of 50, and especially vegans, should be vigilant in having their B12 levels checked annually.

10.4   CALCIUM

More than 99% of total body calcium resides in bones and teeth. Bone tissue serves as a reservoir for calcium as it is constantly remodeling in a dynamic process of resorption and bone formation. Small amounts of calcium also reside in the blood, extracellular fluid, muscle, and other tissues, where it plays an important role in regulating nerve transmission, muscle contraction, vasodilation, and glandular secretion (Food and Nutrition Board, Institute of Medicine, 1997). Clearly, adequate calcium is important to maintain essential body functions. Absorbing adequate levels of calcium and diminishing calcium urinary losses is key to maintaining calcium balance.

While calcium intakes of lacto-ovo vegetarians typically meet recommendations, those of vegans often fall below. Vegans often consume about 20% less calcium than lacto-ovo vegetarians (Craig, 2010). Fractional calcium absorption does increase when calcium intakes are low (Dawson-Hughes et al., 1993). Fractional calcium remains fairly constant throughout most of life but decreases in the elderly. The bioavailability of calcium is a key issue when discussing calcium absorption in vegetarians.

Some plant foods contain a considerable level of phytic acid and oxalic acid, both of which can inhibit calcium absorption. For example, the fractional absorption of calcium from oxalate-rich vegetables, such as spinach (including baby spinach) and Swiss chard, may be as low 5%, while the absorption from almonds, tahini, beans, and fruits such as figs and oranges is substantially lower (20%–25%) than that of dairy products (32%) (Weaver et al., 1999). Soybeans and products such as tofu and soy-based beverages are an exception, as calcium absorption is similar to that of milk (Heaney et al., 1991; Zhao et al., 2005). On the other hand, calcium absorption from low-oxalate vegetables, such as kale, Chinese cabbage, broccoli, collards, and bok choy, can reach as high as 50%–60% (Weaver et al., 1999). Boiling can markedly reduce soluble oxalate content in green leafy vegetables. Boiling is more effective than steaming, while baking has no effect on oxalates. Cooking has less of an effect on insoluble oxalates in vegetables than on the soluble forms (Chai and Liebman, 2005). Soaking green leaves such as taro overnight diminishes the levels of soluble oxalate but not insoluble oxalate forms (Savage and Dubois, 2006).

A considerable number of individuals, especially women, enhance their dietary intake of calcium with calcium supplements. Furthermore, various food and beverage products are enriched with those same calcium compounds. The calcium in calcium carbonate is absorbed to a level similar to that of the calcium in milk, while the fractional calcium absorption rate from tricalcium phosphate is a little less and from calcium citrate malate is significantly higher, at 35% (Miller et al., 1988; Patrick, 1999). Vegans may need to use calcium-fortified foods, such as fortified breakfast cereals, fortified fruit juices, and soy, almond, coconut, and rice beverages, to meet their calcium needs.

Limiting urinary losses of calcium is favorable to an individual's calcium status since this is the major pathway for calcium loss from the body. Vegetarian diets typically report lower urinary calcium excretion levels (Ball and Maughan, 1997). Diets rich in fruits and vegetables, containing high levels of potassium and magnesium, produce a high renal alkaline load, which offsets the calciuric effect of a high renal acid load associated with a diet rich in meat, dairy products, and grains. In addition, a high salt (sodium chloride) intake increases urinary sodium with an accompanying increased obligatory loss of urinary calcium (Kurtz et al., 1987). Hence, a greater use of herbal seasonings, in place of salt, will diminish the urinary calcium losses associated with the high-sodium intake.

The low acid load of vegetarian diets, resulting from a high intake of fruit and vegetables, conveys protection against low bone mineral density and risk of fracture. On the other hand, the diet of Western-style omnivores produces 50–70 mEq of acid daily (Burckhardt, 2016), making the urine more acidic in omnivores (pH 6.2) than in lacto-ovo vegetarians (pH 6.5) or vegans (pH 6.7) (Knurick et al., 2015). Vegan diets have been associated with lower bone mineral density and an increased risk of fracture, but this only appears to be clinically significant when the calcium intake is inadequate (Mangels, 2014). For a detailed discussion of the role of calcium in the risk of osteoporosis in vegetarians, one should refer to Chapter 6.

Analysis of the National Health and Nutrition Examination Survey (NHANES) 2001–2008 data revealed that low-income, overweight, or obese minority populations may be at substantial risk of calcium and vitamin D insufficiency, while calcium and vitamin D intakes from food and supplements were actually unrelated to vegetarian status (Wallace et al., 2013).

10.5   VITAMIN D

In addition to its importance in the maintenance of bone health, vitamin D plays an important role in immune function, reducing inflammation and the risk of chronic diseases. Low vitamin D status has been linked to a wide variety of diseases, including heart disease, type 1 diabetes, colorectal cancer, multiple sclerosis, rheumatoid arthritis, infectious diseases, depression (Holick, 2008), and hypertension (Forman et al., 2008). Serum 25-hydroxyvitamin D (25(OH)D) levels (a measure of vitamin D status) were found to be 24.4% lower in type 2 diabetes mellitus patients than in controls. Glycemic control (measured by HbA1c levels) was inversely related to 25(OH)D levels (Kostoglou-Athanassiou et al., 2013). Many genes encoding proteins regulating cell proliferation, differentiation, and apoptosis are modulated in part by vitamin D. Adequate vitamin D intake is essential since all tissues in the body have vitamin D receptors. Vitamin D plays a role in many metabolic pathways (Holick, 2008). Because cutaneous production of vitamin D from sunlight exposure is not sufficient (especially in the elderly, dark-skinned individuals, and heavy sunscreen users), to meet nutrition needs in populations living in high latitudes (north of 35°N or south of 35°S) especially during the winter months, a regular food source is required; otherwise, a vitamin D supplement is necessary (Mangels, 2014). Recommendations for an optimal serum level of 25(OH)D range from 50 to 75 nmol/L (20 to 30 ng/mL). Depending on one's age, latitude of residence, dietary preferences, body weight, and individual health outcome concerns, a supplemental dose of 10–50 µg (400–2000 IU) of vitamin D per day may be needed to achieve such levels of 25(OH)D year-round (Pludowski et al., 2017).

The intake of vitamin D by vegans tends to be substantially below that of lacto-ovo vegetarians and nonvegetarians (Craig, 2010). Low serum 25(OH)D levels and reduced bone mass have been reported in some vegan groups living in high latitudes

(Parsons et al., 1997; Outila et al., 2000) who did not ingest vitamin D–fortified foods or take vitamin D supplements. For an adequate vitamin D intake, vegetarians, and especially vegans, may need to consume, on a regular basis, fortified plant-based beverages (made from almonds, soy, coconut, rice, or cashew), fortified orange juice, ready-to-eat breakfast cereals, fortified soy yogurt, and margarines. Substantial levels of vitamin D2 (ergocalciferol) may also be obtained from mushrooms that have been exposed to ultraviolet light under controlled conditions (Kamweru and Tindibale, 2016; Keegan et al., 2013). Lacto-ovo vegetarians can also secure vitamin D from fortified dairy products and eggs.

Both vitamin D2 (ergocalciferol, produced from yeast) and, more commonly, vitamin D3 (cholecalciferol, normally derived from lanolin) are used in supplements and for the fortification of foods. At low doses, vitamin D2 appears to be as effective as vitamin D3 in maintaining serum 25(OH)D levels (Holick et al., 2008), but at higher doses, vitamin D2 appears to be less effective than vitamin D3 (Tripkovic et al., 2012).

While vegetarians may be at risk of vitamin D deficiency, it is also true that non-vegetarians are not without risk, based on where they live, their outdoor habits, age, skin pigmentation, and use of sunscreen. In a study of 428 Americans, ethnicity was a major factor determining the serum levels of 25(OH)D, while no significant difference was found in serum 25(OH)D levels between vegetarians and omnivores. The mean value of serum 25(OH)D for blacks (50.7 nmol/L) was 34% lower than that of whites (77.1 nmol/L). Only 16.6% of blacks were found with sufficient vitamin D levels (serum 25(OH)D = 75 nmol/L or above) compared with 52.4% of whites. Factors such as vitamin D supplementation, degree of skin pigmentation, and amount and intensity of sun exposure had a greater influence on serum 25(OH)D than did diet (Chan et al., 2009). In contrast to the American study, plasma 25(OH)D levels were found to be lower in British vegetarians (66.0 nmol/L) and vegans (55.8 nmol/L) than in meat eaters (77.0 nmol/L) in the large EPIC-Oxford study (Crowe et al., 2011).

Foods containing vitamin D are not that abundant, so it is recommended that all persons, especially the elderly, take vitamin D supplements, especially during the winter months (or late autumn to early spring). While vegans are at risk of lower bone mineral density, by paying attention to potential shortfall nutrients (calcium and vitamin D), a careful selection of D-fortified foods, and the use of supplements, one can ensure a healthy bone mineral density in individuals choosing a vegetarian diet (Tucker, 2014).

10.6   ZINC

Zinc acts as a coenzyme for a vast array of enzymes involved with growth, immune function, cognitive function, and bone function, as well as the regulation of gene expression (Saunders et al., 2013). Zinc deficiency results in stunted growth, poor appetite, dermatitis, alopecia, endocrine dysfunction, and impaired immunity (Samman, 2007b; Huang et al., 2015). Although severe zinc deficiency is relatively rare in developed countries, mild deficiency can be a concern in some populations (Wuehler et al., 2005); however, the consequences of marginal zinc intake are not well understood (Hunt, 2002).

Iron-rich plant foods are often also good sources of zinc, including whole-grain cereals, nuts and seeds, legumes, soy products, and fortified breakfast cereals. Dairy and meat products are also sources of zinc. As with iron, there are bioactive substances in plants, such as phytates, that may inhibit the absorption of zinc (Hunt, 2003). Phytic acid is the principal storage form of phosphorus in cereals, legumes, and seeds and therefore abundant in a plant-based diet (Foster and Samman, 2015). The inhibitory effect of phytic acid can be minimized by the normal modern processing and cooking methods (baking, soaking, sprouting, leavening, and fermentation) due to the action of phytases that hydrolyze phytic acid (Gibson et al., 2006; Samman, 2007b; Foster and Samman, 2015). Hence, zinc deficiency is less likely to be a problem where a variety of foods and cooking methods are present (Hunt, 2003; Saunders et al., 2013; Foster and Samman, 2015). Regular consumption of iron supplements may inhibit zinc absorption (Foster and Samman, 2015), while calcium and fiber do not inhibit zinc absorption (Saunders et al., 2013).

Sulfur-containing amino acids (cysteine and methionine) in seeds, nuts, and grains and organic acids (such as citric, malic, tartaric, and lactic acids) will also enhance zinc absorption (Lonnerdal, 2000; Foster and Samman, 2015). Adding garlic or onion to legumes, grains, or seeds may also negate the influence of phytates and enhance zinc absorption (Gautam et al., 2011).

Homeostatic mechanisms regulate plasma zinc levels in spite of diverse zinc intakes and bioavailability. These mechanisms can reduce endogenous zinc losses and increase the efficiency of absorption, maintaining cellular zinc concentrations within a narrow physiologic range as needed (King, 2011; Saunders et al., 2013; Huang et al., 2015). The body can regulate zinc absorption by how much zinc gets excreted (Lim et al., 2013). Considerable amounts of zinc also come from endogenous sources, such as pancreatic secretions (Otten et al., 2006). Zinc absorption also becomes more efficient during pregnancy and other periods of high physiological demand (infancy and lactation) (Krebs and Hambidge, 1986).

Zinc intake of vegetarians is about the same as or slightly lower than that of omnivores, with a compensatory improved efficiency of absorption and retention (less excretion) of zinc (Otten et al., 2006; King, 2011; Foster et al., 2013). Vegans are more likely to show marginal zinc status (Foster et al., 2013).

Overall, studies show that vegetarians do not have a significantly greater risk of low zinc status than nonvegetarians, even during times of greatest demand (pregnancy, lactation, childhood, and elderly) (Ball and Ackland, 2000; Gibson et al., 2014; Foster and Samman, 2015; Foster et al., 2015). While serum zinc levels are a common measure of zinc status, they are recognized as an insensitive indicator of it. Further research is needed to find a more precise parameter (King, 2011).

The Reference Daily Intake (RDI) for zinc for vegetarians is 1.5 times higher than it is for others, due to concerns about availability (Food and Nutrition Board, Institute of Medicine, 2001). However, the RDI does not appear to take into appropriate account that vegetarians seem to adapt to lower zinc intakes by reducing losses and increasing the efficiency of absorption (Saunders et al., 2013). Further research is needed to better understand zinc metabolism and requirements for vegetarians.

10.7 PROTEIN

Contrary to popular opinion, vegetarian and vegan diets typically meet or exceed recommended protein intakes when energy intakes are adequate (Melina et al., 2016).

The best sources of plant protein include legumes (such as beans, soybeans, lentils, and chickpeas), soy foods (including soy milk, soy sausages or burgers, tofu, and tempeh), nuts, and seeds. Whole grains, including quinoa and amaranth, are also good sources of protein. Plant foods rich in proteins are low in saturated fat, free of *trans* fat, and cholesterol-free, and are good sources of iron, zinc, dietary fiber, antioxidants, and phytonutrients. While soy milk has a protein content similar to that of dairy milk, the other plant-based beverages, such as rice, oat, coconut, and almond milk, are much lower in protein content and should not be used by growing children as a milk substitute.

Protein is required by the body to produce vital molecules, such as hormones, enzymes, immunoglobulins, transport proteins, and hemoglobin. It was once thought that plant protein quality was compromised due to one or more of the essential amino acids being limited (soy and quinoa being the exception), suggesting the need to combine proteins to obtain an ideal amino acid profile. Examined over a 24-hour period, a vegetarian or vegan diet that contains a variety of plant foods easily meets that ideal (Mangels et al., 2011; Marsh et al., 2013). In addition to the proteins eaten, there is a constant supply of endogenous proteins available. These derive from desquamated mucosal cells, digestive enzymes, and glycoproteins that provide a level of protein similar to that from exogenous sources (Fuller and Reeds, 1998).

There are no differences between the protein requirements for vegetarians and nonvegetarians for all stages of the life cycle (Food and Nutrition Board, Institute of Medicine, 2005). Only 10% of energy from protein is actually required to meet physiological needs. The recommended daily intake for protein is 0.84/kg body weight for adult males and 0.75g/kg body weight for adult females. It is slightly higher during pregnancy and breastfeeding, as well as for older adults (over 70 years), who all need around 1.0g/kg body weight. Protein requirements for all age groups, including athletes, are easily achieved on a vegetarian and vegan diet (Melina et al., 2016).

Research shows that consuming protein from plant sources rather than animal sources is associated with a lower risk of chronic diseases (including hypertension, type 2 diabetes, and heart disease) and with lower rates of overweight or obesity (Marsh et al., 2012, 2013). The EPIC-Oxford study compared weight gain over 5 years and found that it was lowest in the vegan group, including those who, during follow-up, had changed to a diet containing fewer animal foods. They also found that meat eaters had the highest BMI and vegans the lowest, with high protein and low fiber intakes most strongly associated with increasing BMI (Spencer et al., 2003; Halkjaer et al., 2010). Low-carbohydrate, high-animal protein diets are associated with higher all-cause mortality, but not when protein comes from plant sources, indicating that the protein source is an important factor (Fung et al., 2010).

10.8   OMEGA-3 POLYUNSATURATED FATTY ACIDS

Omega-3 fatty acids have important functions in the body. They reduce the risk of blood clots and arrhythmias, improve vascular endothelial function, lower blood triglyceride levels, and have anti-inflammatory activity (Jacobsen, 2008; Jung et al.,

2008; Kimmig and Karalis, 2013); long-chain omega-3 fatty acids are needed for visual function and brain development; and they may help protect against cognitive decline (Van Gelder et al., 2007; Sarter et al., 2015). This means that an adequate intake (AI) of omega-3 fatty acids can lower the risk of stroke and sudden cardiac death and possibly reduce the pain and stiffness in rheumatoid arthritis. Recent evidence suggests that long-chain omega-3 fatty acids may possibly help alleviate depression (Martins, 2009).

Linoleic acid (LA), found in corn, sunflower, and safflower oils, and alpha-linolenic acid (ALA), found in walnuts, flaxseed, chia seeds, canola, and soy oils, are designated as essential fatty acids and belong to the omega-6 and omega-3 families, respectively. Typically, vegetarians have a high intake of omega-6 and a much lower intake of omega-3. Vegetarians and nonvegetarians, who rarely eat oily fish, may not consume adequate amounts of the long-chain omega-3 polyunsaturated fatty acids, eicosapentaenoic acid (EPA), and docosahexaenoic acid (DHA) (Sanders, 2009; Welch et al., 2010; Saunders et al., 2013).

EPA and DHA can be synthesized in the body by converting ALA to EPA and then to DHA. DHA can also be retroconverted into EPA. Some have reported that the conversion of ALA to EPA may be quite inefficient (Jensen et al., 1997; Makrides et al., 2000; Elorinne et al., 2016), while the conversion to DHA is even less efficient (Williams and Burdge, 2006; Lane et al., 2014; Sanders, 2014). Conversion of ALA may be negatively affected by consuming high levels of omega-6 and too little omega-3 (Saunders et al., 2013). Other factors that may affect conversion include high intakes of saturated fat and *trans* fat, genetics, gender (ALA conversion is promoted by estrogen), aging, diabetes, alcohol, and smoking (Lane et al., 2014). Conversion appears to be greater in those who do not consume EPA and DHA, such as non–fish eaters (Welch et al., 2010) and possibly vegetarians. Consuming marine algal oils (containing DHA) is probably the most effective way for a vegetarian to increase their serum DHA level (Lane et al., 2014).

Vegetarians must be intentional about increasing their omega-3 intake from plant sources (flaxseed, walnuts, chia, and the oils made from such seeds and nuts, canola, and soy oils). Plant sources of DHA include some fortified breakfast foods, some fortified dairy products, eggs, one brand of soymilk, one brand of orange juice, some microalgae, and seaweeds. DHA supplements (derived from marine algal oil) are also available for vegans. Some recommend a DHA supplement of 250 mg to 1 g/day (Lane et al., 2014; Sarter et al., 2015). Others have recommended consuming twice the AI of ALA (i.e., about 2.5 g for men and 1.5 g for women) (Saunders et al., 2013). This is easily achieved by daily consuming 1 tablespoon of chia or flaxseeds.

Although plasma and tissue concentrations of EPA and DHA are lower in vegetarians than in nonvegetarians, a large UK study suggested that endogenous production of EPA and DHA in vegetarians and vegans resulted in low but stable plasma concentrations of these fatty acids over years (Rosell et al., 2005). To date, there is no evidence of adverse effects on health or cognitive function in vegetarians or vegans, despite very low DHA intakes (Sanders, 2009). There appears to be no need for the vegetarian to supplement their diet with EPA and DHA for the prevention of cardiovascular disease, since they already have a low risk (Marsh et al., 2012; Sanders, 2014).

To ensure an adequate omega-3 status, a vegetarian should boost their ALA intake with chia seeds, flaxseeds, or walnuts. In addition, a portion of the LA-rich vegetable oils should be replaced by monounsaturated oils, such as olive oil. For further protection, a DHA and/or EPA supplement derived from microalgae can be regularly consumed. This supplement may be especially beneficial for those with increased needs (pregnant and lactating women) or who may have bigger challenges with the ALA-to-DHA conversion, such as people with diabetes, metabolic syndrome, hypertension, or the elderly.

10.9 CONCLUSIONS

Vegetarian diets can provide considerable health benefits in the prevention of some common chronic diseases. They can also be nutritionally adequate when appropriately planned. Consuming adequate calories in a balanced vegetarian diet usually provides adequate protein quality and quantity. The iron status of all vegetarians, consuming a balanced diet, appears not to be compromised. More research is needed to clarify the essential role of ALA and DHA in providing the omega-3 needs of the vegetarian and the clinical significance of a lower DHA status in vegetarians. While vegetarians may consume diets of lower zinc bioavailability, the significance of this is unclear. There are real dangers that vegetarians, especially vegans, could develop a deficiency of calcium, vitamin D, and especially vitamin B12. Foods fortified with vitamins B12 and D should be given a priority; otherwise, supplementation would be recommended. Vegetarians, especially vegans, should take care to ensure an AI of calcium-rich foods. Vegans who consume only unprocessed foods that are not fortified with the critical nutrients may be nutritionally compromised and show need for a regular intake of appropriate supplements. Micronutrient deficiencies can have serious clinical outcomes, so that appropriate food choices, including the regular use of fortified foods, is an important consideration for all vegetarians.

REFERENCES

Agarwal U. 2013. Rethinking red meat as a prevention strategy for iron deficiency. *Infant Child Adolesc Nutr* 5(4):231–5.
Alexander D, Ball MJ, Mann J. 1994. Nutrient intake and haematological status of vegetarians and age-sex matched omnivores. *Eur J Clin Nutr* 48(8):538–46.
Armah SM, Carriquiry A, Sullivan D, Cook JD, Reddy MB. 2013. A complete diet-based algorithm for predicting nonheme iron absorption in adults. *J Nutr* 143(7):1136–40.
Ball D, Maughan RJ. 1997. Blood and urine acid-base status of premenopausal omnivorous and vegetarian women. *Br J Nutr* 78:683–93.
Ball MJ, Ackland ML. 2000. Zinc intake and status in Australian vegetarians. *Br J Nutr* 83(1):27–33.
Ball MJ, Bartlett MA. 1999. Dietary intake and iron status of Australian vegetarian women. *Am J Clin Nutr* 70(3):353–8.
Beck W. 1991. Neuropsychiatric consequences of cobalamin deficiency. *Adv Intern Med* 36:33–56.
Burckhardt P. 2016. The role of low acid load in vegetarian diet on bone health: A narrative review. *Swiss Med Wkly* 146:w14277. doi: 10.4414/smw.2016.14277.

Carpenter CE, Mahoney AW. 1992. Contributions of heme and nonheme iron to human nutrition. *Crit Rev Food Sci Nutr* 31(4):333–67.

Chai W, Liebman M. 2005. Effect of different cooking methods on vegetable oxalate content. *J Agric Food Chem* 53(8):3027–30.

Chan J, Jaceldo-Siegl K, Fraser GE. 2009. Serum 25-hydroxyvitamin D status of vegetarians, partial vegetarians, and nonvegetarians: The Adventist Health Study-2. *Am J Clin Nutr* 89(Suppl.):1686S–92S.

Chatthanawaree W. 2011. Biomarkers of cobalamin (vitamin B12) deficiency and its application. *J Nutr Hlth Aging* 15:227–31.

Collings R, Harvey LJ, Hooper L, Hurst R, Brown TJ, Ansett J, King M, Fairweather-Tait SJ. 2013. The absorption of iron from whole diets: A systematic review. *Am J Clin Nutr* 98(1):65–81.

Craig WJ. 1994. Iron status of vegetarians. *Am J Clin Nutr* 59(5 Suppl.):1233S–7S.

Craig WJ. 2010. Nutrition concerns and health effects of vegetarian diets. *Nutr Clin Pract* 25:613–20.

Craig WJ, Mangels AR. 2009. Position of the American Dietetic Association: Vegetarian diets. *J Am Diet Assoc* 109(7):1266–82.

Crichton R. 2016. Mammalian iron metabolism and dietary iron absorption. In *Iron Metabolism: From Molecular Mechanisms to Clinical Consequences*. 4th ed. Chichester, UK: John Wiley & Sons.

Cross AJ, Ferrucci LM, Risch A, Graubard BI, Ward MH, Park Y, Hollenbeck AR, Schatzkin A, Sinha R. 2010. A large prospective study of meat consumption and colorectal cancer risk: An investigation of potential mechanisms underlying this association. *Cancer Res* 70(6):2406–14.

Crowe FL, Steur M, Allen NE, Appleby PN, Travis RC, Key TJ. 2011. Plasma concentrations of 25-hydroxyvitamin D in meat eaters, fish eaters, vegetarians, and vegans: Results from the EPIC-Oxford study. *Public Health Nutr* 14(2):340–6.

Davey GK, Spencer EA, Appleby PN, Allen NE, Knox KH, Key TJ. 2003. EPIC-Oxford: Lifestyle characteristics and nutrient intakes in a cohort of 33,883 meat-eaters and 31,546 nonmeat-eaters in the UK. *Public Health Nutr* 6(3):259–69.

Davidsson L. 2003. Approaches to improve iron bioavailability from complementary foods. *J Nutr* 133(5 Suppl. 1):1560S–2S.

Dawson-Hughes B, Harris S, Kramich C, Dallal G, Rasmussen HM. 1993. Calcium retention and hormone levels in black and white women on high- and low-calcium diets. *J Bone Miner Res* 8:779–87.

De Benoist B, McLean E, Egli I, Cogswell M. 2008. Worldwide prevalence of anaemia 1993–2005. Geneva: World Health Organization.

Doscherholmen A, McMahon J, Ripley D. 1975. Vitamin B12 absorption from eggs. *Proc Soc Exp Biol Med* 149:987–90.

Doyle JJ, Langerin AM, Zipursky A. 1989. Nutritional vitamin B12 deficiency in infancy: Three case reports and a review of the literature. *Pediatr Hematol Oncol* 6(2):161–72.

Elorinne AL, Alfthan G, Erlund I, Kivimaki H, Paju A, Salminen I, Turpeinen U, Voutilainen S, Laakso J. 2016. Food and nutrient intake and nutritional status of Finnish vegans and non-vegetarians. *PLoS One* 11(2):e0148235.

Fidler MC, Davidsson L, Zeder C, Hurrell RF. 2004. Erythorbic acid is a potent enhancer of nonheme-iron absorption. *Am J Clin Nutr* 79(1):99–102.

Food and Nutrition Board, Institute of Medicine. 1997. Dietary Reference Intakes for calcium, phosphorus, magnesium, vitamin D and fluoride. Washington, DC: National Academy Press.

Food and Nutrition Board, Institute of Medicine. 1998. Dietary Reference Intakes for thiamin, riboflavin, niacin, vitamin B6, folate, vitamin B12, pantothenic acid, biotin, and choline. Washington, DC: National Academy Press.

Food and Nutrition Board, Institute of Medicine. 2001. Dietary Reference Intakes for vitamin A, vitamin K, arsenic, boron, chromium, copper, iodine, iron, manganese, molybdenum, nickel, silicon, vanadium, and zinc. Washington, DC: National Academy Press.

Food and Nutrition Board, Institute of Medicine. 2005. Dietary Reference Intakes for energy, carbohydrate, fiber, fat, fatty acids, cholesterol, protein, and amino acids. Washington, DC: National Academy Press.

Forman JP, Curhan GC, Taylor EN. 2008. Plasma 25-hydroxyvitamin D levels and risk of incident hypertension among young women. *Hypertension* 52(5):828–32.

Foster M, Chu A, Petocz P, Samman S. 2013. Effect of vegetarian diets on zinc status: A systematic review and meta-analysis of studies in humans. *J Sci Food Agric* 93(10):2362–71.

Foster M, Herulah UN, Prasad A, Petocz P, Samman S. 2015. Zinc status of vegetarians during pregnancy: A systematic review of observational studies and meta-analysis of zinc intake. *Nutrients* 7(6):4512–25.

Foster M. Samman S. 2015. Vegetarian diets across the lifecycle: Impact on zinc intake and status. *Adv Food Nutr Res* 74:93–131.

Fuller MF, Reeds PJ. 1998. Nitrogen cycling in the gut. *Annu Rev Nutr* 18:385–411.

Fung TT, van Dam RM, Hankinson SE, Stampfer M, Willett WC, Hu FB. 2010. Low-carbohydrate diets and all-cause and cause-specific mortality: Two cohort studies. *Ann Intern Med* 153(5):289–98.

Garcia-Casal MN, Layrisse M, Solano L. 1998. Vitamin A and beta-carotene can improve nonheme iron absorption from rice, wheat and corn by humans. *J Nutr* 128:646–50.

Gautam S, Platel K, Srinivasan K. 2011. Influence of combinations of promoter and inhibitor on the bioaccessibility of iron and zinc from food grains. *Int J Food Sci Nutr* 62(8):826–34.

Geissler C, Powers HJ, Garrow JS. 2005. *Human Nutrition.* Edinburgh: Elsevier/Churchill Livingstone.

Gibson RS, Heath A-LM, Szymlek-Gay EA. 2014. Is iron and zinc nutrition a concern for vegetarian infants and young children in industrialized countries? *Am J Clin Nutr* 100(Suppl. 1):459S–68S.

Gibson RS, Perlas L, Hotz C. 2006. Improving the bioavailability of nutrients in plant foods at the household level. *Proc Nutr Soc* 65(2):160–8.

Gilsing AM, Crowe FL, Lloyd-Wright Z, Sanders TA, Appleby PN, Allen NE, Key TJ. 2010. Serum concentrations of vitamin B12 and folate in British male omnivores, vegetarians and vegans: Results from a cross-sectional analysis of the EPIC-Oxford cohort study. *Eur J Clin Nutr* 64(9):933–9.

Haider LM, Schwingshackl L, Hoffmann G, Ekmekcioglu C. 2016. The effect of vegetarian diets on iron status in adults: A systematic review and meta-analysis. *Crit Rev Food Sci Nutr* 23:0. doi: 10.1080/10408398.2016.1259210.

Halkjaer J, Olsen A, Overvad K, Jakobsen MU, Boeing H, Buijsse B, Palli D et al. 2010. Intake of total, animal and plant protein and subsequent changes in weight or waist circumference in European men and women: The Diogenes project. *Int J Obes (Lond)* 35(8):1104–13.

Hallberg L. 1981. Bioavailability of dietary iron in man. *Annu Rev Nutr* 1:123–47.

Hallberg L, Hulthen L. 2000. Prediction of dietary iron absorption: An algorithm for calculating absorption and bioavailability of dietary iron. *Am J Clin Nutr* 71(5):1147–60.

Harvey LJ, Armah CN, Dainty JR, Foxall RJ, John Lewis D, Langford NJ, Fairweather-Tait SJ. 2005. Impact of menstrual blood loss and diet on iron deficiency among women in the UK. *Br J Nutr* 94(4):557–64.

Heaney RP, Weaver CM, Fitzsimmons ML. 1991. Soybean phytate content: Effect on calcium absorption. *Am J Clin Nutr* 53:745–47.

Herrmann W, Schorr H, Purschwitz K, Rassoul F, Richter V. 2001. Total homocysteine, vitamin B12, and total antioxidant status in vegetarians. *Clin Chem* 47:1094–101.

Holick MF. 2008. The vitamin D deficiency pandemic and consequences for nonskeletal health: Mechanisms of action. *Mol Aspects Med* 29:361–8.

Holick MF, Biancuzzo RM, Chen TC, Klein EK, Young A, Bibuld D, Reitz R, Salameh W, Ameri A, Tannenbaum AD. 2008. Vitamin D2 is as effective as vitamin D3 in maintaining circulating concentrations of 25-hydroxyvitamin D. *J Clin Endocrinol Metab* 93:677–81.

Huang L, Drake VJ, Ho E. 2015. Zinc. *Adv Nutr* 6(2):224–6.

Hunt JR. 2002. Moving toward a plant-based diet: Are iron and zinc at risk? *Nutr Rev* 60(5 Pt. 1):127–34.

Hunt JR. 2003. Bioavailability of iron, zinc, and other trace minerals from vegetarian diets. *Am J Clin Nutr* 78(3 Suppl.):633S–9S.

Hunt JR, Roughead ZK. 1999. Nonheme-iron absorption, fecal ferritin excretion, and blood indexes of iron status in women consuming controlled lactoovovegetarian diets for 8 wk. *Am J Clin Nutr* 69(5):944–52.

Hurrell R, Egli I. 2010. Iron bioavailability and dietary reference values. *Am J Clin Nutr* 91(5):1461S–7S.

Hurrell RF, Reddy M, Cook JD. 1999. Inhibition of non-haem iron absorption in man by polyphenolic-containing beverages. *Br J Nutr* 81(4):289–95.

Jacobsen TA. 2008. Role of n-3 fatty acids in the treatment of hypertriglyceridemia and cardiovascular disease. *Am J Clin Nutr* 87(Suppl.):981S–90S.

Jensen CL, Prager TC, Fraley JK, Chen H, Anderson RE, Heird WC. 1997. Effect of dietary linoleic/alpha-linolenic acid ratio on growth and visual function of term infants. *J Pediatr* 131(2):200–9.

Jung UJ, Torrejon C, Tighe AP, Deckelbaum RJ. 2008. n-3 fatty acids and cardiovascular disease: Mechanisms underlying beneficial effects. *Am J Clin Nutr* 87(Suppl.):2003S–9S.

Kamweru PK, Tindibale EL. 2016. Vitamin D and vitamin D from ultraviolet-irradiated mushrooms [review]. *Int J Med Mushrooms* 18(3):205–14.

Keegan RJ, Lu Z, Bogusz JM, Williams JE, Holick MF. 2013. Photobiology of vitamin D in mushrooms and its bioavailability in humans. *Dermatoendocrinology* 5(1):165–76.

Kimmig LM, Karalis DG. 2013. Do omega-3 polyunsaturated fatty acids prevent cardiovascular disease? A review of the randomized clinical trials. *Lipid Insights* 6:13–20.

King JC. 2011. Zinc: An essential but elusive nutrient. *Am J Clin Nutr* 94(2):679S–84S.

Knurick JR, Johnston CS, Wherry SJ, Aguayo I. 2015. Comparison of correlates of bone mineral density in individuals adhering to lacto-ovo, vegan or omnivore diets: A cross-sectional investigation. *Nutrients* 7(5):3416–26. doi: 10.3390/nu7053416.

Kostoglou-Athanassiou I, Athanassiou P, Gkountouvas A, Kaldrymides P. 2013. Vitamin D and glycemic control in diabetes mellitus type 2. *Ther Adv Endocrinol Metab* 4(4):122–8.

Krebs NF, Hambidge KM. 1986. Zinc requirements and zinc intakes of breast-fed infants. *Am J Clin Nutr* 43(2):288–92.

Kurtz TW, Al-Bander HA, Morris RC. 1987. "Salt sensitive" essential hypertension in men. *N Engl J Med* 317:1043–8.

Lane K, Derbyshire E, Li W, Brennan C. 2014. Bioavailability and potential uses of vegetarian sources of omega-3 fatty acids: A review of the literature. *Crit Rev Food Sci Nutr* 54(5):572–9.

Lim KH, Riddell LJ, Nowson CA, Booth AO, Szymlek-Gay EA. 2013. Iron and zinc nutrition in the economically-developed world: A review. *Nutrients* 5(8):3184–211. doi: 10.3390/nu5083184.

Lindenbaum J, Rosenberg IH, Wilson PWF, Stabler SB, Allen RH. 1994. Prevalence of cobalamin deficiency in the Framingham elderly population. *Am J Clin Nutr* 60:2–11.

Lonnerdal B. 2000. Dietary factors influencing zinc absorption. *J Nutr* 130(5S Suppl.):1378S–83S.

Lonnerdal B. 2009. Soybean ferritin: Implications for iron status of vegetarians. *Am J Clin Nutr* 89(5):1680S–5S.

Madry E, Lisowska A, Grebowiec P, Walkowiak J. 2012. The impact of vegan diet on B-12 status in healthy omnivores: Five-year prospective study. *Acta Sci Pol Technol Aliment* 11(2):209–12.

Makrides M, Neumann MA, Jeffrey B, Lien EL, Gibson RA. 2000. A randomized trial of different ratios of linoleic to alpha-linolenic acid in the diet of term infants: Effects on visual function and growth. *Am J Clin Nutr* 71(1):120–9.

Mangels AR. 2014. Bone nutrients for vegetarians. *Am J Clin Nutr* 100(Suppl. 1):469S–75S.

Mangels R, Messina V, Messina M. 2011. The dietitian's guide to vegetarian diets: Issues and applications. Sudbury, MA: Jones & Bartlett Learning.

Marsh KA, Munn EA, Baines SK. 2013. Protein and vegetarian diets. *Med J Aust* 199(4 Suppl.):S7–10.

Marsh KA, Zeuschner C, Saunders A. 2012. Health implications of a vegetarian diet: A review. *Am J Lifestyle Med* 6(3):250–67.

Martins JG. 2009. EPA but not DHA appears to be responsible for the efficacy of omega-3 long chain polyunsaturated fatty acid supplementation in depression: Evidence from a meta-analysis of randomized controlled trials. *J Am Coll Nutr* 28(5):525–42.

Melina V, Craig W, Levin S. 2016. Position of the Academy of Nutrition and Dietetics: Vegetarian diets. *J Acad Nutr Diet* 116(12):1970–80.

Miller JZ, Smith DL, Flora L, Slemenda C, Jiang X, Johnston CC Jr. 1988. Calcium absorption from calcium carbonate and a new form of calcium (CCM) in healthy male and female adolescents. *Am J Clin Nutr* 48:1291–4.

Obeid R, Fedosov SN, Nexo E. 2015. Cobalamin coenzyme forms are not likely to be superior to cyano- and hydroxyl-cobalamin in prevention or treatment of cobalamin deficiency. *Mol Nutr Food Res* 59(7):1364–72.

Obeid R, Geisel J, Schorr H, Hubner U. Herrmann W. 2002. The impact of vegetarianism on some haematological parameters. *Eur J Haematol* 69(5–6):275–9.

O'Connor H, Munas Z, Griffin H, Rooney K, Cheng HL, Steinbeck K. 2011. Nutritional adequacy of energy restricted diets for young obese women. *Asia Pac J Clin Nutr* 20(2):206–11.

Otten JJ, Hellwig JP, Meyers LD. 2006. *DRI, Dietary Reference Intakes: The Essential Guide to Nutrient Requirements.* Washington DC: National Academy Press.

Outila TA, Karkkainen MU, Seppanen RH, Lamberg-Allardt CJ. 2000. Dietary intake of vitamin D in premenopausal, healthy vegans was insufficient to maintain concentrations of serum 25-hydroxyvitamin D and intact parathyroid hormone within normal ranges during the winter in Finland. *J Am Diet Assoc* 100(4):434–41.

Park SK, Ryoo JH, Kim MG, Shin JY. 2012. Association of serum ferritin and the development of metabolic syndrome in middle-aged Korean men: A 5-year follow-up study. *Diabetes Care* 35(12):2521–6.

Parsons TJ, van Dusseldorp M, van der Vliet M, van de Werken K, Schaafsma G, van Staveren WA. 1997. Reduced bone mass in Dutch adolescents fed a macrobiotic diet in early life. *J Bone Miner Res* 12:1486–94.

Patrick L. 1999. Comparative absorption of calcium sources and calcium citrate malate for the prevention of osteoporosis. *Altern Med Rev* 4(2):74–85.

Pludowski P, Holick MF, Grant WB, Konstantynowicz J, Mascarenhas MR, Haq A, Povoroznyuk V et al. 2017. Vitamin D guidelines. *J Steroid Biochem Mol Biol.* doi: 10.1016/j.jsbmb.2017.01.021.

Qi L, van Dam RM, Rexrode K, Hu FB. 2007. Heme iron from diet as a risk factor for coronary heart disease in women with type 2 diabetes. *Diabetes Care* 30(1):101–6.

Rizzo G, Lagana AS, Rapisarda AMC, La Ferrera GMG, Buscema M, Rossetti P, Nigro A et al. 2016. Vitamin B12 among vegetarians: Status, assessment and supplementation. *Nutrients* 8(12):E767. doi: 10.3390/nu8120767.

Rizzo NS, Jaceldo-Siegl K, Sabate J, Fraser GE. 2013. Nutrient profiles of vegetarian and nonvegetarian dietary patterns. *J Acad Nutr Diet* 113(12):1610–9.

Rosell MS, Lloyd-Wright Z, Appleby PN, Sanders TA, Allen NE, Key TJ. 2005. Long-chain n-3 polyunsaturated fatty acids in plasma in British meat-eating, vegetarian, and vegan men. *Am J Clin Nutr* 82(2):327–4.

Samman S. 2007a. Iron. *Nutr Diet* 64:S126–30.

Samman S. 2007b. Zinc. *Nutr Diet* 64:S131–4.

Sanders TA. 2009. DHA status of vegetarians. *Prostaglandins Leukot Essent Fatty Acids* 81(2–3):137–41.

Sanders TA. 2014. Plant compared with marine n-3 fatty acid effects on cardiovascular risk factors and outcomes: What is the verdict? *Am J Clin Nutr* 100(Suppl. 1):453S–8S.

Sarter B, Kelsey KS, Schwartz TA, Harris WS. 2015. Blood docosahexaenoic acid and eicosapentaenoic acid in vegans: Associations with age and gender and effects of an algal-derived omega-3 fatty acid supplement. *Clin Nutr* 34(2):212–8.

Saunders AV, Craig WJ, Baines SK. 2013a. Zinc and vegetarian diets. *Med J Aust* 199(4 Suppl.):S17–21.

Saunders AV, Craig WJ, Baines SK, Posen JS. 2013b. Iron and vegetarian diets. *Med J Aust* 199(4 Suppl.):S11–16.

Saunders AV, Davis BC, Garg ML. 2013c. Omega-3 polyunsaturated fatty acids and vegetarian diets. *Med J Aust* 199(4 Suppl.):S22–6.

Savage GP, Dubois M. 2006. The effect of soaking and cooking on the oxalate content of taro leaves. *Int J Food Sci Nutr* 57(5–6):376–81.

Schupbach R, Wegmuller R, Berguerand C, Bui M, Herter-Aeberli I. 2017. Micronutrient status and intake in omnivores, vegetarians and vegans in Switzerland. *Eur J Nutr* 56(1):283–93. doi: 10.1007/s00394-015-1079-7.

Scientific Advisory Committee on Nutrition. 2011. Iron and health report. Department of Health. Norwich, UK: The Stationery Office.

Spencer EA, Appleby PN, Davey GK, Key TJ. 2003. Diet and body mass index in 38000 EPIC-Oxford meat-eaters, fish-eaters, vegetarians and vegans. *Int J Obes Relat Metab Disord* 27(6):728–34.

Theil EC, Chen H, Miranda C, Janser H, Elsenhans B, Nunez MT, Pizarro F, Schumann K. 2012. Absorption of iron from ferritin is independent of heme iron and ferrous salts in women and rat intestinal segments. *J Nutr* 142(3):478–83.

Tripkovic L, Lambert H, Hart K, Smith CP, Bucca G, Penson S, Chope G, Hyppönen E, Berry J, Vieth R, Lanham-New S. 2012. Comparison of vitamin D2 and vitamin D3 supplementation in raising serum 25-hydroxyvitamin D status: A systematic review and meta-analysis. *Am J Clin Nutr* 95(6):1357–64.

Tucker KL. 2014. Vegetarian diets and bone status. *Am J Clin Nutr* 100(Suppl.):329S–35S.

Van Asselt DZ, van den Broek WJ, Lamers CB, Corstens FH, Hoefnagels WH. 1996. Free and protein-bound cobalamin absorption in healthy middle-aged and older subjects. *J Am Geriatr Soc* 44:949–53.

Van Gelder BM, Tijhuis M, Kalmijn S, Kromhout D. 2007. Fish consumption, n-3 fatty acids, and subsequent 5-y cognitive decline in elderly men: The Zutphen Elderly Study. *Am J Clin Nutr* 85(4):1142–7.

Wallace TC, Reider C, Fulgoni VL. 2013. Calcium and vitamin D disparities are related to gender, age, race, household income level, and weight classification but not vegetarian status in the United States: Analysis of the NHANES 2001–2008 data set. *J Am Coll Nutr* 32(5):321–30.

Watanabe F. 2007. Vitamin B12 sources and bioavailability. *Exp Biol Med* 232(10):1266–74.

Watanabe F, Yabuta Y, Bito T, Teng F. 2014. Vitamin B12-containing plant food sources for vegetarians. *Nutrients* 6:1861–73. doi: 10.3390/nu6051861.

Watanabe F, Yabuta Y, Tanioka Y, Bito T. 2013. Biologically active vitamin B12 compounds in foods for preventing deficiency among vegetarians and elderly subjects. *J Agric Food Chem* 61:6769–75. doi: 10.1021/jf401545z.

Weaver CM, Proulx WR, Heaney R. 1999. Choices for achieving adequate dietary calcium with a vegetarian diet. *Am J Clin Nutr* 70:543S–8S.

Welch AA, Shakya-Shrestha S, Lentjes MA, Wareham NJ, Khaw KT. 2010. Dietary intake and status of n-3 polyunsaturated fatty acids in a population of fish-eating and non-fish-eating meat-eaters, vegetarians, and vegans and the precursor-product ratio of {alpha}-linolenic acid to long-chain n-3 polyunsaturated fatty acids: Results from the EPIC-Norfolk cohort. *Am J Clin Nutr* 92(5):1040–51.

White DL, Collinson A. 2013. Red meat, dietary heme iron, and risk of type 2 diabetes: The involvement of advanced lipoxidation endproducts. *Adv Nutr* 4(4):403–11.

Whittaker PG, Barrett JF, Lind T. 2001. The erythrocyte incorporation of absorbed non-haem iron in pregnant women. *Br J Nutr* 86(3):323–9.

Williams CM, Burdge G. 2006. Long-chain n-3 PUFA: Plant v. marine sources. *Proc Nutr Soc* 65(1):42–50.

Wilson AK, Ball MJ. 1999. Nutrient intake and iron status of Australian male vegetarians. *Eur J Clin Nutr* 53(3):189–94.

World Health Organization. 2001. Iron deficiency anaemia assessment, prevention and control. Geneva: World Health Organization.

Wuehler SE, Peerson JM, Brown KH. 2005. Use of national food balance data to estimate the adequacy of zinc in national food supplies: Methodology and regional estimates. *Public Health Nutr* 8(7):812–9.

Zhao Y, Martin BR, Weaver CM. 2005. Calcium bioavailability of calcium carbonate fortified soymilk is equivalent to cow's milk in young women. *J Nutr* 135:2379–82.

Zielinska-Dawidziak M. 2015. Plant ferritin—A source of iron to prevent its deficiency. *Nutrients* 7(2):1184–201. doi: 10.3390/nu7021184.

Section V

Vegetarian Issues in Ethnic Groups

11 Vegetarian Practices among Asian Indians and Their Risk of Disease

Sudha Raj

CONTENTS

SUMMARY

Asian Indians, one of the fastest-growing immigrant groups in the United States, face an increased risk for diabetes, metabolic syndrome, and coronary artery disease compared with Caucasians and other ethnic populations. Coronary artery disease is the leading cause of death in this ethnic group. The risk profile called the Asian Indian phenotype is prevalent across all socioeconomic strata, with younger adults and the underprivileged being the most vulnerable. The risk profile exists despite the long-standing tradition of a plant-based diet and is characterized by abdominal obesity, glucose intolerance, and atherogenic dyslipidemia exacerbated by an unhealthy lifestyle and dietary practices. Health professionals working with Asian Indians must recognize that the currently consumed Asian Indian vegetarian diet may not be consistent with optimal health and wellness. Nutrition education interventions must be tailored to tackle a wide spectrum of chronic health conditions. The total lifestyle and dietary patterns must be addressed within a familiar sociocultural context.

11.1   INTRODUCTION

The World Health Organization (WHO) projects that the current global burden of nutrition and lifestyle-related chronic diseases and/or health conditions, such as diabetes, cardiovascular disease, hypertension, arthritis, chronic obstructive pulmonary disease, and their associated morbidities, will exponentially increase by 2030 and beyond (Maskari, 2010). The proportion of global deaths due to noncommunicable (chronic) diseases (NCDs) or chronic degenerative diseases is projected to increase to 55 million by 2030 (WHO, 2013). NCDs result in functional disabilities, loss in productivity, a decline in the gross domestic product of the nation, poor quality of life, and compounding healthcare costs (Siegel et al., 2014). Of concern is the fact that NCDs will disproportionately affect large proportions of the world's population, particularly in the developing world, at a very rapid pace, albeit much earlier in life (Popkin, 1994; Ford et al., 2017). Epidemiological surveys point out that noncommunicable chronic diseases account for 63% of all deaths on a global scale; 80% of all NCD-related deaths occur in developing countries (Shetty, 2013).

In 2013, the Institute for Health Metrics and Evaluation (IHME) identified the Indian subcontinent as a high-priority South Asia region (India, Pakistan, Bangladesh, Nepal, Bhutan, Maldives, and Sri Lanka) facing a dichotomy of public health concerns where undernutrition and overnutrition coexist, also termed as the double burden of disease (IHME, 2013). Significant strides have accrued related to the mitigation of long-standing infectious and nutritional deficiency diseases as seen by the achievement of the Millennium Development Goals (MDGs) (Lomazzi et al., 2014); however, the crisis is far from resolution. Rising population challenges, socioeconomic bias, and limited access to quality healthcare for many segments in the population are limitations hindering greater success in the eradication of undernutrition and its associated maladies (Haddad et al., 2015).

Meanwhile, the subcontinent, like many low- and middle-income countries (LMICs), is amidst rapid epidemiological, demographic, and lifestyle transitions that are at least partially responsible for exponential increases in nutrition-related noncommunicable diseases (NR-NCDs), particularly diabetes, obesity, cancer, and cardiovascular disease (Gayathri et al., 2016). The magnitude of these shifts, along with an accelerated pace in the LMICs, the age at which NCDs appear, and their associated morbidities and mortalities compared with similar changes in the industrialized world, is unique (Popkin, 2002). Further, the healthcare infrastructures, although progressive, continue to be limited in resources and personnel in these countries. The healthcare system originally designed to address the burden associated with undernutrition at present is unable to handle the weight of overnutrition simultaneously (Shrivastava et al., 2017). Although several small-scale governmental and nongovernmental programs are underway to address these issues across the life span, their long-term impact is unknown at present (Gayathri et al., 2016).

11.2   ASIAN INDIANS IN THE UNITED STATES

The U.S. Census Bureau first designated the term *Asian Indian* in 1980 to describe immigrants originating from the Asian subcontinent of India (Williams, 1988), consequently avoiding misrepresentation with the indigenous people of the Americas or American Indians (Bhopal, 2004). Credited as among the fastest-growing immigrant groups in the United States, currently more than 3 million Asian Indians live in the United States. Asian Indians account for nearly 5% of the 41.3 million foreign-born people in the United States (New America Media, 2012). The first wave of Asian Indian immigrants came to the United States via Canada in the nineteenth century to work as farmers in California. Subsequently, the liberalization of immigration and naturalization laws in 1965, coupled with legislation that opened opportunities for highly skilled professionals, provided a gateway for a growing number of students pursuing higher education, professionals in the medical and engineering fields, and their dependents (spouses, children, parents, and siblings) (Bagai, 1972; Williams, 1988). While this trend continues, further refinements to the Immigration Act of 1990 broadened the scope of work for temporary skilled workers and increased the number of permanent work-based visas (Zong and Batalova, 2015). Many of these immigrants chose to stay in the United States, while others opted to return to their homeland. Since the 1990s, the accelerated expansion of the information technology sector and the need for service professionals in the hospitality, food, and other service sectors have further contributed to the population's dramatic growth in the United States. The largest settlement of Asian Indian immigrants in the United States is in the state of California (19%), followed by New Jersey (11%) and Texas (9%). Santa Clara County in California and Middlesex, Cook, and Alameda Counties in New Jersey, Illinois, and California, respectively, account for 15% of the total Asian Indian immigrant population in the United States (Zong and Batalova, 2015).

11.3 NONCOMMUNICABLE DISEASES IN ASIAN INDIANS

Regardless of geographic location and ethnicity, NCDs are a global public health challenge in the twenty-first century, accounting for a sizable proportion of morbidity and mortality (Kruk et al., 2015). Nearly two-thirds of worldwide deaths are attributed to NCDs, and obesity continues to plague nearly 600 million with a body mass index (BMI) greater than or equal to 30 (Bauer et al., 2014). In 2015, more than 400 million had diabetes on a worldwide basis, while cardiovascular disease accounted for 31% of global deaths (WHO, 2015). Sixty percent of all deaths and 44% of disability-adjusted life-years (DALYs) in India were lost in 2011 to NCDs, making them a public health challenge demanding immediate attention (Shrivastava et al., 2017). In India, cardiovascular disease accounted for 26% of all deaths; 13%, 7%, and 2% were due to chronic respiratory diseases, cancer, and diabetes, respectively. Twenty million suffer from mental health conditions, while 28% of the population still suffers from communicable, maternal, perinatal, and nutritional conditions (WHO, 2015). Recent reviews indicate that obesity affects more than 135 million individuals in India (Misra and Khurana, 2011; Misra and Shrivastava, 2013); the age-adjusted prevalence of diabetes in India increased from 6.7% in 2006 to 9.3% in 2014 compared with the U.S. prevalence rates of 7.8% and 10.8%, respectively (IDF, 2006, 2015). By 2030, 35% of all cardiovascular disease deaths in India will occur in individuals between 35 and 64 years of age, compared with 12% for the United States (Jaacks et al., 2016).

In the United States, Asian Indian immigrants, compared with Caucasians and other ethnic groups, are at a similar risk for NCDs (type 2 diabetes, coronary artery disease, obesity, and insulin resistance) (Dodani, 2008; Liem et al., 2009). The Multi-Ethnic Study of Atherosclerosis (MESA) reported that Indian immigrants in the United States are at a higher risk for type 2 diabetes and coronary artery disease (Kanaya et al., 2010). Hypertension, fatty liver disease, and visceral adiposity were associated with prediabetes, while increased carotid intima thickness and microalbuminuria were associated with subclinical atherosclerosis. Coronary heart disease is the leading cause of death in Asian Indians regardless of their geographic residence, and it occurs a decade earlier than in other ethnic groups (Nair and Prabhakaran, 2012). This risk profile is prevalent across all socioeconomic strata of the Asian Indian society, with the underprivileged being most vulnerable.

The NCD etiology is complex, interlinked, and multifactorial. A common thread of chronic subclinical inflammation and concomitant oxidative stress underlies its pathology (Baker, 2008). The exacerbated cardiometabolic risk based on pathophysiology and life course–related risk factors for Asian Indians, regardless of geographic residence, has been documented. This translates to a higher risk relative to other ethnic populations and Caucasians (Jayashree et al., 2015). Despite the paucity of large sample studies, this risk profile, termed the "South Asian or Asian Indian phenotype" (Patel et al., 2016), occurs at a lower BMI and younger age than would be considered normal for other populations (Enas et al., 2007; Unnikrishnan et al., 2014).

11.4   ASIAN INDIAN PHENOTYPE AND ITS RELATIONSHIP TO NCD RISK

The South Asian or Asian Indian phenotype profile, or the "thin–fat phenotype" (Narayan, 2016), is marked by a consistent cluster of physiological, anatomical, and/or biochemical anomalies. Abdominal obesity, glucose intolerance, and atherogenic dyslipidemia are its major features. These are precursors for type 2 diabetes, metabolic syndrome, and coronary artery disease (Pandey et al., 2015). Asian Indians at any BMI and age generally have a short stature and higher body fat, visceral fat, and waist circumference, with lower skeletal mass, short legs, and thinner hips. The thin–fat phenotype's body composition features higher centrally distributed body fat and truncal, subcutaneous, and intra-abdominal fat, at a lower lean body mass than that of other populations (Misra and Shrivastava, 2013). Smaller lean body masses contribute to diabetes risk through decreased glucose tolerance and a prematurely compromised beta-cell function (Pandey et al., 2015), often dependent on fetal programming, maternal nourishment, and physiology (Langley-Evans, 2015). The risk exacerbates upon exposure to a milieu featuring higher glycemic loads and decreased physical activity.

Evolutionary biologists describe the pathophysiology of this variability in diabetes risk as the "capacity-load model" (Wells et al., 2016), illustrating the relationship between metabolic capacity and metabolic load. Small stature and compromised beta-cell function are components of metabolic capacity dictated by fetal programming and early infant growth, while adiposity, dietary glycemic load, and degree of physical activity comprise the metabolic load. Based on data from three U.S. cohorts, it is evident that the diabetes risk is minimal, with a low metabolic load, while a high load intensifies this risk (Li et al., 2015). The thin–fat phenotype has an evolutionary basis resulting from a combination of three factors over centuries: (1) the ecological disturbances to the food supply in a primarily agrarian society, contributing to cycles of plenty and want; (2) interactions between these disturbances, population expansion, and access to food; and (3) the expansion of the vegetarian ethic coupled with compromised lactase digestive capacity, leading to nutritional deficiencies resulting from low protein and micronutrient consumption (Mohan et al., 2007; Anjana et al., 2011; Wells et al., 2016). Consequently, genotypes that favored a short stature, lower lean mass, and larger fat stores evolved over the centuries. This translates into a lower metabolic capacity; in other words, the body adapted to traditional, indigenous diets that provided fewer nutritional resources yet were sufficient for survival. Combined with high physical activity characteristic of traditional agrarian societies, this metabolic capacity was efficient at handling dietary glycemic loads within limits and NCDs, for example, diabetes, were in check (Eaton et al., 1988; Moore et al., 2001). However, in modern times the tables have turned.

Lifestyle practices, including nutrition, physical activity, catchup growth in early childhood, and determinants such as family and work life stress, exacerbate the risk (Bosma-den Boer et al., 2012). Nevertheless, it appears that the body composition trajectory is determined at birth as either a genetic predisposition to a short stature or the result of the impact of maternal physiology and anatomy (Elshenawy and Simmons, 2016). The prenatal and infancy windows are critical during fetal development and depend on optimal nutrition and determine lean mass development. Indian women tend to have a short stature and smaller pelvic dimensions than European populations (Kramer, 1987; Martyn et al., 1996). At low BMIs, suboptimal nutrition and/or nutrient deficiencies stemming from a lifelong pattern of vegetarianism, for example protein and vitamin B12, concomitant to these anatomical constraints limit fetal development (Yajnik et al., 2008). Low birth weights; suboptimal fetal organ development, for example, the size and number of beta-cells; and lower lean muscle tissue are consequences as the organism exerts an effort to spare nutrients for critical entities, such as the developing brain (Padmanabhan et al., 2016). Lean mass deficits decrease glucose tolerance, reduce oxidative capacity and fatty acid utilization, and in combination with reduced beta-cell function, contribute to insulin resistance in early adulthood. Cross-sectional studies comparing South Asian neonates with their Caucasian counterparts (Yajnik et al., 2002; Boon et al., 2012; Stanfield et al., 2012) point out that South Asian neonates of normal as well as low birth weight have less fat-free mass and smaller abdominal, midarm, and head circumferences even after accounting for their overall small size—weight and length. However, their higher subscapular skinfold thickness is interpreted as an indicator of future truncal fat deposition and a relatively higher adipose tissue composition in adult life.

Muscle mass is an indicator of insulin sensitivity; the literature supports that a lower muscle mass is generally inefficient in terms of glucose uptake and glycogen synthesis (Pandey et al., 2015). This is especially disconcerting for the Asian Indian phenotype whose high carbohydrate intake is typical of the traditional diet. Consequently, energy fuels from the large carbohydrate meals get routed into hepatic *de novo* lipogenesis (Boden, 1997; McGarry, 2002). Studies comparing insulin-resistant individuals to insulin-sensitive individuals after a high-carbohydrate meal note that hyperinsulinemia is the cellular signaling mechanism that drives the enhanced expression of key lipogenic enzymes (Kodama et al., 2013). Triglycerides are exported as very low-density lipoproteins (LDLs) into the peripheral and visceral adipose tissue, predisposing to an increase in abdominal obesity. Insulin resistance therefore becomes a forbearer of metabolic syndrome by increasing the prevalence of hyperinsulinemia and glucose intolerance while independently influencing abdominal obesity and the associated dyslipidemia that follows (Misra and Khurana, 2009).

11.5 ATHEROGENIC DYSLIPIDEMIA PROFILE IN ASIAN INDIANS

Epidemiological studies on Asian Indians within India (Ghaffar et al., 2004) and elsewhere (Anand et al., 2000; Bainey and Jugdutt, 2009) point out certain pro-atherogenic dyslipidemia patterns unique to this ethnic population. These include a high ratio of total cholesterol to high-density lipoproteins (HDLs), high levels of a small dense fraction of LDLs (lipoprotein A) (Joshi et al., 2007), and nonesterified fatty acids along with low levels of a dysfunctional HDL (Prabhakaran et al., 2005). Nearly 50% of the Asian Indian population has lower than normal HDL levels attributed to their dietary habits (Radhika et al., 2009). This is of significance in the Asian Indian who has an increased susceptibility to insulin resistance and consumes a refined grain-rich, carbohydrate-dense diet. The consequence is a higher glycemic load that is suggested to encourage a pro-atherogenic profile marked by elevated triglyceride, LDL, lipoprotein A concentration, and fatty acid production in the liver and decreased action of lipoprotein lipase through increased apolipoprotein CIII production with decreased HDL concentrations. Further, the HDL functions in a dysfunctional, pro-inflammatory role. It prevents the apolipoprotein A-1 clearance, promoting LDL-derived lipid oxidation (Dodani et al., 2008). Raised plasma levels of fibrinogen, plasminogen activator inhibitor 1 (PAI-1), and lipoprotein A (Bainey and Jugdutt, 2009) further exacerbate the risk. Lipoprotein A modulates coronary artery disease progression by sharing a structural similarity to plasminogen. It attaches to fibrin binding sites by displacing plasminogen, thereby increasing platelet activity while decreasing endogenous fibrinolytic activity (Nair and Prabhakaran, 2012). A potential thrombogenic risk factor is the increased platelet activity in patients with diabetes and coronary artery disease, as shown in the Chennai Urban Population Study (CUPS) (Deepa et al., 2006).

Another feature of the Asian Indian dyslipidemia phenotype is the high levels of the inflammatory marker C-reactive protein (CRP). This association is reported in few studies yet points to the possibility of CRP as an independent risk factor for coronary artery disease (Mohan et al., 2005). The characteristic abdominal obesity is a source of pro-inflammatory cytokines, such as interleukin 6, a determinant of hepatic CRP synthesis (Libby, 2013; Kamath et al., 2015).

Another well-documented risk factor that contributes to the NCD predisposition in Asian Indians is the elevated levels of homocysteine. Hyperhomocysteinemia in Asian Indians results from a widespread deficiency of vitamin B12, suggested as a consequence of the long-term use of a vegetarian diet (Yajnik et al., 2006). A combination of oxidative stress, systemic inflammation, endothelial dysfunction (Chauhan et al., 2012), altered protein functionality (Thaler et al., 2011), and abnormal gene expression is documented to mediate the effects on coronary artery disease and type 2 diabetes. Alterations in the functioning of the methyl tetrahydrofolate reductase (MTHFR) enzyme are a known mechanism in the elevation of homocysteine levels in the folate vitamin B12 metabolic pathway. C677T and A1298C gene variants contribute to defects in the MTHFR gene, resulting in metabolic aberrations with NCD consequences. The effect of these polymorphisms was examined in more than 400 individuals from different subethnic populations in India based on linguistic lineage and geographic location. The predominance of the A1298C polymorphism was identified as a potential risk factor. This etiological factor warrants further investigation to identify contributors to the chronic disease paradigm. An examination of the association between homocysteine levels and the two polymorphisms in hypertensive patients showed that the presence of either allele C677T or 1298CC genotypes increased the risk of hypertension. Patients with the MTHFR 1298CC genotype had significantly higher homocysteine levels than those with the 1298AA genotype (Markan et al., 2007).

A study involving more than 700 Asian Indian women during and 5 years after delivery showed that B12 deficiency with adequate folate status in pregnancy was associated with a higher BMI, insulin resistance, and incidence of gestational diabetes than it was in nondeficient women (Krishnaveni et al., 2009). Although the mechanism is unclear, it is proposed that cellular folate is trapped as inactive 5-methyl tetrahydrofolate in B12 deficiency, consequently limiting the availability of methyl groups. This results in epigenetic changes in the DNA causing altered protein synthesis and accumulation of methyl malonic acid (MMA) levels arising from the impaired conversion of MMA to succinyl coenzyme A (CoA), leading to an increase in lipogenesis (Yajnik et al., 2006). Although folate does not participate in these pathways, a B12 deficiency concomitant to a higher folate status is associated with high concentrations of homocysteine and MMA (Selhub et al., 2007). It is suggested that the neuropathy associated with severe vitamin B12 deficiency exacerbated by folate is mediated by abnormal fatty acids and their metabolic products (Scott, 1992).

This menacing combination of poor insulin sensitivity and an atherogenic dyslipidemia promotes subclinical chronic inflammation and is strongly associated with type 2 diabetes and cardiovascular disease in Asian Indians. Underlying gene variants, polymorphisms, and telomere status (López-Otín et al., 2013) and vitamin D status (Sapkota et al., 2016) further stoke the metabolic fire. For example, (1) the ectonucleotide pyrophosphate phosphodiesterase 1 (ENPP1) 121 Q variant is implicated in South Indians as negatively influencing insulin receptor signaling (Abate et al., 2005); (2) the DOK5 gene variants are modulators of obesity, thereby increasing diabetes risk in North Indians (Tabassum et al., 2010); (3) the angiotensin-converting enzyme (ACE) insertion/deletion (I/D) and apolipoprotein E (Apo E) Hha I gene polymorphisms are mediators in dyslipidemia and blood glucose regulation in Asian Indians (Das et al., 2013); (4) the K153R and A55T polymorphisms in the Myostatin gene, are promoters of abdominal obesity and low lean body mass in genetically predisposed individuals (Bhatt et al., 2012); (5) the AMDI variant in homocysteine metabolism predisposes children to obesity (Tabassum et al., 2012); and (6) the PPAR gamma polymorphisms contributes to nonalcoholic fatty liver disease (Bhatt et al., 2013).

11.6   ROLE OF EARLY LIFE INFLUENCES

While the quest to identify key metabolic genes and their transcriptional control continues, epidemiologists continue to explore the hypothesis that at least partially credits the cardiometabolic predisposition to early life influences and reduced birthweight (Barker, 2007; Tutino et al., 2014). LMICs struggle to simultaneously handle the double burden of disease consequent to demographic and socioeconomic transitions. In this milieu, there is consensus that undernutrition, obesity, and NCDs are not individual entities but rather a consequence of (1) in utero fetal programming and (2) a subsequent metabolic maladaptation due to a mismatch between the in utero and postnatal environments (Padmanabhan et al., 2016).

In 1986, Barker proposed the *developmental origins of adult disease* or *fetal origins of adult onset disease* (FOAD) hypothesis, which stated that "adverse influences early in development and particularly during intra-uterine life can result in permanent changes in physiology and metabolism which results in increased disease risk in adulthood" (Barker, 2007). The hypothesis focuses on two main principles—developmental programming and metabolic adaptation.

First, environmental factors, including nutrition (poor or excess) and chronic stress marked by elevated glucocorticoid levels, can act as either a stimulus or an insult during critical windows of fetal life, altering tissue and organ development, and structure and function with future consequences as food and lifestyle environments change. For instance, in utero stresses during early development alter mitochondrial activity that influences the function of oxidative phosphorylation linked to skeletal muscle insulin resistance in type 2 diabetics (Befroy et al., 2007). Lowered protein availability can modify beta-cell proliferation, causing alterations in glucose homeostasis (Bruce and Hanson, 2010). Recent reports highlight the links between maternal obesity, gestational diabetes, and future risk of diabetes (Tutino et al., 2014).

Second, a compromised nutritional environment induces the development of a thrifty phenotype with an altered metabolism beneficial to the survival of the fetus and anticipatory of a similar postnatal environment. However, a discrepancy in this expectation occurs upon exposure to a food- and nutrient-rich environment, causing a developmental mismatch and a greater susceptibility to develop metabolic disease (Padmanabhan et al., 2016). A large body of evidence exists that highlights mechanisms yet to be elucidated, such as permanent alterations in cell numbers affecting organ structure and function, and inheritable epigenetic changes that affect DNA methylation patterns consequent to an altered maternal nutrient supply and potentially mediate the metabolic priming process very subtly through modulation of gene expressions (Uauy et al., 2011).

Genetic predispositions, epigenetic influences, developmental programming, socioeconomic status, and education either independently or synergistically mediate the inherent atherogenic and thrombogenic risk factors influencing vulnerability, especially under certain environmental conditions, such as an increased metabolic load (Wells et al., 2016). Industrialization, urbanization, migration, acculturation, and demographic and socioeconomic transitions bring about shifts in dietary and physical activity lifestyle patterns (Egger and Dixon, 2014); exposure to environmental toxins, tobacco, medications (Bosma-den Boer et al., 2012), migration, and family, work, and life stressors (Fernandez et al., 2015) trigger constant activation of the central stress axes, thereby mediating the chronic inflammation process. Unhealthy lifestyle choices, poor health-seeking behaviors (Mehrotra et al., 2012), limited access to quality healthcare, and the inability of the healthcare infrastructure to handle the double burden of infectious and NCD further limit the achievement of positive health outcomes (Shrivastava et al., 2017).

The dramatic increase in NCDs among Asian Indians within India, as well as those who have migrated to other countries, is surprising as there is a long-standing tradition of following a vegetarian diet in this population. A vegetarian, plant-based diet is shown to possess several health-promoting benefits that offer advantages such as fewer calories, a lower saturated fat content, a higher source of dietary fiber, and a host of phytochemicals and antioxidants, all features beneficial in mitigating NCDs (Melina et al., 2016). Questions therefore arise as to the nature and practice of the Asian Indian vegetarian diet, its relationship to the NCD occurrence in Asian Indians, and the need for strategies to reinforce the benefits and value of the traditional diet from a NCD prevention perspective.

11.7 VEGETARIAN ETHIC IN INDIA

Contrary to the Western perspective of vegetarianism as an adopted lifestyle by choice, it is a way of life for one-third of India's population. Asian Indians who follow a vegetarian diet do so for cultural, religious, and spiritual reasons (Agrawal et al., 2014). This dietary practice is transmitted across generations, symbolizing familial traditional values. Unlike Western vegetarians, Asian Indians often do not associate the traditional vegetarian diet with potential to benefit chronic disease. Vegetarianism is a codified lifestyle based on the tenet *Ahimsa parmoh dharmah*, or nonviolence toward all living beings (Balagopal, 2000). The concept of *ahimsa* was introduced between 300 BC and 400 AD by Emperor Ashoka, a strong proponent of Buddhism who banned animal sacrifices and sanctioned prohibitions of animal slaughter. It was further reinforced by religious scriptures and beliefs of Hinduism and Jainism (Tobias, 1991). As a branch of Hinduism, Jainism developed around the time of Buddhism's emergence. Orthodox Jains are strict vegetarians who believe all living things have souls and avoid root vegetables, such as potatoes, carrots, and onions. The daily practice of vegetarianism for Asian Indians goes beyond the principle of *ahimsa*, or nonviolence. It is a conscious and ethical way of living and eating believed to contribute to inner self-improvement and physical well-being (Achaya, 1994; Bhattacharya, 2015).

The practice of vegetarianism in the subcontinent entails widespread prohibition of beef based on the reverence to the cow. Harris (1978) discussed the taboo against eating beef as stemming from this reverence. The cow is held in high esteem in an environment where subsistence agriculture prevails; cattle are used for plowing the fields as well as for producing milk. Cattle have always played a central role in the Indian pastoral society; five of its products—milk, curds or yogurt, ghee or clarified butter, urine, and dung—either individually or in combination continue to be used in a variety of Hindu rituals. The consumption of milk, ghee, curds, buttermilk, and other dairy products is an integral component of the Asian Indian vegetarian diet. Lacto-vegetarianism (inclusion of dairy but not meat, fish, or poultry), followed by lacto-ovo vegetarianism (inclusion of dairy and eggs only), is widely followed. According to the results of India's Third National Family Health Survey (2005–2006), one-fourth of the population were lacto-vegetarians, while nearly two-thirds followed a nonvegetarian diet either daily, weekly, or at least occasionally; 3.2% were lacto-ovo vegetarians, 2.2% were pesco-vegetarians, 5.2% were semivegetarians, and 1.6% of the population followed veganism (Agrawal et al., 2014). Vegetarian practices vary widely with the extent of religious observances and regional preferences. For example, Jains abstain from all flesh foods, roots, and tubers; the Brahmin caste abstains from meat as a symbol of piety, although the coastal Brahmins from West Bengal, Orissa, Assam, and parts of Maharashtra and Kerala consider fish as the staple "fruit of the sea." Brahmins in the north, especially from Punjab, Jammu, and Kashmir, are meat eaters; they believe that eating meat is religiously sanctioned (Balagopal, 2000). The western states of Gujrat and Maharashtra have the highest percentage of vegans (Agrawal et al., 2014). The widespread availability of plant foods fostered by geographic location, terrain, and climate in a primarily agrarian country, coupled with the regional and religious diversity in vegetarian practices, has resulted in the evolution of a predominantly plant-based vegetarian cuisine. Further, the ancient Indian medical system of Ayurveda as an adjuvant to the evolution of vegetarianism has provided an extensive knowledge base of plant sources of nutrition, methods of food preparation and preservation, and codes of dietary practice and conduct (Manohar and Kessler, 2016).

There is no single traditional Asian Indian diet, but a number of variations exist based on regional and religious diversity. Like the Mediterranean diet (Dernini and Berry, 2015), the traditional Asian Indian diet is a true expression of the cultural fabric of the subcontinent. A history replete with migrations, invasions, and colonial rule (Sen, 2004); a diversity of the physical landscape and soil conditions; distinct seasonal cycles; a variety of climates; and diverse religious and cultural followings and family values (Mudambi and Rajagopal, 2001) has contributed to four regional culinary traditions in India. Interregional variations exist within these major culinary traditions; a variety of dishes have evolved using locally available staple grains, lentils, fruits, vegetables, and spices (Shridhar et al., 2014). Nevertheless, there are certain standard features in the Asian Indian meal with variations in regional styles of eating (Balagopal, 2000). The typical meal consists of rice and/or bread made from wheat; *dhal*, made from lentils, pulses, or a variety of beans, such as garbanzo beans and kidney beans; stir-fried vegetables and/or vegetables in gravy; meat, poultry, fish, and eggs for nonvegetarians; fried wafers (made from grains or lentils with or without vegetables and spices); condiments such as chutneys and pickles; raw vegetable salads or *raitas* (raw vegetables with yogurt); and plain yogurt and beverages (coffee in the south; spiced tea in north, east, and west; *lassi* or spiced or sweetened buttermilk; and lemon juice or coconut water for warm climates). Regional cuisines build on this basic framework, featuring staples produced within a geographic region based on climate and soil conditions. For example, rice requires alluvial soil found largely in the fertile deltas of the east and south. A variety of steamed and fried rice dishes in the south, east, and west are served in combination with lentils and pulses and vegetables indigenous to the region. Wheat requires a cool climate; it grows well in the Gangetic Plain and is the staple grain in the north, west, and northern plain states, while corn and millets are staples in the desert regions of the northwest states of Gujrat and Rajasthan.

11.8 NUTRITIONAL QUALITY OF THE ASIAN INDIAN VEGETARIAN DIET

Though less publicized, the traditional Asian Indian vegetarian diet shares many unique features with the Mediterranean diet (Trichopoulo et al., 2014), not only with its nutrient-dense food components but also the interactions between food, culture, people, and the biophysical and sociocultural environments. Since prehistoric times, a variety of staples, such as rice, millets, barley, wheat, and lentils, have been integral components of the diet; they are excellent sources of complex carbohydrates, fiber, and moderate amounts of plant proteins (Singh et al., 2014). Cereal–legume–pulse combinations abound in the cuisine, offering complementary sources of protein and ensuring the availability of essential amino acids. Walnuts, almonds, cashews, pistachios, and peanuts grown in India provide good sources of fats, proteins, and B vitamins in the vegetarian diet. Walnuts, pistachio, and almonds are featured in main entrees and desserts; peanuts are popular in the Western states of India, while cashews and coconuts grown in the south and the coastal regions are used as thickeners and flavoring agents (Sen, 2004).

Temperate vegetables, such as cauliflower, carrots, potatoes, tomatoes, turnips, onion, garlic, and their tropical counterparts (for example, plantains, banana flower, bitter melon, coconut, drumstick, green mango, jackfruit, okra and eggplant), and greens (leaves of mustard, fenugreek, radish, and spinach), are featured in the regional cuisines based on availability. Fruits indigenous to the subcontinent, such as mangoes, papayas, jackfruit, gooseberry, coconut, and custard apple, as well as temperate fruits, for example, apples, are part of the cuisine. An extensive portfolio of dairy products, including fluid milk, butter, ghee or clarified butter, khoa (thickened milk), yogurt, buttermilk, and paneer (cottage cheese), are staple dairy products consumed in India. Yogurt or curds (*dahi*), butter, and ghee (clarified butter) carry geographic and religious significance in the subcontinent, directly influenced by the cultural aspects of the Indian cuisine. Considerable attention is also focused on the humoral properties of milk as they relate to its digestibility, purity, and body-building capabilities based on Ayurvedic traditions. The push is to consume milk in a variety of products as a source of good nutrition, particularly proteins and fats, in a vegetarian-friendly environment across the life span (Wiley, 2014).

Native herbs and spices, such as cilantro, mint, turmeric, ginger, onion, garlic, chilies, cumin, coriander, fenugreek, black pepper, cinnamon, and cardamom, individually and in distinct combinations known as *masalas* provide flavor and aesthetic appeal. While Ayurvedic traditions have enumerated their medicinal and digestive properties (Sharma et al., 2007), recent studies endorse the innumerable health benefits of their bioactive compounds with potential antioxidant, anti-inflammatory, antimicrobial, antibacterial, and chemopreventive properties (Lampe, 2003; Tapsell et al., 2006).

A variety of preparation techniques, such as sprouting, fermentation, steaming, boiling, broiling, and frying, are common in the Asian Indian cuisine. Despite these positive attributes, the diet poses several challenges.

11.9 ASIAN INDIAN VEGETARIAN DIET TODAY

Asian Indians value their traditional diet, an indelible mark of their ethnic identity. Regardless of geographic residence, several acculturative changes marked by ingredient substitutions, modifications of traditional recipes with new ingredients, and/or the abandonment of traditional foods or ingredients, are noted. There is an excessive consumption of festival foods symbolic of ethnic identity and nostalgia (Azar et al., 2013) along with Western foods (e.g., pizza). This biculturalism contributes to excess calories (Fernandez et al., 2015). Availability, access, sociocultural beliefs, nutritional or health concerns, and migration-associated stress contribute to these changes.

Since the 1960s, rapid socioeconomic developments fueled by globalization, technology expansion, the Green Revolution (Sebby, 2010), and trade liberalization have resulted in improvements in economic status for many, as well as changed the face of the food system for Asian Indians both in the United States and more recently back home (Raj et al., 1999; Chapman et al., 2011). The introduction of new technologies in agriculture and food processing, foreign direct investments, and the establishment of transnational food corporations (TFCs) encouraged by relaxed tariff and trade agreements have transformed the way food is produced, processed, distributed, marketed, and consumed (Hawkes, 2006). Mass marketing and advertising strategies have concomitantly increased the attractiveness of certain food categories to consumers, ensuring their sustained purchase and consumption (Gayathri et al., 2016). Singh et al. (2014) characterize the resulting nutrition transition picture in the subcontinent in a recent review. Negative features in the dietary pattern include (1) the substitution of refined grains, such as white polished rice and highly polished refined cereals for whole coarse grains (for example, brown rice); (2) an emphasis and overconsumption of refined carbohydrates, particularly potatoes, at the expense of other whole plant foods, such as lentils, vegetables, fruits, nuts and seeds, and whole unrefined grains; (3) the increased use of omega-6-rich hydrogenated vegetable oils, palm oil, and safflower oil, instead of monounsaturated-rich olive oil, groundnut oil, rice bran oil, and mustard oil; and (4) the increased consumption of low-cost fast or processed foods high in caloric intakes and sugar, and sweetened beverages, as well as foods of animal origin (Trichopoulou et al., 2014).

This so-called "contaminated vegetarianism" (Enas, 2007; Raj, 2011) results from (1) a desire to follow Westernized dietary practices, (2) modifying traditional diets by altering specific ingredients or replacing cooking methods, and (3) being unaware of the beneficial qualities of traditional dietary components and negative health effects of acculturative dietary practices (Haddad et al., 2015). Furthermore, a lack of knowledge; the inability to judge appropriate portion sizes; convenience and cost; an increased frequency of eating out; a rigid adherence to cultural mores of cooking and eating; a rising consumption of ethnic fast foods along with Western-type calorie-dense fast foods to maintain ethnic identity and acculturate at the same time, unaware that certain vegetarian food choices can be unhealthy and have large quantities of salt, sugar, and "invisible fats," such as oils, butter, and ghee; and easy access to convenient, prepared, frozen native vegetarian entrees in Asian Indian retail outlets foster negative acculturative dietary practices detrimental to health. Consequently, several food choices within the present-day Asian Indian vegetarian pattern are pro-inflammatory and prone to oxidative stress.

On a positive note, a few studies on Asian Indian immigrants report a variety of health-promoting behaviors, such as the likelihood to follow lower-fat guidelines (Lesser et al., 2014), an increased consumption of fruits and vegetables (Wandel et al., 2008), an increased use of grilling over frying in food preparation (Lesser et al., 2014), and engagement in healthy lifestyle practices and interest in nutrition information (Varghese and Moore-Orr, 2002). Such positive behaviors need to be encouraged alongside making culturally sensitive recommendations to alter negative health behaviors.

11.10   CHANGING PATTERNS OF VEGETARIAN PRACTICE

Over the past four decades, the practice of vegetarianism among Asian Indians appears to have a declining number of followers, in the United States and among natives in India. Studies on the dietary practices of Asian Indian immigrants in the 1970s and 1980s reported that a hallmark of acculturation was an altered vegetarian status (Gupta, 1975; Karim et al., 1986). A third of them became nonvegetarians in a window of 2 months to a year and were eating beef if so inclined by 7 years of residing in the United States. Females are the primary gatekeepers of food and tradition in the Asian Indian household; they hold a higher allegiance to traditional vegetarian dietary practices and consequently acculturate slower than Asian Indian males.

Dietary acculturation studies in the 1990s reported altered vegetarian practices in Asian Indian immigrants (Gupta, 1975; Karim et al., 1986; Raj et al., 1999). Consumption of white bread, roots and tubers, vegetable oils, legumes, and tea changed little, while that of ghee, yogurt, Indian bread, and rice dishes changed from frequent to low–moderate upon migration. There was an increase in the consumption of fruit juice, chips, fruits, margarine, soft drinks, alcoholic beverages, cheese, American breads, breakfast cereal, and coffee. Perhaps modifying the traditional diet is easier than adopting a new diet altogether, yet many Asian Indians are unaware of the pros and cons of these alterations. Participants in a community-based participatory focus group on psychosocial and cultural perceptions made assumptions that vegetarian diets were low fat or healthy and expressed disbelief that vegetarians could suffer from heart disease (Kalra et al., 2004).

At present, the data on dietary habits of immigrant Asian Indians, though based on small samples in different geographic locations in the United States and elsewhere (Jonnalagadda and Diwan, 2002a, 2002b; Jonnalagadda et al., 2005; Arya et al., 2006; Koenig et al., 2012; Mukherjea et al., 2013; Lesser et al., 2014; Osei-Kwasi et al., 2016), provide valuable information on the populations' dietary trends. Dietary transitions in Asian Indian immigrant communities are marked by a high fat intake of ~32%, lower omega-3 fatty acids and a high ratio of omega-6 to omega-3, the continued use of *trans* fats as a cooking medium (Misra and Shrivastava, 2013), and the consumption of large carbohydrate meals made up of refined, processed grains. A recent examination of the dietary practices of 892 South Asians enrolled in the Mediators of Atherosclerosis in South Asians Living in America (MASALA) study identified three predominant dietary patterns. The *animal protein nonvegetarian* dietary pattern was associated with higher BMIs and waist-to-hip ratios, the *vegetarian* pattern consisting of fried snacks and sweets, and the *high-fat dairy food* pattern was associated with greater insulin resistance as measured by biochemical indices, such as homeostatic model assessment–insulin resistance (HOMA-IR) and lower HDL cholesterol (Gadgil et al., 2014). A parallel exploratory examination of dietary patterns in India using eight published studies highlighted the regional and food composition diversity that exists within the vegetarian dietary practice across India (Green et al., 2016). Of the 41 dietary patterns identified, 29 were vegetarian, in which vegetables, cereals, fruits, pulses, and dairy products were predominant. Six of the 41 patterns reported a high consumption of snacks and sweets. A cross-national comparison of vegetarian dietary practices between the U.S. vegetarian population and that of India reported positive health outcomes, such as a lower probability of central obesity for U.S. vegetarian adults than for their South Asian counterparts (Jaacks et al., 2016). The South Asian vegetarian dietary practice was only weakly associated with central obesity. Furthermore, U.S.-based vegetarians consistently made healthier food choices than their Indian counterparts, who had higher intakes of snacks, fried foods, and desserts.

11.11 THE AUTHENTICITY OF THE TRADITIONAL VEGETARIAN PRACTICE AT STAKE

The present-day following of the Asian Indian vegetarian diet, along with decreased physical activity and elevated psychosomatic stress caused by migration, socioeconomic, cultural, family, work life, and other environmental factors (Dixit et al., 2011; Patel et al., 2012), is at odds with optimal health and wellness. It faces a waning in adherence to traditional, whole, minimally processed food components, preparation methods, and consumption patterns. This is of immediate concern because these factors ultimately exacerbate the vulnerability to NCDs and undernutrition posed by genetic susceptibility, fetal programming, and environmental conditions over generations.

This situation is not unique to the Asian Indian vegetarian pattern. Other traditional patterns, such as the Mediterranean (Dernini and Berry, 2015; Donini et al., 2016) and Okinawan (Willcox et al., 2014) dietary patterns, note similar declines in dietary diversity (Nelson et al., 2016) and adherence to their healthy patterns. A sufficient body of evidence points to health benefits accrued from optimal eating, following a wholesome, nutrient-dense diet close to nature (Katz and Meller, 2014) and adhering to a traditional dietary pattern (Lipski, 2010). Efforts are currently underway to reverse these trends by reeducating the younger generation about the health, family, and societal benefits of these dietary patterns.

11.12   NEXT STEPS

Public health professionals, including nutritionists working with the Asian Indian population, can glean lessons from such initiatives to tailor community-based interventions suited for this population. Equally important is to recognize the natural synergy between the traditional diet pattern and the ancient medical system of Ayurveda contributing to its long-term sustainability. First, Ayurveda provides advice on the food components, properties, seasonality, benefits, and risks of different food combinations; strategies to optimize digestion; bioavailability; metabolism; and rejuvenation therapies applicable across different life cycle stages. Second, it offers ancillary lifestyle management skills, for example, rules for eating, fasting, feasting, the quantity and timing of food consumption, variety, balance, and moderation. Third, it advocates for contextualizing nutritional advice based on an individual's constitution (genotype), food requirement, and the biophysical and sociocultural environments in which the individual functions (Morandi et al., 2011; Payyappallimana and Venkatasubramanian, 2016). Although Asian Indians are familiar with many of Ayurveda's nutrition-related principles, they may not recognize the subtleties and relate to its practical lifestyle applications. For instance, a small study on Asian Indian immigrants noted the categorization of foods as "hot" and "cold" based on the humoral properties of Ayurveda that often resulted in inadvertent abstinence or inclusion of certain food groups or ingredients, for example, abstaining from dairy and fruits in winter because of their ability to increase the "cold" humors in the body (Satyamurthy, 2012).

Community and family-based lifestyle intervention programs organized through ethnic, cultural, and faith-based organizations and health fairs can build on this synergism between Ayurveda and the traditional dietary pattern for garnering positive outcomes (Berra et al., 2017). This entails training a corps of native and nonnative Asian Indian health and nutrition professionals on the (1) culture's food ways and vegetarian practices; (2) synergism between diet, Ayurveda, and mind–body practices such as yoga (Bhurji et al., 2016) and meditation (Das et al., 2015); (3) facilitators and barriers to these practices; (4) communication; (5) education to improve knowledge and dispel common misconceptions; and (6) support to improve adherence and compliance (Sohal et al., 2015). Presenting the salient features of the Asian Indian vegetarian diet in tandem with the lifestyle principles of Ayurveda will foster behavior modification in a realistic, person-centered manner that is familiar to participants and not undermine core cultural values (Mukherjea et al., 2013). Nutrition education for appropriate metabolic control (Joshi et al., 2012) should focus on alternative methods of preparation, reducing the frequency of consumption of certain ethnosymbolic calorie-dense preparations and Western foods, and emphasizing the importance of overall calorie density. Dietary modifications should emphasize the (1) reintroduction of coarse and whole grains, for example, millets; (2) use of legumes, beans, lentils, and/or pulses that are good sources of protein and soluble fiber; (3) types of healthy fats and oils, for example, mustard oil, groundnut oil, and rice bran oil; (4) avoidance of *trans* fats and use of the native ghee or clarified butter in moderation; (5) reduced fat versions of dairy products; and (6) healthy food preparation using sprouting, fermentation, steaming, and so forth, providing assistance with recipe modification. The Consensus Dietary Guidelines document (Misra et al., 2011) and the food-based guidelines (FAO, 2017) specifically created for Asian Indians are useful resources that provide practical, nutrient, and food-based guidelines and recommendations. Information provided in the context of a pragmatic, multipronged, integrative lifestyle intervention approach that is translatable into everyday dietary practices will further augment the experience.

Lessons from a recent randomized control trial, the first of its kind with the Asian Indian population in the United States, can offer guidance in this realm. The researchers modified the Diabetes Prevention Program materials from the National Diabetes Education Program's (NDEP) 2P2 program and tailored them to meet the needs of a Gujarati community in the United States. This 12-week program, conducted in a faith-based facility known as the *mandir*, is facilitated by a bilingual healthcare professional focused on nutrition and lifestyle, including physical activity employing social media to aid in data collection (Patel et al., 2017). The study showed positive results with respect to diabetes prevention while endorsing the value of community engagement in prevention programs. Similar programs may be efficacious for communities requiring dietary and lifestyle interventions across other geographical regions while simultaneously facilitating policy-oriented research.

11.13   CONCLUSIONS

The current Asian Indian NCD profile, especially at a younger age, underscores the need for prevention by taking a life course approach that nurtures healthy lifestyle practices for long-term sustainability. There is an ongoing need for longitudinal studies in Asian Indian immigrants to identify and address (1) risk factors and the multigenerational impact of the evolving vegetarian diet on NCDs across the life span and (2) genetic variants, polymorphisms, and the characterization of the Asian Indian gut microbiome in relation to chronic disease etiology (Shetty et al., 2013). This will pave the way for designing and enhancing the quality of evidence-based interventions and facilitating the formulation of policies to address the chronic disease burden for all Asian Indians.

Addressing the totality of the dietary and lifestyle pattern within a familiar sociocultural context by tailoring interventions to ethnic specific needs will address a wide spectrum of chronic health conditions. This will also ensure that our clients are empowered toward adherence, positive decision making, and partnership in a meaningful and positive way with their health professionals.

REFERENCES

Abate N, Chandalia M, Satija P, Adams-Huet B, Grundy SM, Sandeep S, Radha V, Deepa R, Mohan V. 2005. ENPP1/PC-1 K121Q polymorphism and genetic susceptibility to type 2 diabetes. *Diabetes* 54(4):1207–13.

Achaya KT. 1994. *Indian Food: A Historical Companion*. Oxford: Oxford University Press.

Agrawal S, Millett CJ, Dhillon PK, Subramanian SV, Ebrahim S. 2014. Type of vegetarian diet, obesity and diabetes in adult Indian population. *Nutr J* 13:89. doi: 10.1186/1475-2891-13-89.

Anand SS, Yusuf S, Vuksan V, Devanesen S, Teo KK, Montague PA, Kelemen L et al. 2000. Differences in risk factors, atherosclerosis, and cardiovascular disease between ethnic groups in Canada: The Study of Health Assessment and Risk in Ethnic groups (SHARE). *Lancet* 356(9226):279–84.

Anjana RM, Pradeepa R, Deepa M, Datta M, Sudha V, Unnikrishnan R, Bhansali A et al. 2011. Prevalence of diabetes and prediabetes (impaired fasting glucose and/or impaired glucose tolerance) in urban and rural India: Phase I results of the Indian Council of Medical Research-INdia DIABetes (ICMR-INDIAB) study. *Diabetologia* 54(12):3022–7. doi: 10.1007/s00125-011-2291-5.

Arya S, Isharwal S, Misra A, Pandey RM, Rastogi K, Vikram NK, Dhingra V, Chatterjee A, Sharma R, Luthra K. 2006. C-Reactive protein and dietary nutrients in urban Asian Indian adolescents and young adults. *Nutrition* 22(9):865–71.

Azar KM, Chen E, Holland AT, Palaniappan LP. 2013. Festival foods in the immigrant diet. *J Immigr Minor Health* 15(5):953–60. doi: 10.1007/s10903-012-9705-4.

Bagai LB. 1972. *The East Indians and Pakistanis in America*. Minneapolis: Lerner Publications.

Bainey KR, Jugdutt BI. 2009. Increased burden of coronary artery disease in South-Asians living in North America. Need for an aggressive management algorithm. *Atherosclerosis* 204(1):1–10.

Baker SM. 2008. The metaphor of an oceanic disease. *Integr Med* 7(1):40–5.

Balagopal P. 2000. Indian and Pakistani food practices, customs and holidays. Diabetes Care Practice Group of the American Dietetic Association.

Barker DJ. 2007. The origins of the developmental origins theory. *J Intern Med* 261:412–7.

Bauer UE, Briss PA, Goodman RA, Bowman BA. 2014. Prevention of chronic disease in the 21st century: Elimination of the leading preventable causes of premature death and disability in the USA. *Lancet* 384(9937):45–52. doi: 10.1016/S0140-6736(14)60648-6.

Befroy DE, Petersen KF, Dufour S, Mason GF, de Graaf RA, Rothman DL, Shulman GI. 2007. Impaired mitochondrial substrate oxidation in muscle of insulin-resistant offspring of type 2 diabetic patients. *Diabetes* 56(5):1376–81. doi: 10.2337/db06-0783.

Berra K, Franklin B, Jennings C. 2017. Community-based healthy living interventions. *Prog Cardiovasc Dis* 59(5):430–9. doi: dx.doi.org/10.1016/j.pcad.2017.01.002.

Bhatt SP, Nigam P, Misra A, Guleria R, Luthra K, Jain SK, Qadar Pasha MA. 2012. Association of the Myostatin gene with obesity, abdominal obesity and low lean body mass and in non-diabetic Asian Indians in North India. *PLoS One* 7(8):e40977.

Bhatt SP, Nigam P, Misra A, Guleria R, Luthra K, Pandey RM, Pasha MA. 2013. Association of peroxisome proliferator activated receptor-gamma gene with non-alcoholic fatty liver disease in Asian Indians residing in north India. *Gene* 512(1):143–7.

Bhattacharya M. 2015. A historical exploration of Indian diets and a possible link to insulin resistance syndrome. *Appetite* 95:421–54.

Bhopal R. 2004. Glossary of terms relating to ethnicity and race: For reflection and debate. *J Epidemiol Community Health* 58(6):441–5. doi: 10.1136/jech.2003.013466.

Bhurji N, Javer J, Gasevic D, Khan NA. 2016. Improving management of type 2 diabetes in South Asian patients: A systematic review of intervention studies. *BMJ Open* 6(4):e008986. doi: 10.1136/bmjopen-2015-008986.

Boden, G. 1997. Role of fatty acids in the pathogenesis of insulin resistance and NIDDM. *Diabetes* 46(1):3–10.

Boon MR, Karamali NS, de Groot CJ, van Steijn L, Kanhai HH, van der Bent C, Berbée JF, Middelkoop B, Rensen PC, Tamsma JT. 2012. E-Selectin is elevated in cord blood of South Asian neonates compared with Caucasian neonates. *J Pediatr* 160:844–8.e1.

Bosma-den Boer MM, van Wetten ML, Pruimboom L. 2012. Chronic inflammatory diseases are stimulated by current lifestyle: How diet, stress levels and medication prevent our body from recovering. *Nutr Metab (Lond)* 9(1):32. http://doi.org/10.1186/1743-7075-9-32.

Bruce KD, Hanson MA. 2010. The developmental origins, mechanisms, and implications of metabolic syndrome. *J Nutr* 140(3):648–52. doi: 10.3945/jn.109.111179.

Chapman GE, Ristovski-Slijepcevic S, Beagan BL. 2011. Meanings of food, eating and health in Punjabi families living in Vancouver, Canada. *Health Educ J* 70(1):102–12.

Chauhan G, Kaur I, Tabassum R, Dwivedi OP, Ghosh S, Tandon N, Bharadwaj D. 2012. Common variants of homocysteine metabolism pathway genes and risk of type 2 diabetes and related traits in Indians. *Exp Diabetes Res* 2012:960318. doi: 10.1155/2012/960318.

Das M, Pal S, Ghosh A. 2013. Synergistic effects of ACE (I/D) and Apo E (Hha I) gene polymorphisms on obesity, fat mass, and blood glucose level among the adult Asian Indians: A population-based study from Calcutta, India. *Indian J Endocrinol Metab* 17(1):101–4. doi: 10.4103/2230-8210.107816.

Das MK, Kumar S, Deb PK, Mishra S. 2015. History of cardiology in India. *Indian Heart J* 67(2):163–9. doi: 10.1016/j.ihj.2015.04.004.

Deepa R, Mohan V, Premanand C, Rajan VS, Karkuzhali K, Velmurugan K, Agarwal S, Gross MD, Markovitz J. 2006. Accelerated platelet activation in Asian Indians with diabetes and coronary artery disease: The Chennai Urban Population Study (CUPS-13). *J Assoc Physicians India* 54:704–8.

Dernini S, Berry EM. 2015. Mediterranean diet: From a healthy diet to a sustainable dietary pattern. *Front Nutr* 2:15. doi: 10.3389/fnut.2015.00015.

Dixit AA, Azar KMJ, Gardner CD, Palaniappan LP. 2011. Incorporation of whole, ancient grains into a modern Asian Indian diet: Practical strategies to reduce the burden of chronic disease. *Nutr Rev* 69(8):479–88. doi: 10.1111/j.1753-4887.2011.00411.x.

Dodani S. 2008. Excess coronary artery disease risk in South Asian immigrants: Can dysfunctional high-density lipoprotein explain increased risk? *Vasc Health Risk Manag* 4(5):953–61.

Dodani S, Kaur R, Reddy S, Reed GL, Navab M, George V. 2008. Can dysfunctional HDL explain high coronary artery disease risk in South Asians? *Int J Cardiol* 129(1):125–32.

Donini LM, Dernini S, Lairon D, Serra-Majem L, Amiot MJ, Del Balzo V, Giusti AM et al. 2016. A consensus proposal for nutritional indicators to assess the sustainability of a healthy diet: The Mediterranean Diet as a case study. *Front Nutr* 3:37. doi: 10.3389/fnut.2016.00037.

Eaton SB, Konner M, Shostak M. 1988. Stone agers in the fast lane: Chronic degenerative diseases in evolutionary perspective. *Am J Med* 84(4):739–49. doi: 10.1016/0002-9343(88)90113-1.

Egger G, Dixon J. 2014. Beyond obesity and lifestyle: A review of 21st century chronic disease determinants. *Biomed Res Int* 731685. http://doi.org/10.1155/2014/731685.

Elshenawy S, Simmons R. 2016. Maternal obesity and prenatal programming. *Mol Cell Endocrinol* 435:2–6.

Enas EA. 2007. Contaminated vegetarianism. http://www.cadiresearch.org/topic/diet-indian/contaminated-vegetarianism (accessd August 18, 2016).

Enas EA, Mohan V, Deepa M, Farooq S, Pazhoor S, Chennikkara H. 2007. The metabolic syndrome and dyslipidemia among Asian Indians: A population with high rates of diabetes and premature coronary artery disease. *J Cardiometab Syndr* 2(4):267–75.

Fernandez R, Rolley JX, Rajaratnam R, Everett B, Davidson PM. 2015. Reducing the risk of heart disease among Indian Australians: Knowledge, attitudes, and beliefs regarding food practices—A focus group study. *Food Nutr Res* 59:25770. doi: 10.3402/fnr.v59.25770.

FAO (Food and Agriculture Organization of the United States). 2017. Food-based dietary guidelines—India. http://www.fao.org/nutrition/education/food-based-dietary-guidelines/regions/countries/india/en/.

Ford ND, Patel SA, Narayan KM. 2017. Obesity in low- and middle-income countries: Burden, drivers, and emerging challenges. *Annu Rev Public Health* 38:145–64. doi: 10.1146/annurev-publhealth-031816-04460.

Gadgil MD, Anderson CAM, Kandula NR, Kanaya AM. 2014. Dietary patterns in Asian Indians in the United States: An analysis of the Metabolic Syndrome and Atherosclerosis in South Asians Living in America Study (MASALA). *J Acad Nutr Diet* 114(2):238–43. doi: 10.1016/j.jand.2013.09.021.

Gayathri R, Ruchi V, Mohan V. 2016. Impact of nutrition transition and resulting morbidities on economic and human development. *Curr Diabetes Rev* 13. doi: 10.2174/157339981 2666160901095534.

Ghaffar A, Reddy KS, Singhi M. 2004. Burden of non-communicable diseases in South Asia. *BMJ* 328(7443):807–10.

Green R, Milner J, Joy EJ, Agrawal S, Dangour AD. 2016. Dietary patterns in India: A systematic review. *Br J Nutr* 116(1):142–8. doi: 10.1017/S0007114516001598.

Gupta SP. 1975. Changes in the food habits of Asian Indians in the U.S.: A case study. *Social Sco Res* 60(1):87–99.

Haddad L, Cameron L, Barnett I. 2015. The double burden of malnutrition in SE Asia and the Pacific: Priorities, policies and politics. *Health Policy Plan* 30(9):1193–206. doi: 10.1093/heapol/czu110.

Harris M. 1978. India's sacred cow. *Hum Nat* 28–36.

Hawkes C. 2006. Uneven dietary development: Linking the policies and processes of globalization with the nutrition transition, obesity, and diet related chronic diseases. *Global Health* 2:4. doi: 10.1186/1744-8603-2-4.

IDF (International Diabetes Federation). 2006. *Diabetes Atlas*. 3rd ed. Brussels: IDF.

IDF (International Diabetes Federation). 2015. *Diabetes Atlas*. 7th ed. Brussels: IDF. http://www.idf.org/idf-diabetes-atlas-seventh-edition (accessed April 25, 2017).

IHME (Institute for Health Metrics and Evaluation), Human Development Network, the World Bank. 2013. The global burden of disease: Generating evidence, guiding policy—South Asia regional edition. Seattle, WA: IHME.

Jaacks LM, Kapoor D, Singh K, Narayan KM, Ali MK, Kadi MM, Mohan V, Tandon N, Prabhakaran D. 2016. Vegetarianism and cardiometabolic disease risk factors: Differences between South Asian and US adults. *Nutrition* 32(9):975–84.

Jayashree S, Arindam M, Vijay KV. 2015. Genetic epidemiology of coronary artery disease: An Asian Indian perspective. *J Genet* 94(3):539–49.

Jonnalagadda SS, Diwan S. 2002a. Nutrient intake of first generation Gujarati Asian Indian immigrants in the U.S. *J Am Coll Nutr* 21(5):372–80.

Jonnalagadda SS, Diwan S. 2002b. Regional variations in dietary intake and body mass index of first-generation Asian-Indian immigrants in the United States. *J Am Diet Assoc* 102(9):1286–9.

Jonnalagadda SS, Diwan S, Cohen DL. 2005. U.S. Food Guide Pyramid food group intake by Asian Indian immigrants in the U.S. *J Nutr Health Aging* 9(4):226–31.

Joshi P, Islam S, Pais P, Reddy S, Dorairaj P, Kazmi K, Pandey MR, Hague S, Mendis S, Rangarajan S, Yusuf S. 2007. Risk factors for early myocardial infarction in South Asians compared with individuals in other countries. *JAMA* 297(3):286–94.

Joshi SR, Mohan V, Joshi SS, Mechanick JI, Marchetti A. 2012. Transcultural diabetes nutrition therapy algorithm: The Asian Indian application. *Curr Diab Rep* 12(2):204–12. doi: 10.1007/s11892-012-0260-0.

Kalra P, Srinivasan S, Ivey S, Greenlund K. 2004. Knowledge and practice: The risk of cardiovascular disease among Asian Indians. Results from focus groups conducted in Asian Indian communities in Northern California. *Ethn Dis* 14(4):497–504.

Kamath DY, Xavier D, Sigamani A, Pais P. 2015. High sensitivity C-reactive protein (hsCRP) & cardiovascular disease: An Indian perspective. *Indian J Med Res* 142(3):261–68. doi: 10.4103/0971-5916.166582.

Kanaya AM, Wassel CL, Mathur D, Stewart A, Herrington D, Budoff MJ, Ranpura V, Liu K. 2010. Prevalence and correlates of diabetes in South Asian Indians in the United States: Findings from the Metabolic Syndrome and Atherosclerosis in South Asians Living in America Study and the Multi-Ethnic Study of Atherosclerosis. *Metab Syndr Relat Disord* 8(2):157–63. doi: 10.1089/met.2009.0062.

Karim N, Bloch DS, Falciglia G, Murthy L. 1986. Modifications in food consumption patterns reported by people from India, living in Cincinnati, Ohio. *Ecol Food Nutr* 19(1):11–8.

Katz DL, Meller S. 2014. Can we say what diet is best for health? *Annu Rev Public Health* 35:83–103. doi: 10.1146/annurev-publhealth-032013-182351.

Kodama K, Tojjar D, Yamada S, Toda K, Patel CJ, Butte AJ. 2013. Ethnic differences in the relationship between insulin sensitivity and insulin response: A systemic review and meta-analysis. *Diabetes Care* 36(6):1789–96. doi: 10.2337/dc12-1235.

Koenig CJ, Dutta MJ, Kandula N, Palaniappan L. 2012. "All of those things we don't eat": A culture-centered approach to dietary health meanings for Asian Indians living in the United States. *Health Commun* 27(8):818–28. doi: 10.1080/10410236.2011.651708.

Kramer MS. 1987. Determinants of low birth weight: Methodological assessment and meta-analysis. *Bull World Health Organ* 65(5):663–737.

Krishnaveni GV, Hill JC, Veena S, Bhat DS, Wills AK, Karat CL, Yajnik CS, Fall CH. 2009. Low plasma vitamin B12 in pregnancy is associated with gestational 'diabesity' and later diabetes. *Diabetologia* 52(11):2350–58. doi: 10.1007/s00125-009-1499-0.

Kruk ME, Nigenda G, Knaul FM. 2015. Redesigning primary care to tackle the global epidemic of noncommunicable disease. *Am J Public Health* 105(3):431–7. doi: 10.2105/AJPH .2014.302392.

Lampe JW. 2003. Spicing up a vegetarian diet: Chemopreventive effects of phytochemicals *Am J Clin Nutr* 78(3 Suppl.):579S–83S.

Langley-Evans SC. 2015. Nutrition in early life and the programming of adult disease: A review. *J Hum Nutr Diet* 28(Suppl. 1):1–14. doi: 10.1111/jhn.12212.

Lesser IA, Gasevic D, Lear SA. 2014. The association between acculturation and dietary patterns of South Asian immigrants. *PLoS One* 9(2):e88495. doi: 10.1371/journal .pone.0088495.

Li Y, Ley SH, Tobias DK, Chiuve SE, VanderWeele TJ, Rich-Edwards JW, Curhan GC, Willett WC, Manson JE, Hu FB, Qi L. 2015. Birth weight and later life adherence to unhealthy lifestyles in predicting type 2 diabetes: Prospective cohort study. *BMJ* 351:h3672. doi: 10.1136/bmj.h3672.

Libby P. 2013. Mechanisms of acute coronary syndromes and their implications for therapy. *N Engl J Med* 368(21):2004–13.

Liem SS, Oemrawsingh PV, Cannegieter SC, Le Cessie S, Schreur J, Rosendaal FR, Schalij MJ. 2009. Cardiovascular risk in young apparently healthy descendants from Asian Indian migrants in the Netherlands: The SHIVA study. *Neth Heart J* 17(4):155–61.

Lipski E. 2010. Traditional non-Western diets. *Nutr Clin Pract* 25(6):585–93.

Lomazzi M, Borisch B, Laaser U. 2014. The Millennium Development Goals: Experiences, achievements and what's next. *Glob Health Action* 7:23695. doi: 10.3402/gha.v7.23695.

López-Otín C, Blasco MA, Partridge L, Serrano M, Kroemer G. 2013. The hallmarks of aging. *Cell* 153(6):1194–217. doi: 10.1016/j.cell.2013.05.039.

Manohar R, Kessler CS. 2016. Ayurveda's contributions to vegetarian nutrition in medicine. *Forsch Komplementmed* 23(2):89–94. doi: 10.1159/000445400.

Markan S, Sachdeva M, Sehrawat B, Kumari S, Jain S, Khullar M. 2007. MTHFR 677 CT/ MTHFR 1298 CC genotypes are associated with increased risk of hypertension in Indians. *Mol Cell Biochem* 302(1–2):125–31.

Martyn CN, Barker DJ, Osmond C. 1996. Mothers' pelvic size, fetal growth, and death from stroke and coronary heart disease in men in the UK. *Lancet* 348(9037):1264–8. 10.1016/S0140-6736(96)04257-2.

Maskari FL. 2010. Lifestyle diseases: An economic burden on the health services. *UN Chronicle*, July. https://unchronicle.un.org/article/lifestyle-diseases-economic-burden-health-services.

McGarry JD. 2002. Banting lecture 2001: Dysregulation of fatty acid metabolism in the etiology of type 2 diabetes. *Diabetes* 51(1):7–18.

Mehrotra N, Gaur S, Petrova A. 2012. Health care practices of the foreign born Asian Indians in the United States. A community based survey. *J Community Health* 37(2):328–34. doi: 10.1007/s10900-011-9449-4.

Melina V, Craig W, Levin S. 2016. Position of the Academy of Nutrition and Dietetics: Vegetarian diets. *J Acad Nutr Diet* 116(12):1970–80. doi: 10.1016/j.jand.2016.09.025.

Misra A, Khurana L. 2009. The metabolic syndrome in South Asians: Epidemiology, determinants, and prevention. *Metab Syndr Relat Disord* 7(6):497–514. doi: 10.1089/met .2009.0024.

Misra A, Khurana L. 2011. Obesity-related non-communicable diseases: South Asians vs white Caucasians. See comment in PubMed Commons below*Int J Obes (Lond)* 35(2):167–87. doi: 10.1038/ijo.2010.135.

Misra A, Sharma R, Gulati S, Joshi SR, Sharma V, Ghafoorunissa, Ibrahim A et al. 2011. Consensus dietary guidelines for healthy living and prevention of obesity, the metabolic syndrome, diabetes, and related disorders in Asian Indians. *Diabetes Technol Ther* 13(6):683–94. doi: 10.1089/dia.2010.0198.

Misra A, Shrivastava U. 2013. Obesity and dyslipidemia in South Asians. *Nutrients* 5(7):2708–33. doi: 10.3390/nu5072708.

Mohan V, Deepa R, Velmurugan K, Premalatha G. 2005. Association of C-reactive protein with body fat, diabetes and coronary artery disease in Asian Indians: The Chennai Urban Rural Epidemiology Study (CURES-6). *Diabet Med* 22(7):863–70.

Mohan V, Sandeep S, Deepa R, Shah B, Varghese C. 2007. Epidemiology of type 2 diabetes: Indian scenario. *Indian J Med Res* 125(3):217–30.

Moore SE, Halsall I, Howarth D, Poskitt EM, Prentice AM. 2001. Glucose, insulin and lipid metabolism in rural Gambians exposed to early malnutrition. *Diabet Med* 18(8):646–53. doi: 10.1046/j.1464-5491.2001.00565.x.

Morandi A, Tosto C, Roberti di Sarsina P, Dalla Libera D. 2011. Salutogenesis and Ayurveda: Indications for public health management. *EPMA J* 2(4):459–65. doi: 10.1007/s13167 -011-0132-8.

Mudambi S, Rajagopal M, eds. 2001. *Fundamentals of Food and Nutrition*. 4th ed. Madras: New Age International.

Mukherjea A, Underwood KC, Stewart AL, Ivey SL, Kanaya AM. 2013. Asian Indian views on diet and health in the United States: Importance of understanding cultural and social factors to address disparities. *Fam Community Health* 36(4):311–23. doi: 10.1097/FCH .0b013e31829d2549.

Nair M, Prabhakaran D. 2012. Why do South Asians have high risk for CAD? *Glob Heart* 7(4):307–14. doi: 10.1016/j.gheart.2012.09.001.

Narayan KM. 2016. Type 2 diabetes: Why we are winning the battle but losing the war? 2015 Kelly West Award Lecture. *Diabetes Care* 39(5):653–63. doi: 10.2337/dc16-0205.

Nelson ME, Hamm MW, Hu FB, Abrams SA, Griffin TS. 2016. Alignment of healthy dietary patterns and environmental sustainability: A systematic review. *Adv Nutr* 7(6):1005–25. doi: 10.3945/an.116.012567.

New America Media. 2012. Census: Asian Indian population explodes across U.S. http:// newamericamedia.org/2011/05/census-asian-indian-population-explodes-across-us .php.

Osei-Kwasi HA, Nicolaou M, Powell K, Terragni L, Maes L, Stronks K, Lien N, Holdsworth M, DEDIPAC Consortium. 2016. Systematic mapping review of the factors influencing dietary behaviour in ethnic minority groups living in Europe: A DEDIPAC study. *Int J Behav Nutr Phys Act* 13:85. doi: 10.1186/s12966-016-0412-8.

Padmanabhan V, Cardoso RC, Puttabyatappa M. 2016. Developmental programming a pathway to disease. *Endocrinology* 157(4):1328–40.

Pandey A, Chawla S, Guchhait P. 2015. Type 2 diabetes: Current understanding and future perspectives. *IUBMB Life* 67(7):506–13.

Patel M, Phillips-Caesar E, Boutin-Foster C. 2012. Barriers to lifestyle behavioral change in migrant South Asian populations. *J Immigr Minor Health* 14(5):774–85. doi: 10.1007/s10903-011-9550-x.

Patel RM, Misra R, Raj S, Balasubramanyam A. 2017. Effectiveness of a group-based culturally tailored lifestyle intervention program on changes in risk factors for type 2 diabetes among Asian Indians in the United States. *J Diabetes Res* 2017:2751980. doi: 10.1155/2017/2751980.

Patel SA, Shivashankar R, Ali MK, Anjana RM, Deepa M, Kapoor D, Kondal D et al. 2016. Is the "South Asian phenotype" unique to South Asians? Comparing cardiometabolic risk factors in the CARRS and NHANES studies. *Glob Heart* 11(1):89–96.e3. doi: 10.1016/j.gheart.2015.12.010.

Payyappallimana U, Venkatasubramanian P. 2016. Exploring Ayurvedic knowledge on food and health for providing innovative solutions to contemporary healthcare. *Front Public Health* 4:57. doi: 10.3389/fpubh.2016.00057.

Popkin BM. 1994. The nutrition transition in low income countries: An emerging crisis. *Nutr Rev* 52(9):285–98.

Popkin BM. 2002. The shift in stages of the nutrition transition in the developing world differs from past experiences! Part II. What is unique about the experience in lower- and middle income less-industrialized countries compared with the very-high income industrialized countries? *Public Health Nutr* 5(1A):205–14.

Prabhakaran D, Shah P, Chaturvedi V, Ramakrishnan L, Manhapra A, Reddy KS. 2005. Cardiovascular risk factor prevalence among men in a large industry of North India. *Natl Med J India* 18(2):59–65.

Radhika G, Ganesan A, Sathya RM, Sudha V, Mohan V. 2009. Dietary carbohydrates, glycemic load and serum high-density lipoprotein cholesterol concentrations among South Indian adults. *Eur J Clin Nutr* 63(3):413–20.

Raj S. 2011. The practice of vegetarianism in the South Asian sub-continent. *Vegetarian Nutrition Update* 20(1):1–5.

Raj S, Ganganna P, Bowering J. 1999. Dietary habits of Asian Indians in relation to length of residence in the United States. *J Am Diet Assoc* 99(9):1106–8.

Sapkota BR, Hopkins R, Bjonnes A, Ralhan S, Wander GS, Mehra NK, Singh JR, Blackett PR, Saxena R, Sanghera DK. 2016. Genome-wide association study of 25(OH) vitamin D concentrations in Punjabi Sikhs: Results of the Asian Indian diabetic heart study. *J Steroid Biochem Mol Biol* 158:149–56. doi: 10.1016/j.jsbmb.2015.12.014.

Satyamurthy M. 2012. A comparison of traditional beliefs, practices and health seeking behaviors that influence dietary practices during pregnancy of South Asian Indian women in India and the U.S. Master's thesis, Syracuse University.

Scott JM. 1992. Folate-vitamin B12 interrelationships in the central nervous system. *Proc Nutr Soc* 51(2):219–24.

Sebby K. 2010. The Green Revolution of the 1960's and its impact on small farmers in India. Undergraduate thesis, Environmental Studies Undergraduate Student, Paper 10.

Selhub J, Morris MS, Jacques PF. 2007. In vitamin B12 deficiency, higher serum folate is associated with increased total homocysteine and methylmalonic acid concentrations. *Proc Natl Acad Sci U S A* 104(50):19995–20000.

Sen CT. 2004. *Food Culture in India*. Greenwood Publishing Group.

Sharma H, Chandola HM, Singh G, Basisht G. 2007. Utilization of Ayurveda in health care: An approach for prevention, health promotion, and treatment of disease. Part 1—Ayurveda, the science of life. *J Altern Complement Med* 13(9):1011–9.

Shetty P. 2013. Nutrition transition and its health outcomes. *Indian J Pediatr* 80(Suppl. 1): S21–7. doi: 1007/s12098-013-0971-5.

Shetty SA, Marathe NP, Shouche YS. 2013. Opportunities and challenges for gut microbiome studies in the Indian population. *Microbiome* 1(1):24. doi: 10.1186/2049-2618-1-24.

Shridhar K, Dhillon PK, Bowen L, Kinra S, Bharathi AV, Prabhakaran D, Reddy KS, Ebrahim S. 2014. Nutritional profile of Indian vegetarian diets—The Indian Migration Study (IMS). *Nutr J* 13:55. doi: 10.1186/1475-2891-13-55.

Shrivastava U, Misra A, Mohan V, Unnikrishnan R, Bachani D. 2017. Obesity, diabetes and cardiovascular diseases in India: Public health challenges. *Curr Diabetes Rev* 13(1):65–80. doi: 10.2174/1573399812666160805153328.

Siegel KR, Patel SA, Ali MK. 2014. Non communicable diseases in South Asia: Contemporary perspectives. *Brit. Med. Bull.*

Singh PN, Arthur KN, Orlich MJ, James W, Purty A, Job JS, Rajaram S, Sabaté J. 2014. Global epidemiology of obesity, vegetarian dietary patterns, and noncommunicable disease in Asian Indians. *Am J Clin Nutr* 100(1):359S–64S. doi: 10.3945/ajcn.113.071571.

Sohal T, Sohal P, King-Shier KM, Khan NA. 2015. Barriers and facilitators for type-2 diabetes management in South Asians: A systematic review. *PLoS One* 10(9):e0136202. doi: 10.1371/journal.pone.0136202.

Stanfield KM, Wells JC, Fewtrell MS, Frost C, Leon DA. 2012. Differences in body composition between infants of South Asian and European ancestry: The London Mother and Baby Study. *Int J Epidemiol* 41(5):1409–18. doi: 10.1093/ije/dys139.

Tabassum R, Jaiswal A, Chauhan G, Dwivedi OP, Ghosh S, Marwaha RK, Tandon N, Bharadwaj D. 2012. Genetic variant of AMD1 is associated with obesity in urban Indian children. *PLoS One* 7(4):e33162.

Tabassum R, Mahajan A, Chauhan G, Dwivedi OP, Ghosh S, Tandon N, Bharadwaj D. 2010. Evaluation of DOK5 as a susceptibility gene for type 2 diabetes and obesity in North Indian population. *BMC Med Genet* 11:35.

Tapsell LC, Hemphill I, Cobiac L, Patch CS, Sullivan DR, Fenech M, Roodenrys S et al. 2006. Health benefits of herbs and spices: The past, the present, the future. *Med J Aust* 185(4 Suppl.):S4–24.

Thaler R, Agsten M, Spitzer S, Paschalis EP, Karlic H, Klaushofer K, Varga F. 2011. Homocysteine suppresses the expression of the collagen cross-linker lysyl oxidase involving IL-6, Fli1, and epigenetic DNA methylation. *J Biol Chem* 286(7):5578–88.

Tobias M. 1991. *Life Force: The World of Jainism.* Berkeley, CA: Asian Humanities Press.

Trichopoulou A, Martínez-González MA, Tong TY, Forouhi NG, Khandelwal S, Prabhakaran D, Mozaffarian D, de Lorgeril M. 2014. Definitions and potential health benefits of the Mediterranean diet: Views from experts around the world. *BMC Med* 12:112. doi: 10.1186/1741-7015-12-112.

Tutino GE, Tam WH, Yang X, Chan JC, Lao TT, Ma RC. 2014. Diabetes and pregnancy: Perspectives from Asia. *Diabet Med* 31(3):302–18. doi: 10.1111/dme.12396.

Uauy R, Kain J, Corvalan C. 2011. How can the developmental origins of health and disease (DOHaD) hypothesis contribute to improving health in developing countries? *Am J Clin Nutr* 94(6 Suppl.):1759s–64S. doi: 10.3945/ajcn.110.000562.

Unnikrishnan R, Anjana RM, Mohan V. 2014. Diabetes in South Asians: Is the phenotype different? *Diabetes* 63(1):53–5. doi: 10.2337/db13-1592.

Varghese S, Moore-Orr R. 2002. Dietary acculturation and health-related issues of Indian immigrant families in Newfoundland. *Can J Diet Pract Res* 63(2):72–9.

Wandel M, Raberg M, Kumar B, Holmboe-Ottesen G. 2008. Changes in food habits after migration among South Asians settled in Oslo: The effect of demographic, socioeconomic and integration factors. *Appetite* 50(2–3):376–85.

Wells JC, Pomeroy E, Walimbe SR, Popkin BM, Yajnik CS. 2016. The elevated susceptibility to diabetes in India: An evolutionary perspective. *Front Public Health* 4:145. doi: 10.3389/fpubh.2016.00145.

WHO (World Health Organization). 2013. WHO Global Action Plan for the prevention and control of noncommunicable diseases: 2013–2020. Geneva: World Health Organization. http://apps.who.int/iris/bitstream/10665/94384/1/9789241506236_eng.pdf?ua=1.

WHO (World Health Organization). 2015. Global status report on non-communicable diseases 2014. Geneva: World Health Organization. http://www.who.int/nmh/publications /en/.

Wiley AS. 2014. *Cultures of Milk: The Biology and Meaning of Dairy Products in the United States and India.* Cambridge, MA: Harvard University Press.

Willcox DC, Scapagnini G, Willcox BJ. 2014. Healthy aging diets other than the Mediterranean: A focus on the Okinawan diet. *Mech Ageing Dev* 136–37:148–62. doi: 10.1016/j.mad.2014.01.002.

Williams RB. 1988. *Religions of Immigrants from India and Pakistan.* New York: Cambridge University Press.

Yajnik CS, Deshpande SS, Jackson AA, Refsum H, Rao S, Fisher DJ, Bhat DS et al. 2008. Vitamin B12 and folate concentrations during pregnancy and insulin resistance in the offspring: The Pune Maternal Nutrition Study. *Diabetologia* 51(1):29–38. doi: 10.1007 /s00125-007-0793-y.

Yajnik CS, Deshpande SS, Lubree HG, Naik SS, Bhat DS, Uradey BS, Deshpande JA, Rege SS, Refsum H, Yudkin JS. 2006. Vitamin B12 deficiency and hyperhomocysteinemia in rural and urban Indians. *J Assoc Physicians India* 54:775–82.

Yajnik CS, Lubree HG, Rege SS, Naik SS, Deshpande JA, Deshpande SS, Joglekar CV, Yudkin JS. 2002. Adiposity and hyperinsulinemia in Indians are present at birth. *J Clin Endocrinol Metab* 87(12):5575–80.

Zong J, Batalova J. 2015. Indian immigrants in the United States. http://www.migrationpolicy .org/article/indian-immigrants-united-states/ (accessed April 27, 2017).

Section VI

*Vegetarian Diets
for Special Groups*

12 Vegetarian Diets for Pregnancy, Lactation, Infancy, and Early Childhood

Reed Mangels

CONTENTS

SUMMARY

Vegetarian (including vegan) diets can be nutritionally adequate for pregnant and lactating women, infants, and children and may offer significant benefits. Diets during these stages of the life cycle should contain adequate amounts of protein, vitamin B12, calcium, vitamin D, iodine, iron, zinc, and other essential nutrients. In some instances, fortified foods or supplements may be needed to ensure adequacy. Nutritionally adequate vegetarian diets support recommended weight gain in pregnancy, result in infant birth weight within normal limits, and support appropriate growth of infants and children. During the first year after birth, breast milk is the ideal primary beverage, with a commercial infant formula the only recommended alternative. After 6 months of age, most term infants will begin to eat complementary foods. These foods can help to meet needs for energy, protein, iron, zinc, and other micronutrients.

12.1 INTRODUCTION

As of 2016, approximately 8 million people in the United States consistently follow a vegetarian diet, not eating meat, fish, or poultry (The Vegetarian Resource Group, 2016). Of these, approximately 3.7 million follow a vegan diet, which is a vegetarian diet that does not include any animal-based products (The Vegetarian Resource Group, 2016). Little or no information is available about the prevalence of vegetarian diets in pregnancy. Approximately 4% of children and adolescents in the United States age 8–18 years are vegetarian; 1% of U.S. children and adolescents are vegan (The Vegetarian Resource Group, 2014). Limited information is available for younger children and for children in other countries.

The most recent position paper on vegetarian diets from the Academy of Nutrition and Dietetics supports the use of vegetarian diets throughout the life cycle (Melina et al., 2016). The Academy (formerly known as the American Dietetic Association) has endorsed the used of vegetarian diets in the life cycle since at least 1980 (American Dietetic Association, 1980). The *2015–2020 Dietary Guidelines for Americans* has identified a "Healthy Vegetarian Eating Pattern" as one of three examples of healthy eating patterns (U.S. Department of Health and Human Services, U.S. Department of Agriculture, 2015). These *Dietary Guidelines* are for people age 2 years and older. The American Academy of Pediatrics and the Canadian Paediatric Society have concluded that children can be well nourished on vegetarian and vegan diets (American Academy of Pediatrics, 2015; Amit et al., 2010).

Although the number of research papers published annually related to vegetarian nutrition has increased markedly over the past 30 years, few studies have examined the use of vegetarian diets in pregnancy, lactation, and infancy. Studies of these life stages tend to focus on nutritional issues of people new to vegetarianism in the 1970s and 1980s. With changes in knowledge, dietary practices, and availability of fortified foods, these earlier studies often have limited relevance to vegetarians today. Studies of vegetarians during pregnancy, lactation, and infancy tend to be small and may focus on specific dietary practices, such as macrobiotic diets, again, limiting their generalizability. Additional research on vegetarian diets in these life stages should be conducted.

12.2 PREGNANCY

Pregnancy outcome, including the infant's birth weight and health, is affected by the nutritional adequacy of the maternal diet. Evidence-based analysis conducted by the Academy of Nutrition and Dietetics Evidence Analysis Library concluded that there are no significant health differences in babies born to vegetarian (nonvegan) mothers versus nonvegetarians (Academy of Nutrition and Dietetics, 2007). A lack of research prevented this group from reaching conclusions about vegan pregnancy (Academy of Nutrition and Dietetics, 2007). Infant birth weight is an important indicator of nutritional adequacy in pregnancy. Birth weights of infants of vegetarian women are typically similar to those of infants born to nonvegetarian women and to birth weight norms (King et al., 1981; Ward et al., 1988; Drake et al., 1998) provided maternal weight gain is appropriate and energy intake is adequate (Dagnelie et al., 1988, 1989). The neurodevelopment of infants born to vegetarian mothers is similar to that of infants of nonvegetarian mothers (Larsen et al., 2014).

12.2.1 Benefits of a Vegetarian Diet in Pregnancy

A vegetarian diet can be advantageous in pregnancy. For example, the typically higher fiber content of a vegetarian diet can alleviate the constipation that commonly occurs in pregnancy. Pregnant vegetarian women tend to have diets that are higher in folate (Koebnick et al., 2001) and magnesium (Koebnick et al., 2005). One study has found that maternal use of a vegetarian diet in the first trimester resulted in lower risk of excessive gestational weight gain (Stuebe et al., 2009). Since excessive gestational weight gain is associated with an increased risk of gestational diabetes, hypertensive disorders of pregnancy, and type 2 diabetes later in life (Ferraro et al., 2015), a vegetarian diet offers a potential means to reduce risk of these conditions.

In addition to the potentially beneficial effects of lower gestational weight gain, the plant-based nature of vegetarian diets may also contribute to the beneficial effects of these diets. A high consumption of plant-derived foods during pregnancy has been shown to reduce the risk of hypertensive disorders of pregnancy, gestational diabetes, and some pediatric diseases (Pistollato et al., 2015). Maternal diets high in animal protein during pregnancy have been associated with an increased risk of offspring being overweight at age 20 (Maslova et al., 2014).

Vegetarians may choose soy products as alternatives to animal-based products. Exposure to soy in pregnancy may be beneficial to mothers and offspring. Higher urinary concentrations of isoflavones in pregnant women were correlated with self-reported frequency of soy consumption in an analysis of the National Health and Nutrition Examination Survey (NHANES) 2001–2008 surveys (Shi et al., 2014). Women in the highest quartile of urinary isoflavone concentration had significantly lower fasting glucose, insulin, and triglyceride concentrations, suggesting that soy consumption may offer benefits for pregnant women (Shi et al., 2014). Animal studies suggest that maternal consumption of an isoflavone-rich diet during pregnancy, followed by consumption of a similar diet during weaning and postweaning, can reduce the risk of cardiovascular disease late in life (Bonacasa et al., 2011).

12.2.2 Nutritional Needs in Vegetarian Pregnancy

12.2.2.1 Protein

Protein needs increase in pregnancy to support fetal and placental needs, as well as the expansion of maternal blood volume and uterine and breast tissue. Little protein is deposited in maternal or fetal tissue during the first trimester of pregnancy (Butte and King, 2005). Deposition increases through the second trimester and is highest in the third trimester (Butte and King, 2005). During the first trimester, the Recommended Dietary Allowance (RDA) for protein is similar to the RDA for nonpregnant women of 0.8 g/kg/day (Food and Nutrition Board, Institute of Medicine, 2002). In the second and third trimesters, the RDA for protein increases to 1.1 g/kg/day, or 25 g/day of additional protein (Food and Nutrition Board, Institute of Medicine, 2002). Recent research using the indicator amino acid oxidation method suggests the need to revisit protein requirements in pregnancy since requirements appear to be 1.2 g/kg protein in early pregnancy and 1.52 g/kg in late pregnancy (Elango and Ball, 2016). The researchers who conducted studies of protein needs in pregnancy estimate that diets with approximately 14%–18% of energy as protein will be adequate to meet these higher protein recommendations (Elango and Ball, 2016).

Nonpregnant lacto-ovo vegetarian women's diets typically consist of 12%–14% of energy from protein, while vegan women's diets generally are between 10% and 12% of calories from protein (Mangels et al., 2011). During pregnancy, women typically increase both the energy and protein content of their diets, so these ranges may not change significantly. If the higher protein requirements are supported by additional research, pregnant vegetarian women, especially vegan women, may need to add an additional serving or two of protein-rich foods to their diets.

12.2.2.2 Omega-3 Fatty Acids

Docosahexaenoic acid (DHA), a long-chain omega-3 fatty acid, is mainly found in fish and fish oil. Thus, unsupplemented vegetarian diets are very low in DHA and unsupplemented vegan diets contain little or no DHA. Pregnant vegetarians and their infants have lower plasma DHA concentrations than do nonvegetarian women and their infants (Lakin et al., 1998; Sanders, 1999). The fetal brain and retinal tissues accumulate DHA, especially in the third trimester (Martinez, 1992; Martinez and Mougan, 1998). Observational studies suggest that maternal and/or infant DHA supplementation may be beneficial for infant neurodevelopment (Meldrum and Simmer, 2016). However, supplementation with DHA during pregnancy has not been found to enhance development in term infants (De Giuseppe et al., 2014; Meldrum and Simmer, 2016). Maternal supplementation appears promising in reducing the risk of preterm birth (De Giuseppe et al., 2014; Kar et al., 2015) and may play a role in allergy prevention in childhood (De Giuseppe et al., 2014).

DHA can be synthesized to some extent from alpha-linolenic acid (ALA) by fetuses, infants, children, and adults (Leikin-Frenkel, 2016). Rates of synthesis are somewhat higher in pregnancy than at other stages of the life cycle, but total synthesis is quite low (Williams and Burdge, 2006). Use of ALA supplements in pregnancy has not been shown to be effective in increasing maternal or infant DHA concentrations (de Groot et al., 2004). Although it is important to have adequate amounts of the essential fatty acid ALA (Leikin-Frenkel, 2016), it is unlikely that ALA can substitute for DHA (Jensen, 2006).

Pregnant and lactating vegetarians may benefit from direct sources of DHA derived from microalgae (Jensen, 2006; Carlson et al., 2013). Microalgae-derived supplements and foods fortified with DHA from microalgae effectively improve DHA status (Arterburn et al., 2007). Intakes of 200 mg/day of DHA have been suggested in pregnancy (Koletzko et al., 2008).

12.2.2.3   Vitamin B12

Vitamin B12 is required to support neurodevelopment during the perinatal period (Dror and Allen, 2008; Finkelstein et al., 2015). Vitamin B12 deficiency in pregnancy is associated with numerous problems, including impaired cognitive development as well as low birth weight, intrauterine growth restriction, and pregnancy loss (Finkelstein et al., 2015). Marginal vitamin B12 concentrations early in pregnancy are associated with an increased risk of neural tube defects, independent of folate status (Finkelstein et al., 2015).

The mother's current intake of vitamin B12, from diet and supplements, has a stronger influence on the vitamin B12 status of the infant than does maternal stores of vitamin B12 (Dror and Allen, 2008). Pregnant women need daily, reliable sources of vitamin B12. Use of vitamin B12 supplements in pregnancy is correlated with improved maternal vitamin B12 status and higher cord serum vitamin B12 concentrations (Duggan et al., 2014; Visentin et al., 2016).

An estimated 0.1–0.2 µg/day of vitamin B12 is transferred to the fetus throughout pregnancy (Food and Nutrition Board, Institute of Medicine, 1998). Although maternal absorption is more efficient in pregnancy, the RDA for vitamin B12 is increased from 2.4 µg/day in nonpregnant women to 2.6 µg/day during pregnancy due to the higher need for this vitamin (Food and Nutrition Board, Institute of Medicine, 1998). Some have called for a higher RDA for adults, saying that the current RDA might be inadequate for optimal status (Bor et al., 2010). If this is the case, the RDA for pregnancy would also likely need to be raised.

Many prenatal supplements supply vitamin B12. Pregnant women may also choose fortified foods or supplemental vitamin B12. Doses of vitamin B12 below 5 µg are absorbed as well as or better than naturally occurring vitamin B12, with 50% of naturally occurring vitamin B12 absorbed and 60% of low-dose crystalline vitamin B12 absorbed (Food and Nutrition Board, Institute of Medicine, 1998). Higher doses, as may be found in some supplements, are less well absorbed, with about 5% of vitamin B12 in a 25 µg supplement absorbed (Heyssel et al., 1966; Berlin et al., 1968; Adams et al., 1971). A lesser amount, 1% or less, of the vitamin B12 in a supplement containing more than 100 μg of vitamin B12 is absorbed (Berlin et al., 1968; Food and Nutrition Board, Institute of Medicine, 1998).

12.2.2.4   Iron and Zinc

Estimates of iron needs in pregnancy are between 700 and 800 mg (Food and Nutrition Board, Institute of Medicine, 2001). Iron deficiency is associated with numerous complications, including preterm birth and compromised neurological development. One study has found that pregnant vegetarians were less likely to have low dietary iron intakes than nonvegetarians, and that they were more likely to use iron supplements during the first and second trimesters (Alwan et al., 2011). Higher dietary iron intakes, however, may not be enough to compensate for the lower absorption of nonheme iron. Because of iron's importance, the Centers for Disease Control and Prevention recommends the use of a daily low-dose (30 mg) iron supplement for pregnant women (CDC, 1998). The World Health Organization recommends a weekly supplementation of 120 mg of iron for nonanemic women (WHO, 2012). Intermittent iron supplementation, in which women take supplements once or twice a week, appears to be as effective as daily supplementation in reducing the risk of anemia; intermittent iron supplementation was better tolerated with fewer reports of constipation and nausea (Peña-Rosas et al., 2015).

Zinc plays an essential role in pregnancy due to its involvement in cell differentiation and replication. The increased zinc requirement of approximately 100 mg of zinc over the course of pregnancy (Swanson and King, 1987) can be met through a combination of increased intake and higher absorption (King, 2000). A recent meta-analysis found that the zinc intake of pregnant vegetarians was significantly lower than that of nonvegetarians (Foster et al., 2015). No differences in biomarkers of zinc status or in pregnancy outcomes, such as pregnancy duration and birth weight, were found between the groups (Foster et al., 2015).

12.2.2.5   Iodine

Some research suggests that vegetarian diets, especially those not containing iodized salt, sea vegetables, or other good sources of iodine, can be low in iodine (Leung et al., 2011a). Iodine in eggs and cow's milk arises from feed supplements and the iodine solution used for disinfection of bovine teats (Ershow et al., 2016). The amount of iodine found in these foods may be decreasing (Ershow et al., 2016), which could affect the iodine intake of lacto-ovo vegetarians. Iodine plays an important role in fetal brain development (Alexander et al., 2017; Leung et al., 2011b), so it essential that pregnant women have an adequate intake of iodine. While iodized salt can be a major source of iodine, only about 50% of salt sold in the United States is iodized (Alexander et al., 2017). Processed foods do not typically contain iodized salt. With many people reducing their intake of added salt, it may be challenging to meet the RDA of 220 μg/day for pregnancy. The American Thyroid Association recommends that women in the United States supplement their diet with 150 μg/day of iodine in the form of potassium iodide, ideally starting 3 months prior to pregnancy (Alexander et al., 2017). Some, but not all, prenatal supplements contain iodine (Leung et al., 2009). While iodine adequacy is important, excess iodine intake should be avoided. Excessive iodine in pregnancy can lead to congenital hypothyroidism (Leung and

Braverman, 2014). The American Thyroid Association advises against ingesting iodine or kelp supplements containing more than 500 μg of iodine daily in pregnancy and lactation (Leung et al., 2015).

12.2.3   PRACTICAL CONSIDERATIONS IN VEGETARIAN PREGNANCY

12.2.3.1   Weight Gain

Current recommendations in pregnancy call for a weight gain of 25–35 lb for women beginning pregnancy in the normal weight range, 28–40 lb for women underweight prior to pregnancy, 15–25 lb for those categorized as overweight, and 11–20 lb for those whose prepregnancy body mass index is in the obese range (Rasmussen and Yaktine, 2009). These recommendations are based on observational studies that correlated weight gain with pregnancy outcome. The limited research that has been conducted on weight gain in pregnant vegetarians suggests that weight gain of both lacto-ovo vegetarians and vegans is generally adequate (King et al., 1981; Carter et al., 1987; Ward et al., 1988).

12.2.3.2   Use of Supplements

Pregnant women frequently are prescribed a multivitamin and multimineral prenatal supplement. The frequency of use varies depending on age, race and ethnicity, and maternal education (Burris et al., 2015). One study found that 75% of pregnant women attending a Boston perinatal center used a prenatal supplement at least sometimes during pregnancy (Burris et al., 2015). A study that included 223 Danish women who reported being vegetarian during pregnancy, most of whom were lacto-ovo vegetarians, found that 91% of lacto-ovo vegetarians and 95% of vegans used multivitamins during pregnancy; 73% and 57%, respectively, used iron supplements (Larsen et al., 2014). Prenatal supplements that are identified as "vegetarian," "vegan," or "suitable for vegetarians" are available and can be a helpful source of nutrients, such as vitamin B12, calcium, vitamin D, iron, zinc, iodine, and DHA, although content and nutrient amounts vary widely (Mangels, 2008). The Institute of Medicine recommends that all women capable of becoming pregnant consume 400 μg of folate daily from supplements, fortified food, or a combination of fortified food and supplements, and that pregnant women get at least 600 μg of folate (Food and Nutrition Board, Institute of Medicine, 1998). The American College of Obstetricians and Gynecologists recommends a prenatal vitamin supplement for most pregnant women to ensure that they obtain adequate amounts of folic acid and other nutrients (ACOG, 2017).

12.2.3.3   Soy Safety

Many vegetarians choose to use soy-based products, such as tofu, soy milk, and some meat analogues. These products can make significant nutritional contributions, as well as providing dietary variety. Isoflavones found in soy products appear to be transferred to the fetus (Adlercreutz et al., 1999; Todaka et al., 2005). The effects of fetal exposure to isoflavones are uncertain. Although these substances have estrogenic effects, their activity differs from that of natural estrogens (Messina, 2016). A British study found that hypospadias, a congenital malformation of the penis, occurred more frequently in infants whose mothers followed a vegetarian diet during pregnancy (North and Golding, 2000). Although some have attributed these results to the use of soy, there was no significant association between the use of soy milk and other soy products and development of hypospadias (North and Golding, 2000). Another study found a reduced risk of hypospadias associated with higher intakes of phytoestrogens and isoflavones (Carmichael et al., 2013). Since the original study, one other study has reported an association between maternal vegetarian diet and hypospadias, while at least seven studies have found no association between maternal vegetarian diets or low meat and fish intake and hypospadias (Carmichael et al., 2012).

12.3 LACTATION

Many of the nutritional recommendations for lactation are similar to, or slightly higher than, those for pregnancy. Energy needs are higher or pregnant women than for nonpregnant women. The Estimated Energy Requirement for lactation, which allows for a weight loss of 0.8 kg/month for the first 6 months postpartum, calls for an additional 330 kcal above prepregnancy energy needs for the first 6 months of lactation and an additional 400 kcal for the second 6 months (Food and Nutrition Board, Institute of Medicine, 2002). The RDA for protein in lactation is 1.3 g/kg/day (Food and Nutrition Board, Institute of Medicine, 2002).

Vegetarian (including vegan) diets can be used safely during lactation (Melina et al., 2016). Breastfed infants of adequately nourished vegetarian and vegan women grow and develop normally (Melina et al., 2016). Breast milk's nutritional content is most affected by the mother's dietary intake of most of the B vitamins, vitamin C, vitamins A and D, selenium, and iodine (Lönnerdal, 1986; Food and Nutrition Board, Institute of Medicine, 1991; Allen, 2012). Other nutrients, including calcium, iron, zinc, and folate, are generally not affected by maternal diet. Breast milk from vegetarians does not appear to differ in mineral, lactose, or fat concentration compared with breast milk from nonvegetarians (Finley et al., 1985).

12.3.1 NUTRITION IN VEGETARIAN LACTATION

12.3.1.1 Omega-3 Fatty Acids

The omega-3 fatty acid DHA begins to accumulate in the fetal brain in the second trimester of pregnancy and continues to increase until at least age 2 (Martinez and Mougan, 1998). Breast milk supplies some DHA, but as might be expected, in view of low maternal dietary DHA content, the breast milk of lacto-ovo vegetarian and vegan women typically has a lower concentration of DHA than does the breast milk of nonvegetarians (Sanders, 1999). In view of DHA's important roles in growth and development of the brain and retina, questions arise as to whether lactating women should supplement their diet. A recent systematic review concluded that supplementing lactating women with DHA did not appear to have significant beneficial effects on their children's neurodevelopment or visual acuity (Delgado-Noguera et al., 2015). This review did not specifically examine vegetarian women whose DHA intakes may be lower than those of the unsupplemented women who were included in this review. An international consensus recommends that lactating women have a DHA intake of 200 mg/day (Koletzko et al., 2008). This amount of DHA is said to result in milk DHA concentration equivalent to that recommended by the European Food Safety Authority to be included in infant formula if label claims about support of infant visual development are made (Carlson and Colombo, 2016).

Vegetarian women can use microalgae-derived DHA supplements, which are effective in increasing breast milk DHA (Jensen et al., 2005). Some have proposed flaxseed or other sources of ALA as a means of improving DHA status in lactation. Although flaxseed oil supplements increase breast milk concentrations of ALA, no effect was seen on milk DHA concentrations (Francois et al., 2003). In addition, high levels of dietary ALA appear to inhibit the conversion of ALA to DHA (Gibson et al., 2011).

12.3.1.2   Vitamin B12

The adequacy of maternal vitamin B12 is essential throughout pregnancy and lactation. Maternal vitamin B12 status during pregnancy is associated with infant stores of this vitamin at birth (Allen, 2008). A well-nourished newborn infant has stores of 25–30 µg of vitamin B12; lower stores are seen in infants of mothers who are vitamin B12 deficient (Allen, 2008; Food and Nutrition Board, Institute of Medicine, 1998). If the infant's stores are low and exclusive breastfeeding with milk low in vitamin B12 is used, vitamin B12 deficiency symptoms appear around 4–7 months after birth (Allen, 2012), although earlier appearance has been reported (Honzik et al., 2010). Vitamin B12 deficiency can be prevented by adequate maternal intake during pregnancy and lactation. Use of vitamin B12 supplements during pregnancy and lactation is a successful means for increasing breast milk vitamin B12 concentrations in women at risk for inadequate vitamin B12 (Duggan et al., 2014). This maternal supplementation indirectly improves infant vitamin B12 status (Duggan et al., 2014). Supplementation appears to be needed throughout lactation since one study reported a decrease in milk vitamin B12 concentration once supplementation ceased (Duggan et al., 2014).

12.3.1.3   Vitamin D

Breast milk, even from healthy mothers with adequate vitamin D status, is quite low in vitamin D. This means that exclusively breastfed infants typically receive less than 20% of the recommended daily amount of vitamin D during their first year (við Streym et al., 2016). The limited amount of vitamin D in breast milk has led to recommendations for supplemental vitamin D for breastfed infants. The American Academy of Pediatrics calls for the use of a 400 IU/day vitamin D supplement for breastfed infants beginning soon after birth (Wagner et al., 2008). Compliance with this recommendation is low, placing many infants at risk for rickets (Ahrens et al., 2016). An alternative option appears to be higher-dose maternal vitamin D supplements. A daily 6400 IU vitamin D3 supplement given to lactating women resulted in breast milk that contained enough vitamin D to meet infants' needs (Hollis et al., 2015). Lower amounts of vitamin D (400 and 2400 IU) did not increase milk vitamin D enough to meet infants' needs (Hollis et al., 2015).

12.4 INFANCY AND EARLY CHILDHOOD

Common questions with regard to vegetarian diets in infancy and early childhood center on the appropriateness of vegetarian diets for this stage of the life cycle, use of breast milk versus formula, types of weaning foods, and whether supplements are needed.

12.4.1 APPROPRIATENESS OF VEGETARIAN DIETS IN INFANCY AND EARLY CHILDHOOD

As previously stated, the Academy of Nutrition and Dietetics has recently reaffirmed its position statement that "these [vegetarian, including vegan] diets are appropriate for all stages of the life cycle including pregnancy, lactation, infancy, childhood" (Melina et al., 2016). The Canadian Paediatric Society also supports the use of vegetarian diets, saying, "Well-planned vegetarian and vegan diets with appropriate attention to specific nutrient components can provide a healthy alternative lifestyle at all stages of fetal, infant, child and adolescent growth" (Amit et al., 2010).

Case reports of malnutrition in vegetarian infants and children do appear in the medical literature. These reports provide insight into harmful practices that should be avoided. For example, deficiencies of vitamin C, vitamin D, and zinc were reported in an infant whose primary diet from age 2.5–11 months consisted of unfortified almond milk (Vitoria et al., 2016). Rickets, iron deficiency anemia, and severe protein-calorie malnutrition was reported in nine young infants exclusively receiving plant milks for 1–3 months (Le Louer et al., 2014). Poor growth has been reported in young macrobiotic infants with apparently inadequate energy intake (Dagnelie et al., 1989). Vitamin B12 deficiencies are reported in breastfed infants of women with inadequate vitamin B12 status (Allen, 2008). These and similar reports support the importance of providing vegetarian infants with appropriate and adequate food and the need for lactating women to have satisfactory vitamin B12 status.

12.4.2 GROWTH OF VEGETARIAN INFANTS AND CHILDREN

The growth of vegetarian infants is typically similar to that of nonvegetarian infants during the first 6 months after birth (Mangels et al., 2011). This is not surprising in view of recommendations for exclusive breastfeeding for the first 6 months (Section on Breastfeeding, 2012). If vegetarian women are well nourished, their breast milk will be similar to that of nonvegetarian women, so we would expect that infant growth would be similar in these two groups. The growth of both lacto-ovo vegetarian and vegan children is similar to that of their nonvegetarian peers (Sanders, 1988; Nathan et al., 1997; Leung et al., 2001; Yen et al., 2008), although research is limited. Children in Denmark whose mothers were vegetarian during pregnancy walked slightly earlier than and had similar head circumferences as children of nonvegetarians (Larsen et al., 2014).

12.4.3   MILK FOR VEGETARIAN INFANTS

Poor growth in vegetarian infants is associated with inadequate (Dagnelie et al., 1989) or inappropriate (Le Louer et al., 2014) feeding practices. Infants should exclusively receive human milk for the first 6 months with a combination of breast milk and supplemental foods until at least 12 months of age (Section on Breastfeeding, 2012). The benefits of breastfeeding are numerous and include lower risk of obesity, type 1 and type 2 diabetes, and celiac disease; lower rates of postpartum depression; and lower maternal breast and ovarian cancer risk (Section on Breastfeeding, 2012). When exclusive breastfeeding is not possible, commercial infant formula, either fully or partially replacing breast milk, is the only safe option. Commercial or homemade plant milks, fruit or vegetable juices, unmodified cow's or goat's milk, or other products cannot replace breast milk or commercial infant formula (Mangels and Messina, 2001; Mangels and Driggers, 2012).

12.4.4   INTRODUCTION OF COMPLEMENTARY FOODS

After 6 months of age, most term infants will begin to eat complementary foods. These foods can help to meet needs for energy, protein, iron, zinc, and other micronutrients. Either fortified infant cereals or firm tofu can be useful first complementary foods because they supply iron, zinc, and protein without providing excess energy (Mangels and Driggers, 2012). Once feeding patterns have been established, additional foods, such as vegetables, fruits, dried beans, dairy products, and eggs, can be introduced. Food texture should be adjusted to meet the infant's needs. During the first year after birth, breast milk is the ideal primary beverage, with a commercial infant formula the only recommended alternative.

12.4.5   FEEDING YOUNG CHILDREN

The World Health Organization recommends continued breastfeeding along with appropriate complementary foods up to 2 years of age or beyond (WHO, 2017). The American Academy of Pediatrics calls for continuing breastfeeding for at least the first year after birth (Section on Breastfeeding, 2012). While many vegetarians may choose to breastfeed their infants after the infants' first birthday, others will seek an alternative primary beverage. Once breast milk or infant formula is eliminated, a substitute must be found for the energy, protein, fat, calcium, and other nutrients supplied by breast milk or formula. For nonvegan toddlers, whole cow's milk can be used as a primary beverage from age 1–2 years, with reduced fat milk replacing whole milk after 2 years. Cow's milk intake should be limited to 3 cups/day since overconsumption has been associated with an increased risk of impaired growth and iron deficiency (CDC, 1998; Mangels and Driggers, 2012). Vegan toddlers who are no longer using breast milk or infant formula as a primary beverage should use full-fat soy milk fortified with calcium, vitamin D, and vitamin B12, beginning no earlier than age 1 year (Mangels and Driggers, 2012). Cessation of breast milk or infant formula should be delayed if the child's growth is inadequate or if the diet is extremely limited (Mangels and Messina, 2001). Other plant milks, such as rice milk, almond milk, coconut milk, and hemp milk, are low in protein and energy and should not serve as the toddler's primary beverage.

Although vegetarian children's growth is usually appropriate, young children whose diets are very high in fiber from whole grains, beans, fruits, and vegetables may experience poor weight or height growth. The bulky nature of some diets, combined with limited capacity, can lead to early satiety and inadequate energy and nutrient intake. If this occurs, some reduction of fiber is indicated, as well as greater use of energy-dense foods. Fiber can be reduced by replacing some whole grains with refined grains and peeling fruits and vegetables. Nutritious energy-dense foods include avocados, dried fruits, and nut butters.

Vegan children may need somewhat higher amounts of protein than children whose diets contain animal-derived protein because of plant protein's amino acid composition and digestibility (Mangels et al., 2011). Young vegan children, age 1–2 years, may need as much as an additional 30%–35% protein compared with the protein RDA, or about 1.4–1.5 g protein/kg body weight (Messina and Mangels, 2001).

12.4.6 SUPPLEMENTS AND FORTIFIED FOODS FOR VEGETARIAN INFANTS AND YOUNG CHILDREN

Recommendations for supplements for vegetarian infants are similar to those for nonvegetarian infants. A 400 IU/day supplement of vitamin D beginning soon after birth is recommended for all breastfed infants (Wagner et al., 2008). The form of vitamin D does not appear important in infants. Either vitamin D2 or vitamin D3 has been shown to be effective in maintaining vitamin D status in breastfed infants (Gallo et al., 2013). The recommended 400 IU/day of vitamin D, from either diet or supplements, or both, should continue throughout infancy and childhood (Wagner et al., 2008). The American Academy of Pediatrics recommends the use of a 1 mg/kg/day iron supplement for exclusively breastfed infants beginning at 4 months and continuing until iron-containing complementary foods are introduced (Baker et al., 2010). Breastfed infants whose mother's diet is inadequate in vitamin B12 should be given vitamin B12 supplements, orally or intramuscularly, with amounts based on that needed to achieve normal vitamin B12 status (Dror and Allen, 2008). Maternal supplementation is also commonly used, in addition to infant supplementation. There is some evidence that maternal supplementation beginning in lactation in women with a vitamin B12 deficiency may not be effective in increasing milk vitamin B12 concentration (Allen, 2012). In cases of maternal vitamin B12 deficiency, direct supplementation of the breastfed infant seems appropriate. When infants and young children are weaned or partially weaned, vitamin B12 supplements and/or fortified foods will be needed for vegans and may be needed for lacto and lacto-ovo vegetarians to meet recommended intake levels.

Prior to 6 months after birth, term infants who are exclusively breastfed are likely to have their needs for iron and zinc met (Gibson et al., 2014; Foster and Samman, 2015). After this time, complementary foods that supply iron and zinc are needed (Gibson et al., 2014). The RDA for iron for older infants (7–12 months) is 11 mg/day.

No adjustment to the RDA for older infants is needed for the lower bioavailability of iron from a vegetarian diet; the infant iron recommendation was based on a moderate bioavailability of 10%, rather than the usual 18%, since an infant's diet contains little heme iron (Food and Nutrition Board, Institute of Medicine, 2001). The RDA for zinc for older infants is 3 mg/day, with additional zinc needed if the infant's diet is high in unrefined grains and legumes (Food and Nutrition Board, Institute of Medicine, 2001). Infant cereals fortified with electrolytic iron or with ferrous fumarate are effective in protection against iron deficiency (Ziegler et al., 2011). Serving fortified cereals or other iron-rich foods with a vitamin C source enhances iron absorption.

One longitudinal study that compared the zinc status of infants who did not consume meat to that of infants who consumed meat reported no significant difference among the groups in zinc intake or in serum zinc (Taylor et al., 2004). Although frank zinc deficiency is quite uncommon in vegetarian children in industrialized countries, use of practical strategies to enhance zinc absorption is recommended (Gibson et al., 2014). These strategies can be applied to the diets of young vegetarians and include soaking dried beans prior to cooking and discarding the soaking water, using some sprouted legumes, and choosing yeast-raised or sourdough wholegrain breads (Gibson et al., 2014).

12.4.7 BENEFITS OF VEGETARIAN DIETS FOR CHILDREN

A body of research supports the benefits of vegetarian diets for adults. Benefits include a reduced risk of obesity, cardiovascular disease, type 2 diabetes, hypertension, and some types of cancer (Orlich and Fraser, 2014; Melina et al., 2016). Limited research has examined the health benefits of vegetarian diets for children. Vegetarian children appear to eat more fruits and vegetables than do nonvegetarian children (Yen et al., 2008) and are at lower risk for childhood obesity (Sabaté and Wien, 2010). Due to the avoidance of animal products, vegan children appear to have lower intakes of fat, saturated fat, and cholesterol than do their nonvegan peers (Larsson and Johansson, 2002). If these eating behaviors and reduced risk of obesity continue past childhood, the result may be a reduced risk of a number of chronic diseases. In addition, vegetarian diets may expose children to a greater variety of whole plant foods, thus establishing lifelong eating habits.

12.5 MEAL PLANS

A variety of meal plans have been developed for vegetarian pregnancy, lactation, infants, and young children. The *2015–2020 Dietary Guidelines for Americans* (U.S. Department of Health and Human Services, U.S. Department of Agriculture, 2015) include vegetarian food patterns at a variety of energy levels that are appropriate for ages 2 and older. Other patterns have been developed for lacto-ovo vegetarians (Mangels et al., 2011) and vegans (Mangels and Messina, 2001; Mangels and Driggers, 2011; Messina and Mangels, 2001; Norris and Messina, 2011; Davis and Melina, 2014).

12.6 CONCLUSIONS

Major professional organizations have endorsed the use of vegetarian (lacto-ovo, lacto, and vegan) diets throughout the life cycle. Nutritionally adequate vegetarian diets support appropriate weight gain in pregnancy, normal pregnancy duration, and infant birth weights within the normal range. These diets also support successful lactation and the appropriate growth of infants and children. Key nutrients during pregnancy, lactation, infancy, and childhood include protein, omega-3 fatty acids, iron, zinc, iodine, calcium, vitamin D, and vitamin B12. Although most nutrients can be obtained from an adequate, healthful vegetarian diet, supplements and fortified foods may be needed to ensure adequacy.

REFERENCES

Academy of Nutrition and Dietetics. 2007. Evidence analysis library. Pregnancy and nutrition-vegetarian nutrition. http://www.andeal.org/topic.cfm?pcat=3105&menu=5271&cat=3473 (accessed February 16, 2017).

ACOG (American College of Obstetricians and Gynecologists). 2017. Frequently asked questions. Nutrition during pregnancy. http://www.acog.org/~/media/For%20Patients /faq001.pdf?dmc=1&ts=20120515T1154495022 (accessed February 16, 2017).

Adams JF, Ross SK, Mervyn L, Boddy K, King P. 1971. Absorption of cyanocobalamin, coenzyme B12, methylcobalamin, and hydroxocobalamin at different dose levels. *Scand J Gastroenterol* 6:249–52.

Adlercreutz H, Yamada T, Wahala K, Watanabe S. 1999. Maternal and neonatal phytoestrogens in Japanese women during birth. *Am J Obstet Gynecol* 180:737–43.

Ahrens KA, Rossen LM, Simon AE. 2016. Adherence to vitamin D recommendations among US infants aged 0 to 11 months, NHANES, 2009 to 2012. *Clin Pediatr (Phila)* 55(6):555–6.

Alexander EK, Pearce EN, Brent GA, Brown RS, Chen H, Dosiou C, Grobman WA et al. 2017. 2017 guidelines of the American Thyroid Association for the diagnosis and management of thyroid disease during pregnancy and the postpartum. *Thyroid*. doi: 10.1089/thy.2016.0457.

Allen LH. 2008. Causes of vitamin B12 and folate deficiency. *Food Nutr Bull* 29(2 Suppl.):S20–34; discussion S35–7.

Allen LH. 2012. B vitamins in breast milk: Relative importance of maternal status and intake, and effects on infant status and function. *Adv Nutr* 3(3):362–9.

Alwan NA, Greenwood DC, Simpson NA, McArdle HJ, Godfrey KM, Cade JE. 2011. Dietary iron intake during early pregnancy and birth outcomes in a cohort of British women. *Hum Reprod* 26(4):911–9.

American Academy of Pediatrics. 2015. Vegetarian diets for children. https://www.healthy children.org/English/ages-stages/gradeschool/nutrition/Pages/Vegetartian-Diet-for -Children.aspx (accessed February 15, 2017).

American Dietetic Association. 1980. Position paper on the vegetarian approach to eating. *J Am Diet Assoc* 77:61–8.

Amit M, Canadian Paediatric Society. 2010. Position statement: Vegetarian diets in children and adolescents. *Paediatr Child Health* 15(5):303–14.

Arterburn LM, Oken HA, Hoffman JP, Bailey-Hall E, Chung G, Rom D, Hamersley J, McCarthy D. 2007. Bioequivalence of docosahexaenoic acid from different algal oils in capsules and in a DHA-fortified food. *Lipids* 42:1011–24.

Baker RD, Greer FR, Committee on Nutrition American Academy of Pediatrics. 2010. Diagnosis and prevention of iron deficiency and iron-deficiency anemia in infants and young children (0–3 years of age). *Pediatrics* 126(5):1040–50.

Berlin H, Berlin R, Brante G. 1968. Oral treatment of pernicious anemia with high doses of vitamin B12 without intrinsic factor. *Acta Med Scand* 184:247–58.

Bonacasa B, Sio RC, Mann GE. 2011. Impact of dietary soy isoflavones in pregnancy on fetal programming of endothelial function in offspring. *Microcirculation* 18:270–85.

Bor MV, von Castel-Roberts KM, Kauwell GP, Stabler SP, Allen RH, Maneval DR, Bailey LB, Nexo E. 2010. Daily intake of 4 to 7 mg dietary vitamin B-12 is associated with steady concentrations of vitamin B-12-related biomarkers in a healthy young population. *Am J Clin Nutr* 91:571–7.

Burris HH, Thomas A, Zera CA, McElrath TF. 2015. Prenatal vitamin use and vitamin D status during pregnancy, differences by race and overweight status. *J Perinatol* 35(4):241–5.

Butte NF, King JC. 2005. Energy requirements during pregnancy and lactation. *Public Health Nutr* 8:1010–27.

Carlson SE, Colombo J. 2016. Docosahexaenoic acid and arachidonic acid nutrition in early development. *Adv Pediatr* 63(1):453–71.

Carlson SE, Colombo J, Gajewski BJ, Gustafson KM, Mundy D, Yeast J, Georgieff MK, Markley LA, Kerling EH, Shaddy DJ. 2013. DHA supplementation and pregnancy outcomes. *Am J Clin Nutr* 97(4):808–15.

Carmichael SL, Cogswell ME, Ma C, Gonzalez-Feliciano A, Olney RS, Correa A, Shaw GM, National Birth Defects Prevention Study. 2013. Hypospadias and maternal intake of phytoestrogens. *Am J Epidemiol* 178:434–40.

Carmichael SL, Ma C, Feldkamp ML, Munger RG, Olney RS, Botto LD, Shaw GM, Correa A. 2012. Nutritional factors and hypospadias risks. *Paediatr Perinat Epidemiol* 26(4):353–60.

Carter JP, Furman T, Hutcheson HR. 1987. Preeclampsia and reproductive performance in a community of vegans. *South Med J* 80:692–7.

CDC (Centers for Disease Control and Prevention). 1998. Recommendations to prevent and control iron deficiency in the United States. *Morb Mortal Wkly Rep* 47(RR-3):1–29.

Dagnelie PC, van Staveren WA, van Klaveren JD, Burema J. 1988. Do children on macrobiotic diets show catch-up growth? *Eur J Clin Nutr* 42:1007–16.

Dagnelie PC, van Staveren WA, Vergot FJVRA, Burema J, van't Hof MA, van Klaveren JD, Hautvast JG. 1989. Nutritional status of infants aged 4 to 18 months on macrobiotic diets and matched omnivorous control infants: A population-based mixed-longitudinal study. II. Growth and psychomotor development. *Eur J Clin Nutr* 43:325–38.

Davis B, Melina V. 2014. *Becoming Vegan: Comprehensive Edition.* Summertown, TN: Book Publishing Co.

De Giuseppe R, Roggi C, Cena H. 2014. n-3 LC-PUFA supplementation: Effects on infant and maternal outcomes. *Eur J Nutr* 53(5):1147–54.

de Groot RH, Hornstra G, van Houwelingen AC, Roumen F. 2004. Effect of alpha-linolenic acid supplementation during pregnancy on maternal and neonatal polyunsaturated fatty acid status and pregnancy outcome. *Am J Clin Nutr* 79(2):251–60.

Delgado-Noguera MF, Calvache JA, Bonfill Cosp X, Kotanidou EP, Galli-Tsinopoulou A. 2015. Supplementation with long chain polyunsaturated fatty acids (LCPUFA) to breastfeeding mothers for improving child growth and development. *Cochrane Database Syst Rev* (7):CD007901. doi: 10.1002/14651858.CD007901.pub3.

Drake R, Reddy S, Davies J. 1998. Nutrient intake during pregnancy and pregnancy outcome of lactoovo-vegetarians, fish-eaters and non-vegetarians. *Veg Nutr* 2:45–52.

Dror DK, Allen LH. 2008. Effect of vitamin B12 deficiency on neurodevelopment in infants: Current knowledge and possible mechanisms. *Nutr Rev* 66(5):250–5.

Duggan C, Srinivasan K, Thomas T, Samuel T, Rajendran R, Muthayya S, Finkelstein JL et al. 2014. Vitamin B-12 supplementation during pregnancy and early lactation increases maternal, breast milk, and infant measures of vitamin B-12 status. *J Nutr* 144(5):758–64.

Elango R, Ball RO. 2016. Protein and amino acid requirements during pregnancy. *Adv Nutr* 15;7(4):839S–44S.

Ershow AG, Goodman G, Coates PM, Swanson CA. 2016. Research needs for assessing iodine intake, iodine status, and the effects of maternal iodine supplementation. *Am J Clin Nutr* 104(Suppl. 3):941S–9S.

Ferraro ZM, Contador F, Tawfiq A, Adamo KB, Gaudet L. 2015. Gestational weight gain and medical outcomes of pregnancy. *Obstet Med* 8(3):133–7.

Finkelstein JL, Layden AJ, Stover PJ. 2015. Vitamin B-12 and perinatal health. *Adv Nutr* 6:552–63.

Finley DA, Lönnerdal B, Dewey KG, Grivetti LE. 1985. Inorganic constituents of breast milk from vegetarian and nonvegetarian women: Relationships with each other and with organic constituents. *J Nutr* 115(6):772–81.

Food and Nutrition Board, Institute of Medicine. 1991. *Nutrition during Lactation.* Washington, DC: National Academy Press.

Food and Nutrition Board, Institute of Medicine. 1998. *Dietary Reference Intakes for Thiamin, Riboflavin, Niacin, Vitamin B_6, Folate, Vitamin B_{12}, Pantothenic Acid, Biotin, and Choline.* Washington, DC: National Academy Press.

Food and Nutrition Board, Institute of Medicine. 2001. *Dietary Reference Intakes for Vitamin A, Vitamin K, Arsenic, Boron, Chromium, Copper, Iodine, Iron, Manganese, Molybdenum, Nickel, Silicon, Vanadium, and Zinc.* Washington, DC: National Academy Press.

Food and Nutrition Board, Institute of Medicine. 2002. *Dietary Reference Intakes for Energy, Carbohydrate, Fiber, Fat, Fatty Acids, Cholesterol, Protein, and Amino Acids.* Washington, DC: National Academy Press.

Foster M, Herulah UN, Prasad A, Petocz P, Samman S. 2015. Zinc status of vegetarians during pregnancy: A systematic review of observational studies and meta-analysis of zinc intake. *Nutrients* 7(6):4512–25.

Foster M, Samman S. 2015. Vegetarian diets across the lifecycle: Impact on zinc intake and status. *Adv Food Nutr Res* 74:93–131.

Francois CA, Connor SL, Bolewicz LC, Connor WE. 2003. Supplementing lactating women with flaxseed oil does not increase docosahexaenoic acid in their milk. *Am J Clin Nutr* 77(1):226–33.

Gallo S, Phan A, Vanstone CA, Rodd C, Weiler HA. 2013. The change in plasma 25-hydroxyvitamin D did not differ between breast-fed infants that received a daily supplement of ergocalciferol or cholecalciferol for 3 months. *J Nutr* 143(2):148–53.

Gibson RA, Muhlhausler B, Makrides M. 2011. Conversion of linoleic acid and alpha-linolenic acid to long-chain polyunsaturated fatty acids (LCPUFAs), with a focus on pregnancy, lactation and the first 2 years of life. *Matern Child Nutr* 7(Suppl. 2):17–26.

Gibson RS, Heath AL, Szymlek-Gay EA. 2014. Is iron and zinc nutrition a concern for vegetarian infants and young children in industrialized countries? *Am J Clin Nutr* 100(Suppl. 1):459S–68S.

Heyssel RM, Bozian RC, Darby WJ, Bell MC. 1966. Vitamin B12 turnover in man: The assimilation of vitamin B12 from natural foodstuff by man and estimates of minimal daily dietary requirements. *Am J Clin Nutr* 18:176–84.

Hollis BW, Wagner CL, Howard CR, Ebeling M, Shary JR, Smith PG, Taylor SN, Morella K, Lawrence RA, Hulsey TC. 2015. Maternal versus infant vitamin D supplementation during lactation: A randomized controlled trial. *Pediatrics* 136(4):625–34.

Honzik T, Adamovicova M, Smolka V, Magner M, Hruba E, Zeman J. 2010. Clinical presentation and metabolic consequences in 40 breastfed infants with nutritional vitamin B12 deficiency—What have we learned? *Eur J Paediatr Neurol* 14(6):488–95.

Jensen CL 2006. Effects of n-3 fatty acids during pregnancy and lactation. *Am J Clin Nutr* 83(Suppl. 6):1452S–7S.

Jensen CL, Voigt RG, Prager TC, Zou YL, Fraley JK, Rozelle JC, Turcich MR, Llorente AM, Anderson RE, Heird WC. 2005. Effects of maternal docosahexaenoic acid on visual function and neurodevelopment in breastfed term infants. *Am J Clin Nutr* 82:125–32.

Kar S, Wong M, Rogozinska E, Thangaratinam S. 2015. Effects of omega-3 fatty acids in prevention of early preterm delivery: A systematic review and meta-analysis of randomized studies. *Eur J Obstet Gynecol Reprod Biol* 198:40–6.

King JC. 2000. Determinants of maternal zinc status during pregnancy. *Am J Clin Nutr* 71(Suppl.):1334S–43S.

King JC, Stein T, Doyle M. 1981. Effect of vegetarianism on the zinc status of pregnant women. *Am J Clin Nutr* 34:1049–55.

Koebnick C, Heins UA, Hoffmann I, Dagnelie PC, Leitzmann C. 2001. Folate status during pregnancy in women is improved by long-term high vegetable intake compared with the average Western diet. *J Nutr* 131:733–9.

Koebnick C, Leitzmann R, Garcia AL, Heins UA, Heuer T, Golf S, Katz N, Hoffmann I, Leitzmann C. 2005. Long-term effect of a plant-based diet on magnesium status during pregnancy. *Eur J Clin Nutr* 59:219–25.

Koletzko B, Lien E, Agostoni C, Böhles H, Campoy C, Cetin I, Decsi T et al. 2008. The roles of long chain polyunsaturated fatty acids in pregnancy, lactation and infancy: Review of current knowledge and consensus recommendations. *J Perinat Med* 36:5–14.

Lakin V, Haggarty P, Abramovich DR, Ashton J, Moffat CF, McNeill G, Danielian PJ, Grubb D. 1998. Dietary intake and tissue concentration of fatty acids in omnivore, vegetarian and diabetic pregnancy. *Prostaglandins Leukot Essent Fatty Acids* 59(3):209–20.

Larsen PS, Andersen AN, Uldall P, Bech BH, Olsen J, Hansen AV, Strandberg-Larsen K. 2014. Maternal vegetarianism and neurodevelopment of children enrolled in the Danish National Birth Cohort. *Acta Paediatr* 103(11):e507–9. doi: 10.1111/apa.12761.

Larsson CL, Johansson GK. 2002. Dietary intake and nutritional status of young vegans and omnivores in Sweden. *Am J Clin Nutr* 76:100–6.

Leikin-Frenkel A. 2016. Is there a role for alpha-linolenic acid in the fetal programming of health? *J Clin Med* 5(4):E40. doi: 10.3390/jcm5040040.

Le Louer B, Lemale J, Garcette K, Orzechowski C, Chalvon A, Girardet JP, Tounian P. 2014. Severe nutritional deficiencies in young infants with inappropriate plant milk consumption. *Arch Pediatr* 21(5):483–8.

Leung AM, Avram AM, Brenner AV, Duntas LH, Ehrenkranz J, Hennessey JV, Lee SL et al. 2015. Potential risks of excess iodine ingestion and exposure: Statement by the American Thyroid Association Public Health Committee. *Thyroid* 25(2):145–6.

Leung AM, Braverman LE. 2014. Consequences of excess iodine. *Nat Rev Endocrinol* 10(3):136–42.

Leung AM, LaMar A, He X, Braverman LE, Pearce EN. 2011a. Iodine status and thyroid function of Boston-area vegetarians and vegans. *J Clin Endocrin Metab* 96:E1303–7. doi: 10.1210/jc.2011-0256.

Leung AM, Pearce EN, Braverman LE. 2009. Iodine content of prenatal multivitamins in the United States. *N Engl J Med* 360:939–40.

Leung AM, Pearce EN, Braverman LE. 2011b. Iodine nutrition in pregnancy and lactation. *Endocrinol Metab Clin North Am* 40:765–77.

Leung SSF, Lee R, Sung S, Luo HY, Kam CW, Yuen MP, Hjelm M, Lee SH. 2001. Growth and nutrition of Chinese vegetarian children in Hong Kong. *J Paediatr Child Health* 37:247–53.

Lönnerdal B. 1986. Effects of maternal dietary intake on human milk composition. *J Nutr* 116(4):499–513.

Mangels AR. 2008. Vegetarian diets in pregnancy. In *Handbook of Nutrition and Pregnancy*, ed. Lammi-Keefe CJ, Couch SC, Philipson EH, 215–31. Totowa, NJ: Humana Press.

Mangels AR, Messina V. 2001. Considerations in planning vegan diets: Infants. *J Am Diet Assoc* 101(6):670–7.

Mangels R, Driggers J. 2012. The youngest vegetarians: Vegetarian infants and toddlers. *Infant Child Adolesc Nutr* 4:8–20.

Mangels R, Messina V, Messina M. 2011. *The Dietitian's Guide to Vegetarian Diets: Issues and Applications*. 3rd ed. Sudbury, MA: Jones & Bartlett Learning.

Martinez M. 1992. Tissue levels of polyunsaturated fatty acids during early human development. *J Pediatr* 120(4 Pt. 2):S129–38.

Martinez M, Mougan I. 1998. Fatty acid composition of human brain phospholipids during normal development. *J Neurochem* 71(6):2528–33.

Maslova E, Rytter D, Bech BH, Henriksen TB, Rasmussen MA, Olsen SF, Halldorsson TI. 2014. Maternal protein intake during pregnancy and offspring overweight 20 y later. *Am J Clin Nutr* 100(4):1139–48.

Meldrum S, Simmer K. 2016. Docosahexaenoic acid and neurodevelopmental outcomes of term infants. *Ann Nutr Metab* 69(Suppl. 1):22–8.

Melina V, Craig W, Levin S. 2016. Position of the Academy of Nutrition and Dietetics: Vegetarian diets. *J Acad Nutr Diet* 116:1970–80.

Messina M. 2016. Soy and health update: Evaluation of the clinical and epidemiologic literature. *Nutrients* 8(12):E754.

Messina V, Mangels AR. 2001. Considerations in planning vegan diets: Children. *J Am Diet Assoc* 101:661–9.

Nathan I, Hackett AF, Kirby S. 1997. A longitudinal study of the growth of matched pairs of vegetarian and omnivorous children, aged 7–11 years, in the north-west of England. *Eur J Clin Nutr* 51:20–5.

Norris J, Messina V. 2011. *Vegan for Life*. Boston: Da Capo Press.

North K, Golding J. 2000. A maternal vegetarian diet in pregnancy is associated with hypospadias. The ALSPAC Study Team. Avon Longitudinal Study of Pregnancy and Childhood. *BJU Int* 85:107–13.

Orlich MJ, Fraser GE. 2014. Vegetarian diets in the Adventist Health Study 2: A review of initial published findings. *Am J Clin Nutr* 100(Suppl. 1):353S–8S.

Peña-Rosas JP, De-Regil LM, Gomez Malave H, Flores-Urrutia MC, Dowswell T. 2015. Intermittent oral iron supplementation during pregnancy. *Cochrane Database Syst Rev* (10):CD009997. doi: 10.1002/14651858.CD009997.

Pistollato F, Sumalla Cano S, Elio I, Masias Vergara M, Giampieri F, Battino M. 2015. Plant-based and plant-rich diet patterns during gestation: Beneficial effects and possible shortcomings. *Adv Nutr* 6(5):581–91.

Rasmussen KM, Yaktine AL, eds. 2009. *Weight Gain during Pregnancy: Reexamining the Guidelines*. Washington, DC: National Academies Press.

Sabaté J, Wien M. 2010. Vegetarian diets and childhood obesity prevention. *Am J Clin Nutr* 91:1525S–9S.

Sanders TA. 1988. Growth and development of British vegan children. *Am J Clin Nutr* 48(3 Suppl.):822–5.

Sanders TA. 1999. Essential fatty acid requirements of vegetarians in pregnancy, lactation, and infancy. *Am J Clin Nutr* 70(3 Suppl.):555S–9S.

Section on Breastfeeding. 2012. Breastfeeding and the use of human milk. *Pediatrics* 129(3):e827–41.

Shi L, Ryan HH, Jones E, Simas TA, Lichtenstein AH, Sun Q, Hayman LL. 2014. Urinary isoflavone concentrations are inversely associated with cardiometabolic risk markers in pregnant U.S. women. *J Nutr* 144(3):344–51.

Stuebe AM, Oken E, Gillman MW. 2009. Associations of diet and physical activity during pregnancy with risk for excessive gestational weight gain. *Am J Obstet Gynecol* 201(1):58.e1–8.

Swanson CA, King JC. 1987. Zinc and pregnancy outcome. *Am J Clin Nutr* 46:763–71.

Taylor A, Redworth EW, Morgan JB. 2004. Influence of diet on iron, copper, and zinc status in children under 24 months of age. *Biol Trace Elem Res* 97(3):197–214.

Todaka E, Sakurai K, Fukata H, Miyagawa H, Uzuki M, Omori M, Osada H, Ikezuki Y, Tsutsumi O, Iguchi T, Mori C. 2005. Fetal exposure to phytoestrogens—The difference in phytoestrogen status between mother and fetus. *Environ Res* 99(2):195–203.

U.S. Department of Health and Human Services, U.S. Department of Agriculture. 2015. *2015–2020 Dietary Guidelines for Americans.* 8th ed. http://health.gov/dietaryguidelines/2015/guidelines/ (accessed February 15, 2017).

The Vegetarian Resource Group. 2014. How many teens and other youth are vegetarian and vegan? The Vegetarian Resource Group Blog, May 30. http://www.vrg.org/blog/2014/05/30/how-many-teens-and-other-youth-are-vegetarian-and-vegan-the-vegetarian-resource-group-asks-in-a-2014-national-poll/ (accessed February 14, 2017).

The Vegetarian Resource Group. 2016. How many adults in the U.S are vegetarian and vegan? http://www.vrg.org/nutshell/Polls/2016_adults_veg.htm (accessed February 14, 2017).

við Streym S, Højskov CS, Møller UK, Heickendorff L, Vestergaard P, Mosekilde L, Rejnmark L. 2016. Vitamin D content in human breast milk: A 9-mo follow-up study. *Am J Clin Nutr* 103(1):107–14.

Visentin CE, Masih SP, Plumptre L, Schroder TH, Sohn KJ, Ly A, Lausman AY et al. 2016. Low serum vitamin B-12 concentrations are prevalent in a cohort of pregnant Canadian women. *J Nutr* 146(5):1035–42.

Vitoria I, López B, Gómez J, Torres C, Guasp M, Calvo I, Dalmau J, 2016. Improper use of a plant-based vitamin C-deficient beverage causes scurvy in an infant. *Pediatrics* 137:1–5.

Wagner CL, Greer FR, American Academy of Pediatrics Section on Breastfeeding, American Academy of Pediatrics Committee on Nutrition. 2008. Prevention of rickets and vitamin D deficiency in infants, children, and adolescents. *Pediatrics* 122(5):1142–52.

Ward RJ, Abraham R, McFadyen IR, Haines AD, North WR, Patel M, Bhatt RV. 1988. Assessment of trace metal intake and status in a Gujerati pregnant Asian population and their influence of the outcome of pregnancy. *Br J Obstet Gynecol* 95:676–82.

WHO (World Health Organization. 2012. Guideline: Intermittent iron and folic acid supplementation in non-anaemic pregnant women. Geneva: World Health Organization.

WHO (World Health Organization). 2017. Breastfeeding. http://www.who.int/topics/breastfeeding/en/ (accessed February 14, 2017).

Williams CM, Burdge G. 2006. Long-chain n-3 PUFA: Plant v. marine sources. *Proc Nutr Soc* 65:42–50.

Yen C-E, Yen C-H, Huang M-C, Cheng CH, Huang YC. 2008. Dietary intake and nutritional status of vegetarian and omnivorous preschool children and their parents in Taiwan. *Nutr Res* 28:430–6.

Ziegler EE, Fomon SJ, Nelson SE, Jeter JM, Theuer RC. 2011. Dry cereals fortified with electrolytic iron or ferrous fumarate are equally effective in breast-fed infants. *J Nutr* 141(2):243–8.

13 Nutritionally Adequate Vegetarian Diets and Athletic Performance

D. Enette Larson-Meyer

CONTENTS

SUMMARY

Although vegetarian diets have many health benefits, available evidence supports neither a beneficial or detrimental effect of a vegetarian diet on physical performance capacity. Vegetarian diets, however, can support the energy and nutrient needs of all athletes—from recreational to elite. To ensure optimal performance, athletes following vegetarian diets should consume adequate energy and select foods rich in the "red-flag" nutrients, which either are found less abundantly in vegetarian foods or are less well absorbed from plant than animal sources. These nutrients include iron, zinc, iodine, vitamin B12, calcium, and vitamin D. Compromised intake of these and other nutrients has the potential to negatively impact exercise performance.

13.1   INTRODUCTION

Athletes at all levels—from recreational to elite—may opt for vegetarian diets for any number of reasons, including health, ethical, environmental, ecological, philosophical, religious, or spiritual reasons, or simply due to food aversion or dislike of meat. While performance advantages are typically not a reason, there are many aspects of a nutritionally adequate plant-based diet that may help the athlete optimize training and performance while also reducing risk for chronic diseases (Craig and Mangels, 2009; Yokoyama et al., 2014; Dinu et al., 2017; Melina et al., 2016). Depending on the extent of dietary limitations, however, athletes need to ensure that they consume adequate amounts of the nutrients that either are found less abundantly in vegetarian foods or are less well absorbed from plant than animal sources. Like most athletes, vegetarian athletes may benefit from education about food choices to optimize their health and peak performance (Larson-Meyer, 2007). The dietitian or health professional working with vegetarian athletes should understand the athletes' reason for being vegetarian and educate them on nutrient sources that fit their personal beliefs and values (Melina et al., 2016; Thomas et al., 2016).

This chapter reviews the potential benefits of vegetarian diets on performance and the specific energy, macronutrient, vitamin, and mineral requirements of vegetarian athletes at all levels of sports performance—from the casual exerciser to the competitive athlete. Specific tips for meeting energy and nutrient needs are also provided.

13.2   POTENTIAL PERFORMANCE BENEFITS OF VEGETARIAN DIETS

As noted in previous chapters in this text, vegetarian and vegan diets may have many health advantages over the typical Westernized diet, namely, reducing risk for chronic disease. Whether such diets can affect training or sports performance has not been adequately explored (Nieman, 1988; Craddock et al., 2016; Thomas et al., 2016). This may be due to a general lack of interest in the influence of diet on athletic performance by funding agencies, such as the National Institutes of Health or the U.S. Department of Agriculture, and/or the limited population size; that is, vegetarian athletes make up only a small portion of an already limited number. One of the few surveys conducted in athletes at the international level found that as many as 8% of athletes from various international commonwealth countries report following vegetarian diets, with 1% of those being vegan (Pelly and Burkhart, 2014).

Apart from the health benefits, vegetarian diets have the potential to improve performance but—if food choices are consistently suboptimal—also impair it. Plausible theories suggest that the high carbohydrate and high phytochemical content of the vegetarian diet, along with its potential to induce a slight serum alkalinity, may offer performance advantages. The high carbohydrate content, as will be further discussed later in this chapter, may lead to improved glycogen stores and endurance performance capacity (Nieman, 1988, 1999). The higher content of phytochemicals, including antioxidants, may additionally help reduce oxidative stress associated with prolonged exercise and modulate immune function and inflammation (Trapp et al., 2010). The vegetarian diet is more likely to promote higher intakes of the antioxidant vitamins (vitamin C, vitamin E, and beta-carotene) and other phytochemicals

(Rauma and Mykkanen, 2000; Krajcovicova-Kudlackova et al., 2003b). Muscular exercise promotes the production of free radicals and other reactive oxygen species that are thought to be responsible for exercise-induced protein oxidation and the promotion of muscle fatigue (Powers et al., 2004). Research, however, is needed to determine whether a plant-based diet naturally high in antioxidants and phytochemicals enhances recovery, prevents inflammatory (or overuse) injury, and attenuates the oxidative damage that occurs with heavy training. Furthermore, the high fruit and vegetable intake common in the vegetarian diet may have an alkaline effect on acid–base levels (Deriemaeker et al., 2010; Hietavala et al., 2015), thereby helping to buffer acid production during intense exercise in a manner similar to that of bicarbonate ingestion (Carr et al., 2011). The potential detriments of a vegetarian diet due to low nutrient intake and/or lower muscle creatine content are reviewed later in this chapter.

Despite the promise of performance improvements, little evidence supports a performance advantage of vegetarian diets in athletes. Interestingly, in the early 1900s a handful of studies investigated the value of a vegetarian diet as a means of increasing physical capacity. Most of these studies, however, were not adequately controlled (based on today's standards) and, in a few cases, may have resulted in the answer the investigators or athletes desired—namely, that a vegan or vegetarian diet was superior to a meat-containing diet (Nieman, 1988). Indeed, in his interpretation of these studies, Nieman (1988) suggested that the superior performance of some of the early vegetarian athletes is explained by their high-carbohydrate diet (relative to the diet of other athletes at the time) and their motivation to demonstrate the superiority of the vegetarian diet. More recent cross-sectional studies have found no differences in the aerobic or anaerobic capacities of male and female athletes following vegetarian compared with meat-based diets (Hanne et al., 1986), or in their performance during a 1000 km endurance run (Eisinger et al., 1994). A randomly assigned crossover study additionally found that performance was not altered in male omnivorous athletes placed on a lacto-ovo vegetarian diet, compared with a meat-rich macronutrient-controlled diet, for 6 weeks (Richter et al., 1991; Raben et al., 1992). Although total testosterone decreased slightly on the vegetarian diet, training and performance indicators were not affected (Raben et al., 1992). The authors speculated that the decrease in testosterone was most likely temporary and related to the high fiber intake on the vegetarian compared with the meat-based diet (98 vs. 47 g). A recent analysis that explored the effect of an exclusive vegetarian-based diet on aerobic and anaerobic performance using a rigorous systematic approach (Craddock et al., 2016) further concluded, as Nieman did nearly 20 years ago (Nieman, 1999), that vegetarian diets do not seem to benefit or impair performance. Due to the limited studies in athletes and the high noted variability among athletes of different sports and body sizes, however, the authors conclude that further research is warranted (Craddock et al., 2016).

13.3 OVERVIEW OF ENERGY UTILIZATION DURING EXERCISE AND MACRONUTRIENT GUIDELINES

A fundamental understanding of how the interaction between training and macronutrient intake affects energy systems, substrate availability, training adaptations, and performance is necessary for understanding the macronutrient-specific guidelines for athletes

(Thomas et al., 2016). These guidelines form the basics of the sports nutrition guidelines for all athletes, including those following vegetarian diets. Exercise is fueled by an integrated series of energy systems that include the phosphagen, glycolytic, and aerobic systems, using substrates that are from both endogenous (body stores) and exogenous (recent dietary intake) sources (Thomas et al., 2016). These pathways are modulated primarily by exercise intensity and duration, but also by the athletes' training status and nutritional intake (Hargreaves, 2000; Maughan and Gleeson, 2010). During exercise, the immediate source of energy is the disruption of the high-energy phosphate bonds of adenosine triphosphate (ATP) and creatine phosphate (CP). Existing ATP and CP stores in skeletal muscle are expended within ~10 seconds of exercise initiation and must be regenerated from energy stored within the chemical bonds of carbohydrate, fat, and protein substrates. CP and muscle glycogen are the main fuels for short-duration, high-intensity exercise, where performance capacity is limited by lactate accumulation and muscle cell acidosis (by-products of the rapid generation of energy from carbohydrate, commonly called "fast" or "anaerobic" glycolysis). Oxidation of glucose, glycogen, and free fatty acids (from muscle triglyceride and adipose tissue) supplies energy for exercise lasting longer than about 2 minutes. The relative contribution increases almost exponentially with the intensity of the exercise, whereas the relative contribution of fat increases with longer duration or lower intensity of muscular work (Romijn et al., 1993, 2000; Hargreaves, 2000; Maughan and Gleeson, 2010). Muscle and liver glycogen and muscle triglycerides may be almost completely depleted in exercise lasting longer than about 2–3 hours. Under these conditions, gluconeogenesis from specific amino acids, and adipose tissue triglycerides serve as the major source of fuel, but they cannot be used rapidly enough to support moderate to intense bouts of exercise. The contribution of protein as a fuel during exercise is minimal (~5%–10% of total energy) but increases in latter stages of exhaustive exercise if gluconeogenesis is present. Diets that are higher in carbohydrates increase muscle and liver glycogen stores, increase carbohydrate oxidation, and spare protein, as will be reviewed in detail in the following sections.

13.4 REQUIREMENTS FOR ENERGY AND ENERGY-GENERATING MACRONUTRIENTS

13.4.1 ENERGY

Meeting energy needs is a nutrition priority for all athletes (Thomas et al., 2016). The energy needs of athletes and active individuals vary considerably and are dependent on sex, body size, body composition, training regimen, and general (nontraining) physical activity patterns. Exposure to environmental extremes during training or competition, including hot and cold temperatures and high altitude, also impacts energy requirement. Using doubly labeled water, energy expenditure has been shown to range from ~2600 kcal/day in female swimmers to ~8500 kcal/day in male cyclists participating in the Tour de France bicycle race (Goran, 1995). Daily energy requirements, however, are likely to be lower in smaller and/or less active individuals and during times of less intense training. Although vegetarianism does not necessarily affect energy needs, higher resting energy expenditure (REE), along with higher basil sympathetic nervous system activity, has been observed in male vegetarians and vegans compared with male omnivores (of similar weight, body composition, and fitness); this effect is thought to be mediated by the higher carbohydrate content of the vegetarian diet (Toth and Poehlman, 1994).

In practice, total daily energy expenditure (TDEE) of vegetarian athletes can be estimated using a variety of methods. One method is to estimate REE using an appropriate prediction equation, including the Cunningham (Cunningham, 1980) and Harris–Benedict (Harris and Benedict, 1919) equations, or predictive equations from the Dietary Reference Intakes, and then multiply the estimated REE by an activity factor of between 1.4 and 2.5, depending on the estimated physical activity level. Typical activity factors include 1.5 (range = 1.4–1.59) for low physical activity, 1.75 (1.6–1.89) for active athletes (athletes who exercise approximately 1 hour/day), and 2.2 (1.9–2.5) for very active athletes (competitive athletes engaging in several hours of vigorous exercise training) (Manore and Thompson, 2000; Brooks et al., 2004). Use of either the Cunningham (Cunningham, 1980) or Harris–Benedict (Harris and Benedict, 1919) equations may provide better estimates of REE in athletic populations unless population-specific equations are available. Another approach, outlined in Table 13.1,

TABLE 13.1
Estimation of Total Daily Energy Needs Using the Factorial Method. Example: 22-Year-Old Male Collegiate Soccer Player who Practices for 90 Minutes and Strength Trains for 30 Minutes; He is 176 cm with a BM of 75 kg

Energy Expenditure	Formula	
REE (resting energy expenditure)	$66 + 13.7 \times$ BM (kg) $+ 5 \times$ height (cm) $- 6.8 \times$ age	Harris–Benedict: $66 + (13.7 \times 75) + (5 \times 176) - (6.8 \times 22) = 1824$ kcal/day
Harris–Benedict (men)	$655 + 9.6 \times$ BM (kg) $+ 1.7 \times$	
Harris–Benedict (women)	height (cm) $- 4.7 \times$ age	
Cunningham[a]	$22 \times$ fat-free mass (kg)[a]	
NEAT (energy expenditure during nonexercise training activity)	Light activity: $0.3 \times$ REE Moderate activity: $0.5 \times$ REE Heavy activity: $0.7 \times$ REE	Occupation = student; assume light activity when not training $1824 \times 0.3 = 547$ kcal/day
ExEE (energy expenditure during exercise training)	Refer to the physical activity tables found in many nutrition or exercise physiology texts for approximate caloric expenditure per minute for various physical activities	A 70 kg athlete uses 7.8 net kcal/ minute (above rest) for soccer and 6.6 kcal/minute for weight training: 7.8 kcal/minute $\times$ 90 minutes $= 702 +$ 6.6 kcal/minute $\times$ 30 minutes $= 198 =$ 900 kcal/day
TDEE (total daily energy expenditure)	REE + NEAT + ExEE = kcal/ day	$1824 + 547 + 900 = 3270$ kcal/day[b]

[a] The Cunningham equation for estimating REE has been shown to closely estimate REE in male and female endurance athletes (Manore and Thompson, 2000), such as distance runners and cyclists, but is dependent on obtaining an accurate estimate of body fat.

[b] Some sources suggest that total daily energy needs are 6%–10% higher than TDEE to account for the thermic effect of food.

is to sum the estimates of the components of TDEE, which include REE (Cunningham, 1980), the energy cost of training or organized physical exercise (TrEE), and the energy cost of occupational and spontaneous physical activity (nontraining energy expenditure [NTrEE]). Energy expenditure from training and occupation can be estimated from activity logs with subjective estimates of intensity using activity codes (Williams et al., 2013) or metabolic equivalents (Ainsworth et al., 2000). Although estimation of TDEE from its components may be more cumbersome, it accounts for greater variation in training and daily activity patterns and can also serve as an educational tool when calculated in the athlete's presence. Estimates of TDEE may be useful when developing meal plans and/or when evaluating the adequacy of energy intake (along with body mass [BM] changes and dietary intake assessments).

As previously mentioned, meeting nutrient needs is a priority (Thomas et al., 2016). Inadequate energy intake relative to energy expenditure negates the benefits of training, compromises performance, and may result in health complications, including loss of muscle mass, menstrual cycle dysfunction, loss of or failure to gain bone density, and an increased risk of fatigue, injury, and illness. Some athletes who follow vegetarian and vegan diets may have difficulty meeting energy requirements. This may be due to excessively high energy requirements, food choices that are high in fiber and/or of low energy density, and hectic schedules that do not allow adequate time to eat. Striving to eat frequent meals and snacks, that is, about six to eight meals or snacks per day, and adequate planning ("brown-bag" lunches, snacks packed in the gym bag or kept in a desk drawer, etc.) may help athletes meet energy needs and maintain BM. When appropriate, athletes can increase energy intake by selecting energy-dense foods, such as nuts, seeds, and avocado, and limiting fiber-rich foods. For example, consuming only one-third to one-half of grain and fruit servings in the whole, unprocessed form will reduce excessive fiber intake and reduce early onset of satiety (Larson-Meyer, 2007). Other vegetarian athletes, in contrast, may require lower energy intakes to promote weight reduction for health and/or performance. These athletes may benefit from an emphasis on whole, unprocessed food choices to promote satiety and help in achievement of a healthy BM (see Chapter 14 for additional information geared toward weight concerns in the vegetarian athlete). Both MyPlate, which has adjustments of energy requirements and tips for vegetarians (U.S. Department of Agriculture, https://www.choosemyplate.gov/), and the guidelines developed by Larson-Meyer specifically for vegetarian athletes (Larson-Meyer, 2007) may be useful in educating athletes about healthy eating patterns. Eating plans developed for individuals who consume vegetarian or vegan diets (Messina et al., 2003, 2004) may also provide a useful framework if the number of servings is increased appropriately to the higher energy demands of many athletes. A sample menu for a 3200 kcal vegetarian and a 3200 kcal vegan diet based off of MyPlate is shown in Table 13.2. Energy intake of 3200 kcal and even higher may be required to meet the needs of individuals who train or exercise regularly, as was outlined in Table 13.1 for a collegiate soccer player.

13.4.2 CARBOHYDRATES

Carbohydrates are an important fuel for muscle during exercise and for the central nervous system and should make up the greater part of the athlete's diet. Although carbohydrates, fat, and, to a lesser extent, protein, serve as energy substrates during physical

TABLE 13.2
Sample Day's Menu for a Vegetarian and Vegan Athlete Requiring 3200 kcal/day Using MyPlate

Food group amounts: 2.5 cups fruit, 4 cups vegetables, 10 oz grains, 7 oz protein, 3 cups dairy (or calcium foods)

	Vegetarian	Vegan
Breakfast	**Oatmeal with fruit and nuts**	
½ cup fruit		
2 oz grains	1 cup oatmeal with raisins	1 cup oatmeal with raisins
1 protein equivalent	½ oz toasted walnuts	½ oz toasted walnuts
1 cup dairy/calcium foods	1 cup milk	1 cup soy milk
Lunch	**Pasta salad with vinegar and oil**	
1 cup vegetables	1 cup mixed vegetables	1 cup mixed vegetables
3 oz grains	1½ cups pasta	1½ cups pasta
2 protein equivalents	1 oz mozzarella cheese + ¼ cup chick peas	½ cup chick peas
1 cup fruit	1 large apple	1 large apple
Snack	**Peanut butter sandwich**	
2 oz grains	2 slices whole-grain bread	2 slices whole-grain bread
2 protein equivalents	2 tbsp peanut butter	2 tbsp peanut butter
1 cup dairy/calcium foods	1 tbsp honey	1 tbsp fruit preserves
1 cup fruit	1 cup fresh fruit in season	1 cup fresh fruit in season
Dinner	**Stir-fry**	
2 cups vegetables	2 cups vegetables (broccoli, bok	2 cups vegetables (broccoli, bok
3 oz grains	choy, carrots, sprouts)	choy, carrots, sprouts)
2 protein equivalents	1½ cups brown rice	1½ cups brown rice
	4 oz tofu	4 oz tofu
	Lemon, sesame, ginger sauce	Lemon, sesame, ginger sauce
Bedtime snack		
1 cup vegetables	1 cup milk	1 cup calcium-fortified juice
1 cup dairy/calcium foods	1 cup edamame peas	1 cup edamame peas

activity, carbohydrates are the only fuel that can sustain the moderate- to high-level activity required by most sports and athletic endeavors. Carbohydrates are also the only fuel used by the brain and central nervous system without adaptation to ketone body utilization. Carbohydrate stores as liver and muscle glycogen become depleted during prolonged exercise lasting longer than ~90 minutes and during intense intermittent activities, which include the stop-and-go running efforts of many team sports. Adequate carbohydrate intake maintains muscle and liver glycogen stores, helping to optimize performance during prolonged, moderate-intensity exercise (Brewer et al., 1988; O'Keeffe et al., 1989; Spencer et al., 1991; Coggan and Swanson, 1992; Achten et al., 2004) and intermittent and short-duration, high-intensity exercise (Hargreaves et al., 1984; Sugiura and Kobayashi, 1998). Performance benefits include delayed time to fatigue during training or competition and/or better sprinting potential at the end of a race or sporting event. Dietary carbohydrate further optimizes mood (Achten et al., 2004) and may be important

TABLE 13.3

Carbohydrate Recommendations for Athletes

Low intensity or skill based: 3–5 g CHO/kg BW

Moderate exercise (~1 hour/day): 5–7 g CHO/kg BW

Endurance program (moderate to high intensity of 1–3 hours/day): 6–10 g CHO/kg BW

Extreme program (moderate to high intensity of 4–5 hours/day): 8–12 g CHO/kg BW

Goal: Optimize liver and muscle glycogen stores

Note: BW = body weight; CHO = carbohydrate.

for the maintenance of Krebs cycle intermediates (Spencer et al., 1991) and preservation of the bioenergetic state of the muscle phosphagen system (i.e., the ratio of high-energy CP to its breakdown products) during intense exercise (Larson et al., 1994).

The carbohydrate needs of athletes are easily met by consuming a variety of carbohydrate-rich plant foods, such as cereals, grains, legumes, starchy vegetables, and fruits. The carbohydrate recommendations for athletes are summarized in Table 13.3 and range from as low as 3–5 g/kg BM/day to as high as 12 g/kg BM/day (Burke et al., 2011; Thomas et al., 2016). The recommended amount within this range depends on the athlete's TDEE, training intensity, training goals, and competitive season. For example, competitive, elite-level athletes undergoing intensive training (>4–5 hours/day) may benefit from a higher carbohydrate intake within the upper range (8–12 g/kg BM/day), whereas athletes participating at a level that demands less training (e.g., skill-based activity or recreational exercisers) likely have lower carbohydrate needs (3–5 g/kg BM/day).

Although the typical vegetarian diet is packed with carbohydrates, label reading skills along with a working knowledge of carbohydrate sources (Larson-Meyer, 2007) may help athletes achieve carbohydrate intake recommendations in the overall diet and before, during, and after exercise (as will be reviewed in Chapter 14). The estimated carbohydrate and protein content of vegetarian and vegan foods is included in Chapter 14 (Table 14.2). Having the athlete count carbohydrate intake at a meal, snack, or over the course of a day may be a particularly useful tool for educating the athlete on the importance of dietary carbohydrates—particularly when intake is compared with a training log or feedback from a coach. As an example, an athlete who notices that low carbohydrate intake on a particular day was associated with lightheadedness or "dead" legs after training may then make the connection between carbohydrate intake and performance.

13.4.3   PROTEIN

The protein requirements for athletes are generally higher than the Recommended Dietary Allowance (RDA) and vary according to the sport or activity, intensity of training, level of experience, and carbohydrate and energy availability (Phillips and Van Loon, 2011). The protein needs of active vegetarians who engage in light to moderate activity several times per week will likely be met by the RDA of 0.8 g/kg BM/day, whereas the requirement for those who train more intensely may be higher than the RDA, in the range from 1.2 to 2.0 g/kg BM/day

(Thomas et al., 2016). The protein needs of athletes vary according to the sport or activity, intensity of training, and level of experience (Phillips and Van Loon, 2011). Additional protein and essential amino acids during routine endurance and strength training are required to cover the enhanced protein deposition during muscle development and the increased protein utilization as an auxiliary fuel during exercise (Tipton et al., 2007).

Furthermore, inadequate intake of total energy and/or carbohydrates increases the protein requirement. During prolonged endurance activity, for example, athletes with low glycogen stores metabolize twice as much protein as those with adequate stores, primarily due to increased amino acid utilization as a source for gluconeogenesis (Lemon and Mullin, 1980). Recent research has also found that dietary protein, namely, the amino acid leucine, serves as a trigger for muscle protein synthesis induced by training (Phillips and Van Loon, 2011)—a role beyond the supply of amino acids for building blocks or energy. More specifically, it is thought that leucine must be increased to a critical concentration after a meal or snack in order to "turn on" muscle protein synthesis. Research further shows that the peak in leucine concentration varies by content and absorbability from protein-rich foods. Whey, for example, induces a much greater spike in plasma leucine than soy or casein proteins. As is summarized in Table 13.4, soy, particularly fiber-free isolated protein, is a rich source of leucine, as are

TABLE 13.4
Leucine Content of Selected Protein Foods

Food	Protein, g	Leucine, g
Cheese, cheddar, 1 oz	7.1	0.68
Cheese, cottage, ½ cup	13.4	1.34
Cheese, Swiss, 1 oz	7.6	0.84
Cottage cheese, 2%	13.4	1.34
Egg, 1 large whole	6.3	0.54
Milk, fat-free (skim)	8.3	0.80
Milk, reduced fat (2%)	8.1	0.81
Yogurt, low-fat vanilla	12.1	1.2
Whey, sweet fluid	2.1	0.19
Whey, sweet dry	3.9	0.36
Black beans, ½ cup	7.6	0.61
Chick peas, ½ cup	7.3	0.52
Lentils, ½ cup	8.9	0.65
Peanut butter, 2 tbsp	8.0	0.49
Pinto beans, ½ cup	7.7	0.65
Soy beans, mature	14.3	1.17
Tofu, firm, ½ cup	19.9	1.51
Tofu, soft, ½ cup	8.1	0.62
Soy protein isolate, 1 oz	22.9	1.9

most legumes. The leucine in soy foods and legumes is not as absorbable as the leucine in whey and therefore may not serve as big of a trigger as whey. A recent study, however, found that consumption of pea protein was just as effective as whey in promoting gains in muscle mass and strength during 12 weeks of resistance training (Babault et al., 2015). After the initial leucine-mediated stimulation of muscle protein synthesis, increased activation may be dependent on adequate provision of other essential amino acids.

The protein recommendations for athletes following vegetarian diets are no different than those of athletes following omnivorous diets. While it has been suggested that vegetarians may need approximately 10% more protein than omnivores to account for the lower digestibility of plant than animal proteins (Rodriguez et al., 2009), the Institute of Medicine does not believe there is sufficient evidence to support a higher protein requirement for vegetarians consuming complementary plant proteins (Otten et al., 2006). In support, a meta-analysis of nitrogen balance studies found that the source of dietary protein did not significantly impact the protein requirement of healthy individuals (Rand et al., 2003). The protein needs of athletes whose food choices most exclusively consist of less-well digested plant sources (legumes and unprocessed grains), rather than well-digested sources (including tofu, isolated soy protein, dairy, and eggs), however, may have higher requirements to account for the lower amino acid digestibility (FAO/WHO/UNU, 2002).

Vegetarian diets contain an average of 12.5% of energy from protein, whereas vegan diets contain 11% (Messina et al., 2004). Thus, a 75 kg male athlete consuming 3200 kcal, for example, would receive 1.33 and 1.17 g protein/kg BM from the average vegetarian and vegan diets, respectively. Similarly, a 50 kg female athlete consuming 2200 kcal would receive 1.38 g/kg BM from a vegetarian diet and 1.21 g/kg from a vegan diet. Vegetarian athletes would therefore meet the lower range of the recommendation without additional planning. Athletes actively engaged in strength training, muscle building, or high-frequency or interval training (Rand et al., 2003), or those purposely restricting energy intake to reduce BM, however, may need to focus on incorporating more protein-rich foods to achieve intakes in the upper range of the recommendations. This is accomplished by incorporating more protein-rich vegetarian foods in meals or snacks. Specific examples include adding chickpeas or cottage cheese to a salad, soy milk or Greek yogurt to a fruit snack, lentils to spaghetti sauce, or tofu or quinoa to a stir-fry. Not all milk alternates, including almond and rice milks, however, are rich sources of proteins. The approximate protein content of selected vegetarian protein sources is shown in Tables 13.4 and 14.2.

Recent research has also suggested an additional benefit to protein consumption in close proximity to strength or endurance exercise (Tipton et al., 2001; Tipton and Witard, 2007), as will be reviewed in further detail in Section 14.2.2, and to the spreading of protein throughout the course of the day (i.e., consuming 15–25 g [0.25–0.3 g/kg BM/day]) at regular meals and snacks versus all in an evening meal (Mamerow et al., 2014). The need to complement proteins at every meal, that is, eating specific combinations of plant-based proteins, however, is not necessary (Young and Pellett, 1994; Craig and Mangels, 2009; Melina et al., 2016). Emphasizing amino acid balance at individual meals is not necessary because "limiting amino acids" in one meal are buffered by amino acid pools (Young and Pellett, 1994) found primarily in skeletal muscle and supported by the turnover of endogenous gut proteins (Bergstrom et al., 1990). The only exception may be in the postexercise period, where a certain concentration of leucine and about 10 g of essential acids are thought to be necessary to optimize muscle protein synthesis in the immediate postexercise period. Furthermore, although some plant foods tend to be low in certain amino acids—including methionine and lysine—usual combinations of protein, such as rice and beans or grains and nuts, tend to be "complete" (Young and Pellett, 1994). It is important to note, however, that because cereals tend to be low in lysine, athletes who do not consume dairy and/or eggs should incorporate beans and soy products into their diets to ensure adequate lysine intake.

13.4.4   FAT

Dietary fat is a necessary component of a healthy diet and should make up the remainder of energy needs after carbohydrate and protein requirements are met. Recent guidelines from the Academy of Nutrition and Dietetics, the American College of Sports Medicine, and Dietitians of Canada recommend that intake of fat by athletes should be in accordance with public health guidelines and be individualized based on training and body composition goals (Thomas et al., 2016). These guidelines emphasize that the proportion of energy from saturated fats should be limited to less than 10% and that sources of essential fatty acids should be included to meet the adequate intake recommendations (U.S. Department of Health and Human Services and U.S. Department of Agriculture, 2011).

The recommendations for athletes further discourage chronic implementation of fat intakes below 20% of energy and strategies that promote low-carbohydrate, high-fat diets for purported performance benefits (Thomas et al., 2016). While the extremely low-fat vegetarian diets (<10% energy from fat) recommended by Ornish et al. (1990) and Barnard et al. (2009a) have been shown to promote regression of coronary atherosclerosis (Ornish et al., 1990; Gould et al., 1992, 1995) and improve glycemic control (Barnard et al., 2009a, 2009b) in nonathletes, such diets may be too restrictive for athletes during heavy training. In athletes, consumption of less than 20% of energy from fat has the potential to impair endurance performance (Muoio et al., 1994; Hoppeler et al., 1999; Horvath et al., 2000), unfavorably alter lipid profile (Thompson et al., 1984; Brown and Cox, 1998; Larson-Meyer et al., 2002, 2008), reduce absorption of fat-soluble vitamins, and compromise muscle triglyceride stores (Decombaz et al., 2001; Larson-Meyer et al., 2002)—an important fuel source during prolonged, moderate-intensity exercise (Romijn et al., 1993, 2000). In contrast, the recently revised craze of chronic adaptation to high-fat, low-carbohydrate diets to enhance fat oxidation capacity downregulates carbohydrate metabolism and compromises exercise performance during the high-intensity efforts needed for most sports (Havemann et al., 2006; Burke, 2015).

Athletes can ensure fat intake within the guidelines through judicious incorporation of vegetarian fat sources, including nuts, seeds, avocado, vegetable oils, and low- or full-fat dairy products. In general, however, vegetarian diets are rich in sources of omega-6 polyunsaturated fatty acids but may be low in omega-3 fatty acids (Reid et al., 2013). Lacto-ovo diets may also provide excessive saturated fat if large servings of eggs and full-fat dairy products are consumed regularly. Since omega-3 fatty acids may be important for controlling inflammation (Jeromson et al., 2015), vegetarian athletes may benefit from incorporating more omega-3-rich foods (walnuts, flaxseed, canola, flax, hemp, and walnut oils) into their diet in place of some omega-6-rich oils (corn, cotton seed, sunflower, and safflower). Although less than 10% of alpha-linolenic acid is elongated to eicosapentaenoic acid (EPA) in humans (Williams and Burdge, 2006), its conversion may be improved when omega-6 concentrations in the diet or blood are low (Williams and Burdge, 2006). Athletes may benefit from increased omega-3 consumption, including pregnant athletes and those with chronic inflammatory injuries; these athletes may want to consider docosahexaenoic acid (DHA)–rich microalgae supplements (Geppert et al., 2005), which are well absorbed and increase circulating concentrations of both DHA and EPA (Conquer and Holub, 1996). Athletes habitually obtaining more than 10% of energy from saturated fat should replace some servings of full-fat dairy and/or eggs with plant-based oils.

13.5   MINERALS AND VITAMINS

Most athletes—including vegetarian athletes—can meet their vitamin and mineral requirements by consuming a diet that provides adequate energy and consists of a variety of wholesome foods. Because of hectic training and work or school schedules, athletes in general may be prone to make poor food choices, which can result in suboptimal intakes of many vitamins and minerals. The restrictions added on top of this by the vegetarian diet can further increase the athlete's risk for deficiency, specifically for "red-flag nutrients" that are found less abundantly in vegetarian foods or are less well absorbed from plant than animal sources. These red-flag nutrients include iron, zinc, calcium, vitamin B12 (Thomas et al., 2016), and iodine. Compromised intake of these and other vitamins and minerals has the potential to impact exercise performance.

13.5.1   IRON

Iron depletion is one of the most prevalent nutrient deficiencies in athletes in general (Malczewska et al., 2000, 2001; Woolf et al., 2009) and may be more common in female athletes and some athletes following vegetarian diets than in the general population. Iron depletion with (stage III) and without (stage II) anemia can impair maximal oxygen uptake and muscle function (Zhu and Haas, 1997) and decrease endurance performance (Lamanca and Haymes, 1992; Brownlie et al., 2004). In athletes, iron depletion is most commonly attributed to insufficient energy and/or low iron intakes (Thomas et al., 2016), but it can also be impacted by acute inflammation (Peeling et al., 2008) and increased iron losses through gastrointestinal bleeding (Robertson et al., 1987), heavy sweating (Waller and Haymes,1996), footstrike or intravascular hemolysis (Eichner, 1985), high-altitude training, hematuria (Jones and Newhouse, 1997), heavy menstrual blood loss in female athletes (Malczewska et al., 2000), and/or rapid growth in young athletes (Thomas et al., 2016).

As reviewed in Chapter 10, most of the iron in a vegetarian diet is nonheme iron, which has a lower absorption rate (2%–20%) than heme iron (15%–35%) (Craig, 1994) and is sensitive to dietary factors that inhibit and enhance its absorption.

Thus, vegetarian athletes need to consume iron-rich plant sources with foods or beverages that contain iron enhancers, such as vitamin C and other organic acids, and avoid their consumption with dietary components that dampen iron absorption, such as phytates, polyphenolics (e.g., tannins found in tea, coffee, herb teas, and cocoa), and excess calcium (Melina et al., 2016). Due to increased iron losses with training and the lower bioavailability of iron from a vegetarian diet, however, there is some suggestion that vegetarians and athletes may have iron requirements that are 1.3–1.8 times higher than the RDA, respectively. Therefore, it may be prudent that vegetarian athletes aim for intakes that are slightly higher than the RDA.

In most cases, vegetarians who eat a varied and well-balanced diet rich in pulses, whole grains, iron-fortified cereals, nuts, seeds, and green leafy vegetables can achieve adequate iron status (Saunders et al., 2013) without the need for supplementation. Iron-rich plant foods are listed in Table 13.5. Studies in both vegetarian athletes (Snyder et al., 1989) and nonathletes (Ball and Bartlett, 1999; Messina et al., 2004) have found that vegetarians have iron intakes that are on average similar to or higher than those of nonvegetarians but often have lower iron status. These findings support the importance of education not only on the plant sources of iron but also on the factors that enhance and interfere with iron absorption. While supplementation has been shown to improve energetic efficiency and endurance performance in

TABLE 13.5
Vegetarian Sources of Selected Vitamins and Minerals

Nutrient	Good Food Choices
Iron	Pulses, nuts, seeds, whole/enriched grains, enriched/fortified cereals and pasta, leafy green and root vegetables, dried fruits, egg yolk
Zinc	Pulses, nuts, seeds, whole-grain products, fortified ready-to-eat cereal, soy products, commercial meat analogues
Calcium	Calcium-set tofu, calcium-fortified beverages (orange juice and other fruit juices, soy and rice milks), broccoli, Chinese cabbage, kale, collard, mustard and turnip greens, almonds, tahini, texturized vegetable protein, blackstrap molasses, cow's milk, certain cheeses, pulses
Vitamin D[a]	Fatty fish (salmon, sardines, mackerel), fortified foods (cow's milk, some brands of soymilk, other milk alternatives, orange juice, ready-to-eat breakfast cereals, margarines, yogurt), egg yolks, sun-dried mushrooms
Iodine	Iodized salt and sea vegetables (seaweed, kombu, arame, dulse); dairy, vegetables, and bread contain small amounts
Magnesium	Legumes, nuts and seeds, whole grains, green leafy vegetables, blackstrap molasses
Vitamin B12	Eggs, dairy foods, Red Star Nutritional Yeast T6635 (Universal Foods, Milwaukee, Wisconsin), fortified foods (meat analogues, some types/brands of soy and rice milks, ready-to-eat cereal)

Source: Data are from the U.S. Department of Agriculture Research Service National Nutrient Database. The Dietary Reference Intakes are from Otten JJ et al., *The Dietary Reference Intakes: The Essential Guide to Nutrient Requirements*, Food and Nutrition Board, Institute of Medicine Washington, DC, 2006.

[a] Holick MF, *J Nutr* 135 (11):2739S–48S, 2005.

iron-depleted nonanemic athletes (Hinton et al., 2000; Hinton and Sinclair, 2007), iron supplements should be recommended only in those with compromised stores (as indicated by a low-serum ferritin or elevated total iron binding capacity, serum transferrin receptor, or zinc pyrophosphate) (Woolf et al., 2009). Reduced hemoglobin, hematocrit, and/or red blood cell concentrations in athletes are not good indicators of iron status in endurance athletes due to exercise-induced plasma volume expansion (Schumacher et al., 2002; Thomas et al., 2016).

13.5.2 ZINC

Like iron, suboptimal zinc status may be fairly prevalent in some athletes, including female athletes and athletes following vegetarian diets. Zinc is a component of many enzymes in the body, including those involved in protein synthesis, immune function, and energy metabolism, including lactate dehydrogenase, which is an important enzyme in glycolysis. Studies have found that serum zinc concentration—a marker of zinc status—is frequently on the lower end of the normal range or below normal in vegetarian athletes, female athletes, and athletes in heavy training (Lukaski, 1995; Micheletti et al., 2001). In vegetarians, lower zinc status may be attributed to the selection of zinc-poor foods or the reduced bioavailability of zinc from plant compared with animal foods (Melina et al., 2016) (see Chapter 10). The lower bioavailability of zinc in plant foods likely increases the dietary zinc requirements for vegetarian athletes by as much as 50%, particularly those whose major food staples are unrefined grains and legumes (Otten et al., 2006). While overt zinc deficiency is not typically found in Western vegetarians (Melina et al., 2016), the significance of marginal deficiency in the athlete is not known due to the difficulty of evaluating zinc status and the variable symptoms associated with suboptimal status (Otten et al., 2006). Serum zinc concentration, for example, has been found to decrease with the onset of intense training and may not reflect tissue zinc stores or zinc status (Manore et al., 1993; Micheletti et al., 2001; Lukaski, 2004). Although more research is needed, zinc supplementation is not shown to influence serum zinc concentration during training or offer performance benefits (Singh et al., 1992; Manore et al., 1993). Vegetarians who eat a varied and well-balanced diet that contains many zinc-rich plant foods (Table 13.5) can achieve adequate zinc status without the need to supplement.

13.5.3 CALCIUM AND VITAMIN D

Low calcium intake can be associated with restricted energy intake, disordered eating, and/or the specific avoidance of dairy products or other calcium-rich foods. Depending on food choices, low calcium intake and increased risk of low bone mineral density and stress fracture are possible in athletes following vegan and vegetarian diets (Thomas et al., 2016). Calcium intake is especially important in athletes for growth, maintenance, and repair of bone tissue; regulation of muscle contraction; nerve conduction; and normal blood clotting.

In general, vegetarian athletes can meet calcium requirements by incorporating several servings of calcium-containing plant foods and/or several servings of dairy daily (Melina et al., 2016). Plant foods that are rich in well-absorbable calcium are listed in Table 13.5. The calcium bioavailability of most of these plant foods is as good as or better than that of cow's milk, which has a fractional absorption of 32% (Weaver and Plawecki, 1994; Weaver et al., 1999; Heaney et al., 2000; Zhao et al., 2005). Exceptions include soy milk fortified with tricalcium phosphate, most legumes, nuts, and seeds, which have a lower fractional absorption of 17%–24% (Zhao et al., 2005).

Although it is possible to maintain calcium balance on a plant-based diet in a Western lifestyle, some athletes may prefer fortified foods or calcium supplements to achieve calcium balance, particularly when requirements are elevated due to amenorrhea or menopause. Athletes, for example, with restricted intake and amenorrhea (i.e., low energy availability, which is discussed in Chapter 13) may require as much as 1500 mg calcium/day along with 1500–2000 IU of vitamin D to optimize bone health (Thomas et al., 2016). Because vitamin D is also required for adequate calcium absorption and bone health, a calcium supplement that contains vitamin D is advised if vitamin D status is suboptimal. Research has shown that about 10%–15% of dietary calcium is absorbed in the vitamin D–deficient state, whereas about 30%–35% is absorbed when vitamin D status is sufficient (Heaney et al., 2003; Holick, 2004). Higher calcium bioavailability with higher vitamin D status is promoted by vitamin D–induced expression of calbindin (an intestinal calcium binding protein) and an epithelial calcium channel protein (Holick, 2005), which increases intestinal calcium (and phosphorus) absorption efficiency.

Because vitamin D deficiency is prevalent among the general population, its status should be carefully monitored in all athletes. Accumulating evidence suggests that maintaining adequate vitamin D status is important for athletes due to its potential role in the athlete's health (Larson-Meyer and Willis, 2010; Larson-Meyer, 2013) and performance (Cannell et al., 2009) beyond bone health. These functions include skeletal muscle function (Hamilton, 2009), immune function, and inflammatory modulation (Cannell and Hollis, 2008; Willis et al., 2012). Athletes who live at distances away from the equator (>32° N or S latitude), have dark pigmented or light skin, have excess body fat, or who train primarily indoors or in the early morning or late afternoon throughout the year are at risk for poor vitamin D status (Hamilton et al., 2010; Larson-Meyer and Willis, 2010; Larson-Meyer, 2013; Halliday et al., 2011; Heller et al., 2015). Vegetarians and vegans may also be at risk due to lower dietary intake (Crowe et al., 2011), but factors such as vitamin D supplementation, degree of skin pigmentation, and amount and intensity of sun exposure play a more important role than diet in predicting vitamin D status (Chan et al., 2009).

Athletes at risk for low status would benefit from supplementation with enough vitamin D3 (cholecalciferol) or D2 (ergocalciferol) to maintain serum 25-hydroxyvitamin D (25(OH)D) concentration within the optimal range of 40–70 ng/mL (Cannell and Hollis, 2008). Both vitamin D3 and D2 are used in supplements and to fortify foods, including cow's milk and some brands or types of soy and rice milks, orange juice, breakfast cereals, margarines, and yogurt. Vitamin D3 is obtained through UV radiation of 7-dehydrocholesterol from lanolin (and is therefore not vegan), whereas vitamin D3 derived from lichen (Wang et al., 2001) and D2 produced from irradiation of ergosterol from yeast (Holick, 2004) is acceptable to vegans. Research has suggested that vitamin D2 is as effective as vitamin D3 at lower doses (i.e., 1000 IU) (Holick et al., 2008) but is less effective at increasing and maintaining serum

25(OH)D concentration when taken in higher doses (>4000 IU) (Trang et al., 1998; Armas et al., 2004). Sensible sun exposure, defined as 10–30 minutes of exposure to the arms, torso, and legs twice a week at close to solar noon (Hossein-nezhad and Holick, 2013), is also a way to ensure status in individuals without photosensitivity or a strong family or personal history of skin cancer. Cutaneous skin synthesis, however, is not possible in winter months at latitudes >32° N or S. Additional information on vitamin D assessment of athletes is available (Larson-Meyer and Willis, 2010).

13.5.4 IODINE

Iodine is not typically a trace element of concern for the vegetarian athlete (Thomas et al., 2016). Emerging evidence, however, suggests that iodine deficiency is prevalent in certain subpopulations, including vegetarians and vegans (Lightowler and Davies, 1998; Remer et al., 1999; Krajcovicova-Kudlackova et al., 2003a; Waldmann et al., 2003; Leitzmann, 2005) and those who do not use iodized salt. One study assessed the iodine status of 81 nonathletic adults and found that 25% of the vegetarians and 80% of the vegans had iodine deficiency (urinary iodine excretion value below 100 µg/L) compared with 9% in nonvegetarians (Krajcovicova-Kudlackova et al., 2003a). The higher prevalence of iodine deficiency among vegetarians is attributed to the prevailing (or exclusive) consumption of plant foods grown in soil with low iodine content (Remer et al., 1999; Krajcovicova-Kudlackova et al., 2003a), limited consumption of cow's milk (Lightowler and Davies, 1998), no intake of fish or sea products, and reduced use of iodized salt (Remer et al., 1999; Krajcovicova-Kudlackova et al., 2003a). Additional evidence suggests that athletes who sweat heavily may be at increased risk due to iodine loss in sweat (Smyth and Duntas, 2005). These studies have exposed a need for more research on the possible effect of iodine deficiency on the health and performance of athletic individuals. Iodine is a critical trace element for the athlete due to its role in thyroid hormone, which is key in controlling metabolism, heart rate, and gene expression. Vegetarian athletes can ensure adequate iodine status by consuming half a teaspoon of iodized salt in the diet daily. Sea salt, kosher salt, and salty seasonings, including tamari, are generally not iodized. Neither are most high-sodium processed foods. While many plant foods, such as cruciferous vegetables, sweet potatoes, and soybeans, naturally contain goitrogens, these foods have not been associated with hypothyroid or thyroid insufficiency unless iodine status is compromised (Messina and Redmond, 2006).

13.5.5 MAGNESIUM

Suboptimal magnesium status is thought to be widespread in the United States due to the intake of processed foods (Rude et al., 2009). Although the magnesium status of athletes eating a whole-food, plant-based diet would be expected to be more than adequate, athletes participating in weight class, gravitational, and aesthetic sports often requiring weight control and food restriction (e.g., wrestling, ballet, and gymnastics) are vulnerable to an inadequate magnesium status (Nielsen and Lukaski, 2006). Athletes participating in strenuous exercise may also be at risk due to increased magnesium losses through urine and sweat that may increase their magnesium requirement by 10%–20%. Marginal magnesium deficiency impairs exercise performance and amplifies the negative consequences of strenuous exercise, including oxidative stress. In athletes with suboptimal status, increased dietary intake of magnesium (or magnesium supplementation as needed) will have beneficial effects on exercise performance (Nielsen and Lukaski, 2006). Foods rich in magnesium are listed in Table 13.5.

13.5.6   VITAMIN B12

Because cobalamin, the active form of vitamin B12, is found exclusively in animal products (Herrmann and Geisel, 2002; Melina et al., 2016), athletes who follow vegan or near-vegan diets may be at risk for low vitamin B12 status (Pawlak et al., 2013). As with vegan diets in general, vegan athletes should consume vitamin B12–fortified foods daily or take a vitamin B12–containing supplement (or multivitamin). Vegetarian athletes should also consider taking a supplemental source if their intake of dairy products and/or eggs is limited. For example, an 8 oz glass of milk provides ~50% of the RDA for vitamin B12, while an egg provides ~20%. Vegan sources of vitamin B12 are listed in Table 13.5.

TABLE 13.6
Summary of Guidelines for Vegetarian and Vegan Athletes

- Available evidence supports neither a beneficial or detrimental effect of a vegetarian diet on physical performance capacity. More research is needed to determine if diets rich in antioxidants reduce muscle fatigue or improve recovery.
- Vegetarian diets can meet the energy and nutrition needs of all athletes, from the casual and recreational participant to the elite athlete.
- A good sports diet obtains the bulk of calories from carbohydrate-rich grains, fruits, and vegetable, and contains several servings of protein-rich foods, calcium-containing plant or dairy foods, nuts, and vegetable oils.
- An athlete's energy requirements can vary from 2000 to more than 6000 kcal/day, depending on body size, sex, age, and training and nontraining physical activity. Carbohydrates are the main energy source for high-intensity exercise. The carbohydrate needs of vegetarian athletes vary according to training intensity and range between 3 and 5 g carbohydrates/kg BM/day with light or skill-based training to as high as 12 g/kg BM/day with ultraendurance training. Before, during, and after exercise, food selections should include adequate amounts of familiar, easily digested, high-carbohydrate foods.
- Fat is used primarily during prolonged exercise of moderate intensity and during low-level activity. In general, dietary fat should contribute about 20%–35% of energy and provide sources of omega-3 as well as omega-6 fatty acids.
- The protein needs of athletes can easily be met on a vegetarian diet providing energy intake is also adequate. Athletes concerned about meeting their protein requirements should select more protein-rich foods, such as legumes and soy products. Protein in the postexercise meal may enhance recovery.
- Vegetarian athletes should take care to select foods rich in iron, zinc, calcium, and B12, and to ensure that their iron and vitamin D status is normal. A multivitamin and mineral supplement is usually necessary only if the athlete is restricting energy intake or making poor food choices.

13.6 CONCLUSION

Athletes at all levels of performance can meet their energy and nutrient needs on a vegetarian diet that contains a variety of plant foods, including grain products, fruits, vegetables, protein-rich plant foods, and (if desired) dairy products and eggs. Depending on food preferences, eating patterns, and exercise intensity, however, the diet of some athletes may be lacking in certain key nutrients, including total energy, carbohydrates, protein, fat, calcium, vitamin D, iron, zinc, iodine, magnesium, and vitamin B12. In these cases, athletes can generally improve nutrient status and maybe even performance by consistently making an effort to select foods containing the nutrient(s) they lack. Table 13.6 summarizes tips for meeting energy and macronutrient and micronutrient requirements on a vegetarian diet and for meeting sports-specific guidelines. Although research strongly suggests that a plant-based diet may offer many health benefits to athletes and nonathletes alike, there is little evidence to suggest that vegetarian diets per se are better than omnivorous diets for improving athletic training and performance.

REFERENCES

Achten J, Halson SL, Moseley L, Rayson MP, Casey A, Jeukendrup AE. 2004. Higher dietary carbohydrate content during intensified running training results in better maintenance of performance and mood state. *J Appl Physiol* 96 (4):1331–40.

Ainsworth BE, Haskell WL, Whitt MC, Irwin ML, Swartz AM, Strath SJ, O'Brien WL et al. 2000. Compendium of physical activities: An update of activity codes and MET intensities. *Med Sci Sports Exerc* 32 (9 Suppl.):S498–504.

Armas LA, Hollis BW, Heaney RP. 2004. Vitamin D2 is much less effective than vitamin D3 in humans. *J Clin Endocrinol Metab* 89 (11):5387–91.

Babault N, Paizis C, Deley G, Guerin-Deremaux L, Saniez MH, Lefranc-Millot C, Allaert FA. 2015. Pea proteins oral supplementation promotes muscle thickness gains during resistance training: A double-blind, randomized, placebo-controlled clinical trial vs. whey protein. *J Int Soc Sports Nutr* 12 (1):3. doi: 10.1186/s12970-014-0064-5.

Ball MJ, Bartlett MA. 1999. Dietary intake and iron status of Australian vegetarian women. *Am J Clin Nutr* 70 (3):353–8.

Barnard ND, Cohen J, Jenkins DJ, Turner-McGrievy G, Gloede L, Green A, Ferdowsian H. 2009a. A low-fat vegan diet and a conventional diabetes diet in the treatment of type 2 diabetes: A randomized, controlled, 74-wk clinical trial. *Am J Clin Nutr* 89 (5):1588S–96S.

Barnard ND, Katcher HI, Jenkins DJ, Cohen J, Turner-McGrievy G. 2009b. Vegetarian and vegan diets in type 2 diabetes management. *Nutr Rev* 67 (5):255–63.

Bergstrom J, Furst P, Vinnars E. 1990. Effect of a test meal, without and with protein, on muscle and plasma free amino acids. *Clin Sci (Lond)* 79 (4):331–7.

Brewer J, Williams C, Patton A. 1988. The influence of high carbohydrate diets on endurance running performance. *Eur J Appl Physiol Occup Physiol* 57:698–706.

Brooks GA, Butte NF, Rand WM, Flatt JP, Caballero B. 2004. Chronicle of the Institute of Medicine physical activity recommendation: How a physical activity recommendation came to be among dietary recommendations. *Am J Clin Nutr* 79 (5):921S–30S.

Brown RC, Cox CM. 1998. Effects of high fat versus high carbohydrate diets on plasma lipids and lipoproteins in endurance athletes. *Med Sci Sports Exerc* 30 (12):1677–83.

Brownlie T, Utermohlen V, Hinton PS, Haas JD. 2004. Tissue iron deficiency without anemia impairs adaptation in endurance capacity after aerobic training in previously untrained women. *Am J Clin Nutr* 79 (3):437–43.

Burke LM. 2015. Re-examining high-fat diets for sports performance: Did we call the 'nail in the coffin' too soon? *Sports Med* 45 (Suppl. 1):S33–49. doi: 10.1007/s40279-015-0393-9.

Burke LM, Hawley JA, Wong SH, Jeukendrup AE. 2011. Carbohydrates for training and competition. *J Sports Sci* 29 (Suppl. 1):S17–27. doi: 10.1080/02640414.2011.585473.

Cannell JJ, Hollis BW. 2008. Use of vitamin D in clinical practice. *Altern Med Rev* 13 (1):6–20.

Cannell JJ, Hollis BW, Sorenson MB, Taft TN, Anderson JJ. 2009. Athletic performance and vitamin D. *Med Sci Sports Exerc* 41 (5):1102–10.

Carr AJ, Hopkins WG, Gore CJ. 2011. Effects of acute alkalosis and acidosis on performance: A meta-analysis. *Sports Med* 41 (10):801–14. doi: 10.2165/11591440-000000000-00000.

Chan J, Jaceldo-Siegl K, Fraser GE. 2009. Serum 25-hydroxyvitamin D status of vegetarians, partial vegetarians, and nonvegetarians: The Adventist Health Study-2. *Am J Clin Nutr* 89 (5):1686S–92S. doi: 10.3945/ajcn.2009.26736X.

Coggan AR, Swanson SC. 1992. Nutritional manipulations before and during endurance exercise: Effects on performance. *Med Sci Sports Exerc* 24 (4):S331–5.

Conquer JA, Holub BJ. 1996. Supplementation with an algae source of docosahexaenoic acid increases (n-3) fatty acid status and alters selected risk factors for heart disease in vegetarian subjects. *J Nutr* 126 (12):3032–9.

Craddock JC, Probst YC, Peoples GE. 2016. Vegetarian and omnivorous nutrition—Comparing physical performance. *Int J Sport Nutr Exerc Metab* 26 (3):212–20. doi: 10.1123/ijsnem.2015-0231.

Craig WJ. 1994. Iron status of vegetarians. *Am J Clin Nutr* 59 (Suppl.):1233S–7S.

Craig WJ, Mangels AR. 2009. Position of the American Dietetic Association: Vegetarian diets. *J Am Diet Assoc* 109 (7):1266–82.

Crowe FL, Steur M, Allen NE, Appleby PN, Travis RC, Key TJ. 2011. Plasma concentrations of 25-hydroxyvitamin D in meat eaters, fish eaters, vegetarians and vegans: Results from the EPIC-Oxford study. *Public Health Nutr* 14 (2):340–6. doi: 10.1017/S1368980010002454.

Cunningham JJ. 1980. A reanalysis of the factors influencing basal metabolic rate in normal adults. *Am J Clin Nutr* 33:2372–4.

Decombaz J, Schmitt B, Ith M, Decarli B, Diem P, Kreis R, Hoppeler H, Boesch C. 2001. Postexercise fat intake repletes intramyocellular lipids but no faster in trained than in sedentary subjects. *Am J Physiol Regul Integr Comp Physiol* 281 (3):R760–9.

Deriemaeker P, Aerenhouts D, Hebbelinck M, Clarys P. 2010. Nutrient based estimation of acid-base balance in vegetarians and non-vegetarians. *Plant Foods Hum Nutr* 65 (1):77–82. doi: 10.1007/s11130-009-0149-5.

Dinu M, Abbate R, Gensini GF, Casini A, Sofi F. 2017. Vegetarian, vegan diets and multiple health outcomes: A systematic review with meta-analysis of observational studies. *Crit Rev Food Sci Nutr* 57 (17):3640–9. doi: 10.1080/10408398.2016.1138447.

Eichner ER. 1985. Runner's macrocytosis: A clue to footstrike hemolysis. *Am J Med* 78:321–5.

Eisinger M, Plath M, Jung L, Leitzmann C. 1994. Nutrient intake of endurance runners with ovo-lacto-vegetarian diet and regular Western diet. *Z Ernahrungswiss* 33 (3):217–29.

FAO/WHO/UNU (Food and Agriculture Organization/World Health Organization/United Nations University). 2002. Expert consultation on protein and amino acid requirements in human nutrition. Report of a Joint FAO/WHO/UNU Expert Consultation, WHO Technical Report Series No. 935. Geneva: World Health Organization.

Geppert J, Kraft V, Demmelmair H, Koletzko B. 2005. Docosahexaenoic acid supplementation in vegetarians effectively increases omega-3 index: A randomized trial. *Lipids* 40 (8):807–14.

Goran MI. 1995. Variation in total energy expenditure in humans. *Obesity Res* 3 (1):59–66.

Gould KL, Ornish D, Kirkeeide R, Brown S, Stuart Y, Buchi M, Billings J, Armstrong W, Ports T, Scherwitz L. 1992. Improved stenosis geometry by quantitative coronary arteriography after vigorous risk factor modification. *Am J Cardiol* 69 (9):845–53.

Gould KL, Ornish D, Scherwitz L, Brown S, Edens RP, Hess MJ, Mullani N et al. 1995. Changes in myocardial perfusion abnormalities by positron emission tomography after long-term, intense risk factor modification. *JAMA* 274 (11):894–901.

Halliday TM, Peterson NJ, Thomas JJ, Kleppinger K, Hollis BW, Larson-Meyer DE. 2011. Vitamin D status relative to diet, lifestyle, injury, and illness in college athletes. *Med Sci Sports Exerc* 43 (2):335–43. doi: 10.1249/MSS.0b013e3181eb9d4d.

Hamilton B. 2009. Vitamin D and human skeletal muscle. *Scand J Med Sci Sports* 20 (2):182–90.

Hamilton B, Grantham J, Racinais S, Chalabi H. 2010. Vitamin D deficiency is endemic in Middle Eastern sportsmen. *Public Health Nutr* 13 (10):1528–34.

Hanne N, Dlin R, Rotstein A. 1986. Physical fitness, anthropometric and metabolic parameters in vegetarian athletes. *J Sports Med Phys Fitness* 26 (2):180–5.

Hargreaves M. 2000. Skeletal muscle metabolism during exercise in humans. *Clin Exp Pharmacol Physiol* 27 (3):225–8.

Hargreaves M, Costill DL, Coggan A, Fink WJ, Nishibata I. 1984. Effect of carbohydrate feedings on muscle glycogen utilization and exercise performance. *Med Sci Sports Exerc* 16 (3):219–22.

Harris J, Benedict F. 1919. *A Biometric Study of Basal Metabolism in Man*. Washington, DC: Carnegie Institute of Washington.

Havemann L, West SJ, Goedecke JH, MacDonald IA, St. Clair Gibson A, Noakes TD, Lambert EV. 2006. Fat adaptation followed by carbohydrate loading compromises high-intensity sprint performance. *J Appl Physiol* 100 (1):194–202.

Heaney RP, Dowell MS, Hale CA, Bendich A. 2003. Calcium absorption varies within the reference range for serum 25-hydroxyvitamin D. *J Am Coll Nutr* 22 (2):142–6.

Heaney RP, Dowell MS, Rafferty K, Bierman J. 2000. Bioavailability of the calcium in fortified soy imitation milk, with some observations on method. *Am J Clin Nutr* 71 (5):1166–9.

Heller JE, Thomas JJ, Hollis BW, Larson-Meyer DE. 2015. Relation between vitamin D status and body composition in collegiate athletes. *Int J Sport Nutr Exerc Metab* 25 (2):128–35. doi: 10.1123/ijsnem.2013-0250.

Herrmann W, Geisel J. 2002. Vegetarian lifestyle and monitoring of vitamin B-12 status. *Clin Chim Acta* 326 (1–2):47–59.

Hietavala EM, Stout JR, Hulmi JJ, Suominen H, Pitkanen H, Puurtinen R, Selanne H, Kainulainen H, Mero AA. 2015. Effect of diet composition on acid-base balance in adolescents, young adults and elderly at rest and during exercise. *Eur J Clin Nutr* 69 (3):399–404. doi: 10.1038/ejcn.2014.245.

Hinton PS, Giordano C, Brownlie T, Haas JD. 2000. Iron supplementation improves endurance after training in iron-depleted, nonanemic women. *J Appl Physiol* 88 (3):1103–11.

Hinton PS, Sinclair LM. 2007. Iron supplementation maintains ventilatory threshold and improves energetic efficiency in iron-deficient nonanemic athletes. *Eur J Clin Nutr* 61 (1):30–9.

Holick MF. 2004. Sunlight and vitamin D for bone health and prevention of autoimmune diseases, cancers, and cardiovascular disease. *Am J Clin Nutr* 80 (6 Suppl.):1678S–88S.

Holick MF. 2005. The vitamin D epidemic and its health consequences. *J Nutr* 135 (11):2739S–48S.

Holick MF, Biancuzzo RM, Chen TC, Klein EK, Young A, Bibuld D, Reitz R, Salameh W, Ameri A, Tannenbaum AD. 2008. Vitamin D2 is as effective as vitamin D3 in maintaining circulating concentrations of 25-hydroxyvitamin D. *J Clin Endocrinol Metab* 93 (3):677–81.

Hoppeler H, Billeter R, Horvath PJ, Leddy JJ, Pendergast DR. 1999. Muscle structure with low- and high-fat diets in well trained male runners. *Int J Sports Med* 20:522–6.

Horvath PJ, Eagen CK, Fisher NM, Leddy JJ, Pendergast DR. 2000. The effects of varying dietary fat on performance and metabolism in trained male and female runners. *J Am Coll Nutr* 19 (1):52–60.

Hossein-nezhad A, Holick MF. 2013. Vitamin D for health: A global perspective. *Mayo Clin Proc* 88 (7):720–55. doi: 10.1016/j.mayocp.2013.05.011.

Jeromson S, Gallagher IJ, Galloway SD, Hamilton DL. 2015. Omega-3 fatty acids and skeletal muscle health. *Mar Drugs* 13 (11):6977–7004. doi: 10.3390/md13116977.

Jones GR, Newhouse I. 1997. Sport-related hematuria: A review. *Clin J Sport Med* 7 (2):119–25.

Krajcovicova-Kudlackova M, Buckova K, Klimes I, Sebokova E. 2003a. Iodine deficiency in vegetarians and vegans. *Ann Nutr Metab* 47 (5):183–5.

Krajcovicova-Kudlackova M, Ursinyova M, Blazicek P, Spustova V, Ginter E, Hladikova V, Klvanova J. 2003b. Free radical disease prevention and nutrition. *Bratisl Lek Listy* 104 (2):64–8.

Lamanca J, Haymes E. 1992. Effects of low ferritin concentrations on endurance performance. *Int J Sports Med* 2:376–85.

Larson DE, Hesslink RL, Hrovat MI, Fishman RS, Systrom DM. 1994. Dietary effects on exercising muscle metabolism and performance by ^{31}P-MRS. *J Appl Physiol* 77 (3):1108–15.

Larson-Meyer DE. 2007. *Vegetarian Sports Nutrition. Food Choices and Eating Plans for Fitness and Performance.* Champaign, IL: Human Kinetics.

Larson-Meyer DE, Borkhsenious ON, Gullett JC, Russell RR, Devries MC, Smith SR, Ravussin E. 2008. Effect of dietary fat on serum and intramyocellular lipids and running performance. *Med Sci Sports Exerc* 40 (5):892–902.

Larson-Meyer DE, Hunter GR, Newcomer BR. 2002. Influence of endurance running and recovery diet on intramyocellular lipid content in women: A ^{1}H-NMR study. *Am J Physiol* 282:E95–106.

Larson-Meyer DE, Willis KS. 2010. Vitamin D and athletes. *Curr Sports Med Rep* 9 (4):220–6. doi: 10.1249/JSR.0b013e3181e7dd45.

Larson-Meyer E. 2013. Vitamin D supplementation in athletes. *Nestle Nutr Inst Workshop Ser* 75:109–21. doi: 10.1159/000345827.

Leitzmann C. 2005. Vegetarian diets: What are the advantages? *Forum Nutr* (57):147–56.

Lemon PWR, Mullin JP. 1980. Effect of initial muscle glycogen levels on protein catabolism during exercise. *J Appl Physiol* 48 (4):624–9.

Lightowler HJ, Davies GJ. 1998. Iodine intake and iodine deficiency in vegans as assessed by the duplicate-portion technique and urinary iodine excretion. *Br J Nutr* 80 (6):529–35.

Lukaski HC. 1995. Micronutrients (magnesium, zinc, and copper): Are mineral supplements needed for athletes? *Int J Sport Nutr* 5 (Suppl.):S74–83.

Lukaski HC. 2004. Vitamin and mineral status: Effects on physical performance. *Nutrition* 20 (7–8):632–44.

Malczewska J, Raczynski G, Stupnicki R. 2000. Iron status in female endurance athletes and in non-athletes. *Int J Sport Nutr* 10 (3):260–76.

Malczewska J, Szczepanska B, Stupnicki R, Sendecki W. 2001. The assessment of frequency of iron deficiency in athletes from the transferrin receptor-ferritin index. *Int J Sport Nutr Exerc Metab* 11 (1):42–52.

Mamerow MM, Mettler JA, English KL, Casperson SL, Arentson-Lantz E, Sheffield-Moore M, Layman DK, Paddon-Jones D. 2014. Dietary protein distribution positively influences 24-h muscle protein synthesis in healthy adults. *J Nutr* 144 (6):876–80. doi: 10.3945/jn.113.185280.

Manore MM, Helleksen JM, Merkel J, Skinner JS. 1993. Longitudinal changes in zinc status in untrained men: Effects of two different 12-week exercise training programs and zinc supplementation. *J Am Diet Assoc* 93 (10):1165–8.

Manore M, Thompson J. 2000. *Sport Nutrition for Health and Performance*. Champaign, IL: Human Kinetics.

Maughan RJ, Gleeson M. 2010. *The Biochemical Basis of Sports Performance*. New York: Oxford University Press.

Melina V, Craig W, Levin S. 2016. Position of the Academy of Nutrition and Dietetics: Vegetarian diets. *J Acad Nutr Diet* 116 (12):1970–80. doi: 10.1016/j.jand.2016.09.025.

Messina M, Redmond G. 2006. Effects of soy protein and soybean isoflavones on thyroid function in healthy adults and hypothyroid patients: A review of the relevant literature. *Thyroid* 16 (3):249–58.

Messina V, Mangels AR, Messina M. 2004. *A Dietitian's Guide to Vegetarian Diets: Issues and Applications*. 2nd ed. Boston: Jones & Bartlett Publishers.

Messina V, Melina V, Mangels AR. 2003. A new food guide for North American vegetarians. *J Am Diet Assoc* 103 (6):771–5.

Micheletti A, Rossi R, Rufini S. 2001. Zinc status in athletes: Relation to diet and exercise. *Sports Med* 31 (8):577–82.

Muoio DM, Leddy JJ, Horvath PJ, Awad AB, Pendergast DR. 1994. Effect of dietary fat on metabolic adjustments to maximal VO_2 and endurance in runners. *Med Sci Sports Exerc* 26 (1):81–8.

Nielsen FH, Lukaski HC. 2006. Update on the relationship between magnesium and exercise. *Magnes Res* 19 (3):180–9.

Nieman DC. 1988. Vegetarian dietary practices and endurance performance. *Am J Clin Nutr* 48 (3 Suppl.):754–61.

Nieman DC. 1999. Physical fitness and vegetarian diets: Is there a relation? *Am J Clin Nutr* 70 (3 Suppl.):570S–5S.

O'Keeffe KA, Keith RE, Wilson GD, Blessing DL. 1989. Dietary carbohydrate intake and endurance exercise performance of trained female cyclists. *Nutr Res* 9:819–30.

Ornish D, Brown SE, Scherwitz LW, Billings JH, Armstrong WT, Ports TA, McLanahan SM, Kirkeeide RL, Brand RJ, Gould KL. 1990. Can lifestyle changes reverse coronary heart disease? The Lifestyle Heart Trial. *Lancet* 336:129–33.

Otten JJ, Hellwig JP, Meyers LD. 2006. *The Dietary Reference Intakes: The Essential Guide to Nutrient Requirements*. Washington, DC: Food and Nutrition Board, Institute of Medicine.

Pawlak R, Parrott SJ, Raj S, Cullum-Dugan D, Lucus D. 2013. How prevalent is vitamin B(12) deficiency among vegetarians? *Nutr Rev* 71 (2):110–7. doi: 10.1111/nure.12001.

Peeling P, Dawson B, Goodman C, Landers G, Trinder D. 2008. Athletic induced iron deficiency: New insights into the role of inflammation, cytokines and hormones. *Eur J Appl Physiol Occup Physiol* 103 (4):381–91.

Pelly FE, Burkhart SJ. 2014. Dietary regimens of athletes competing at the Delhi 2010 Commonwealth Games. *Int J Sport Nutr Exerc Metab* 24 (1):28–36. doi: 10.1123 /ijsnem.2013-0023.

Phillips SM, Van Loon LJ. 2011. Dietary protein for athletes: From requirements to optimum adaptation. *J Sports Sci* 29 (Suppl. 1):S29–38. doi: 10.1080/02640414.2011.619204.

Powers SK, DeRuisseau KC, Quindry J, Hamilton KL. 2004. Dietary antioxidants and exercise. *J Sports Sci* 22 (1):81–94.

Raben A, Kiens B, Richter EA, Rasmussen LB, Svenstrup B, Micic S, Bennett P. 1992. Serum sex hormones and endurance performance after a lacto-ovo vegetarian and a mixed diet. *Med Sci Sports Exerc* 24 (11):1290–7.

Rand WM, Pellett PL, Young VR. 2003. Meta-analysis of nitrogen balance studies for estimating protein requirements in healthy adults. *Am J Clin Nutr* 77 (1):109–27.

Rauma AL, Mykkanen H. 2000. Antioxidant status in vegetarians versus omnivores. *Nutrition* 16 (2):111–9.

Reid MA, Marsh KA, Zeuschner CL, Saunders AV, Baines SK. 2013. Meeting the nutrient reference values on a vegetarian diet. *Med J Aust* 199 (4 Suppl.):S33–40.

Remer T, Neubert A, Manz F. 1999. Increased risk of iodine deficiency with vegetarian nutrition. *Br J Nutr* 81 (1):45–9.

Richter EA, Kiensn B, Raben A, Tvede N, Pedersen BK. 1991. Immune parameters in male atheletes after a lacto-ovo vegetarian diet and a mixed Western diet. *Med Sci Sports Exerc* 23 (5):517–21.

Robertson J, Maughan RJ, Davidson R. 1987. Faecal blood loss in response to exercise. *Br Med J* 295:303–5.

Rodriguez NR, DiMarco NM, Langley S. 2009. Position of the American Dietetic Association, Dietitians of Canada, and the American College of Sports Medicine: Nutrition and athletic performance. *J Am Diet Assoc* 109 (3):509–27.

Romijn J, Coyle EF, Sidossis LS, Gastaldelli A, Horowitz JF, Endert E, Wolfe RR. 1993. Regulation of endogenous fat and carbohydrate metabolism in relation to exercise intensity and duration. *Am J Physiol Endocrinol Metab* 265 (28):E380–91.

Romijn JA, Coyle EF, Sidossis LS, Rosenblatt J, Wolfe RR. 2000. Substrate metabolism during different exercise intensities in endurance-trained women. *J Appl Physiol* 88 (5):1707–14.

Rude RK, Singer FR, Gruber HE. 2009. Skeletal and hormonal effects of magnesium deficiency. *J Am Coll Nutr* 28 (2):131–41.

Saunders AV, Craig WJ, Baines SK, Posen JS. 2013. Iron and vegetarian diets. *Med J Aust* 199 (4 Suppl.):S11–6.

Schumacher YO, Schmid A, Grathwohl D, Bultermann D, Berg A. 2002. Hematological indices and iron status in athletes of various sports and performances. *Med Sci Sports Exerc* 34 (5):869–75.

Singh A, Moses FM, Deuster PA. 1992. Vitamin and mineral status in physically active men: Effects of a high-potency supplement. *Am J Clin Nutr* 55 (1):1–7.

Smyth PP, Duntas LH. 2005. Iodine uptake and loss—Can frequent strenuous exercise induce iodine deficiency? *Horm Metab Res* 37 (9):555–8. doi: 10.1055/s-2005-870423.

Snyder AC, Dvorak LL, Roepke JB. 1989. Influence of dietary iron source on measures of iron status among female runners. *Med Sci Sports Exerc* 21 (1):7–10.

Spencer MK, Yan Z, Katz A. 1991. Carbohydrate supplementation attenuates IMP accumulation in human muscle during prolonged exercise. *Am J Physiol* 261 (1 Pt. 1):C71–6.

Sugiura K, Kobayashi K. 1998. Effect of carbohydrate ingestion on sprint performance following continuous and intermittent exercise. *Med Sci Sports Exerc* 30 (11):1624–30.

Thomas DT, Erdman KA, Burke LM. 2016. Position of the Academy of Nutrition and Dietetics, Dietitians of Canada, and the American College of Sports Medicine: Nutrition and athletic performance. *J Acad Nutr Diet* 116 (3):501–28. doi: 10.1016/j.jand.2015.12.006.

Thompson PD, Cullinane EM, Eshleman R, Kantor MA, Herbert PN. 1984. The effects of high-carbohydrate and high-fat diets on the serum lipid and lipoprotein concentrations of endurance athletes. *Metab Clin Exp* 33 (11):1003–10.

Tipton KD, Elliott TA, Cree MG, Aarsland AA, Sanford AP, Wolfe RR. 2007. Stimulation of net muscle protein synthesis by whey protein ingestion before and after exercise. *Am J Physiol Endocrinol Metab* 292 (1):E71–6.

Tipton KD, Rasmussen BB, Miller SL, Wolf SE, Owens-Stovall SK, Petrini BE, Wolfe RR. 2001. Timing of amino acid-carbohydrate ingestion alters anabolic response of muscle to resistance exercise. *Am J Physiol Endocrinol Metab* 281 (2):E197–206.

Tipton KD, Witard OC. 2007. Protein requirements and recommendations for athletes: Relevance of ivory tower arguments for practical recommendations. *Clin Sports Med* 26 (1):17–36.

Toth MJ, Poehlman ET. 1994. Sympathetic nervous system activity and resting metabolic rate in vegetarians. *Metabolism* 43 (5):621–5.

Trang HM, Cole DE, Rubin LA, Pierratos A, Siu S, Vieth R. 1998. Evidence that vitamin D3 increases serum 25-hydroxyvitamin D more efficiently than does vitamin D2. *Am J Clin Nutr* 68 (4):854–8.

Trapp D, Knez W, Sinclair W. 2010. Could a vegetarian diet reduce exercise-induced oxidative stress? A review of the literature. *J Sports Sci* 28 (12):1261–8. doi: 10.1080/02640414.2010.507676.

U.S. Department of Health and Human Services and U.S. Department of Agriculture. 2011. *Dietary Guidelines for Americans, 2015–2020.* 8th ed. https://health.gov /dietaryguidelines/2015/guidelines/ (last modified January 31, 2011).

Waldmann A, Koschizke JW, Leitzmann C, Hahn A. 2003. Dietary intakes and lifestyle factors of a vegan population in Germany: Results from the German Vegan Study. *Eur J Clin Nutr* 57 (8):947–55.

Waller MF, Haymes EM. 1996. The effects of heat and exercise on sweat iron loss. *Med Sci Sports Exerc* 28 (2):197–203.

Wang T, Bengtsson G, Karnefelt I, Bjorn LO. 2001. Provitamins and vitamins D(2)and D(3)in *Cladina* spp. over a latitudinal gradient: Possible correlation with UV levels. *J Photochem Photobiol B* 62 (1–2):118–22.

Weaver CM, Plawecki KL. 1994. Dietary calcium: Adequacy of a vegetarian diet. *Am J Clin Nutr* 59 (Suppl.):1238S–41S.

Weaver CM, Proulx WR, Heaney R. 1999. Choices for achieving adequate dietary calcium with a vegetarian diet. *Am J Clin Nutr* 70 (3 Suppl.):543S–8S.

Williams CM, Burdge G. 2006. Long-chain n-3 PUFA: Plant v. marine sources. *Proc Nutr Soc* 65 (1):42–50.

Williams MH, Anderson DE, Rawson ES. 2013. *Nutrition for Health, Fitness & Sport.* 10th ed. Boston: McGraw-Hill.

Willis KS, Smith DT, Broughton KS, Larson-Meyer DE. 2012. Vitamin D status and biomarkers of inflammation in runners. *Open Access J Sports Med* 3:35–42. doi: 10.2147 /OAJSM.S31022.

Woolf K, St. Thomas MM, Hahn N, Vaughan LA, Carlson AG, Hinton P. 2009. Iron status in highly active and sedentary young women. *Int J Sport Nutr Exerc Metab* 19 (5):519–35.

Yokoyama Y, Nishimura K, Barnard ND, Takegami M, Watanabe M, Sekikawa A, Okamura T, Miyamoto Y. 2014. Vegetarian diets and blood pressure: A meta-analysis. *JAMA Intern Med* 174 (4):577–87. doi: 10.1001/jamainternmed.2013.14547.

Young VR, Pellett PL. 1994. Plant proteins in relation to human protein and amino acid nutrition. *Am J Clin Nutr* 59 (Suppl.):1203S–12S.

Zhao Y, Martin BR, Weaver CM. 2005. Calcium bioavailability of calcium carbonate fortified soymilk is equivalent to cow's milk in young women. *J Nutr* 135 (10):2379–82.

Zhu YI, Haas JD. 1997. Iron depletion without anemia and physical performance. *Am J Clin Nutr* 66:334–41.

14 Optimizing Performance on a Vegetarian Diet

D. Enette Larson-Meyer

CONTENTS

SUMMARY

Athletes of all abilities are encouraged to follow sports nutrition strategies that optimize mental and physical performance and support good health. In addition to following a general healthy diet, these strategies include nutrient intake before, during, and immediately after training or competition and maintenance of a healthy body weight for the athlete's chosen sport. The timing of the intake of carbohydrate, protein, and fluid according to exercise and competition helps optimize exercise performance, ensures adequate recovery, and promotes muscle protein synthesis. When weight or body fat reduction is required, weight loss should be accomplished slowly, and not during competitive season. Certain supplements, which include creatine, caffeine, and dietary nitrate, may be of interest to the vegetarian athlete; nutritional supplements should not be used in lieu of good food choices.

14.1 INTRODUCTION

All athletes—including those following vegetarian diets—are encouraged to follow sports nutrition strategies to optimize mental and physical performance and support good health (Maughan and Shirreffs, 2011). These strategies include eating an overall healthy diet that provides adequate energy to meet the carbohydrate, protein, fat, and micronutrient requirements of exercise training and, if appropriate, competition (as reviewed in Chapter 13). In addition to a general overall healthy diet, however, adopting specific nutritional strategies before, during, and after training (or competition) also helps optimize performance, as does maintaining a healthy body weight and/or body composition that is appropriate for that athlete's sport (Maughan and Shirreffs, 2011; Thomas et al., 2016). Judicious use of specific dietary supplements (or ergogenic aids) may also enhance sports performance in some athletes. Use of dietary supplements, however, should be in conjunction with a healthy eating and training regimen and not a substitution for a healthy diet. This chapter addresses the strategies beyond those of a healthy diet that are important for optimizing performance in vegetarian athletes. These strategies include the timing of carbohydrate, protein, and fluid in relation to exercise; the maintenance of a healthy body weight; and the use of specific dietary supplements.

14.2 NUTRITION BEFORE, DURING, AND AFTER EXERCISE

14.2.1 Nutrient Intake before and during Exercise

The timing of fluid and macronutrient intake in association with exercise has long been known to impact performance. Fluid intake ensures adequate hydration and, along with carbohydrates, has a cumulative effect on optimizing performance (Nicholas et al., 1995). Fluid deficits of greater than 2% of body mass (BM) (i.e., 1 kg in a 50 kg female runner or 3 kg in a 150 kg male wrestler) can compromise cognitive function and aerobic performance, particularly in hot environments (Thomas et al., 2016). Additionally, carbohydrate intake before and during exercise has the potential to improve performance particularly during events lasting for an hour or longer (Jeukendrup, 2014). Studies show that ingestion of between 1 and 5 g carbohydrate/kg body weight in the period 1–4 hours before endurance exercise has the potential to improve endurance performance by as much as 14% compared with the fasting state (Sherman et al., 1989; Wright et al., 1991; Coyle et al., 1992). Ingestion of between 30 and 90 g of carbohydrate during exercise also has the potential to improve performance in endurance events by an average of about 2%–6% improvement (Stellingwerff and Cox, 2014). The magnitude of the performance improvements is influenced by factors such as the duration and type of exercise, the athlete's training status, and carbohydrate consumption in the pre-event meal. Similarly, carbohydrate ingestion also optimizes performance during variable-intensity exercise (Ball et al., 1995; Below et al., 1995; Nicholas et al., 1995)—which includes soccer (Currell et al., 2009) and other team sports. The performance benefit is thought to be due to factors including both cognitive stimulation of the central nervous system (CNS) by oral exposure of carbohydrates in shorter events, and metabolic stimulation resulting in maintenance of blood glucose concentration and preservation of carbohydrate oxidation in longer events (Stellingwerff and Cox, 2014). Additionally, more recent research has suggested that "mouth rinsing" with a carbohydrate-containing solution may enhance performance in events lasting less than an hour via CNS stimulation (Burke et al., 2011; Jeukendrup, 2013).

The fluid and carbohydrate required in the period surrounding exercise depends on a variety of factors, including the mode, intensity, and duration of the event; the environmental temperature; and the carryover effect (if any) of previous exercise training (Burke et al., 2011; Thomas et al., 2016). The guidelines for fluid and nutrient intake before, during, and after exercise are summarized in Table 14.1. While these guidelines apply to all athletes, the food preferences and tolerances of vegetarian athletes may dictate individual strategies within the guidelines. For example, although it is generally recommended that carbohydrate-rich sources be low in fiber or residue to avoid gut discomfort during exercise (Thomas et al., 2016), many higher-fiber foods, such as pulses and whole grains, may be well tolerated by the vegetarian athlete who is accustomed to eating these foods. Some whole food sources, such as lentils and other pulses, also have a low glycemic index (GI) that may offer a performance advantage when consumed before exercise (Thomas et al., 1991)—particularly prolonged submaximal exercise—compared with higher GI foods, such as potatoes (Wu and Williams, 2006). Studies, however, have not consistently found performance benefits of consuming low-GI foods in the pre-event meal (Mondazzi and Arcelli, 2009). Although commercial sport drinks and sports nutrition products, such as gels, blocks, bars, and sport beans, consumed with water, work well for delivering easily absorbed carbohydrates (Pfeiffer et al., 2010a, 2010b), some vegetarian athletes may prefer natural or noncommercial carbohydrate sources. In this case, fruit juices diluted with water (4 oz juice in 4 oz water = 6% solution); low-sodium vegetable juices, including carrot juice (7% solution); and honey or solid foods ingested with water (8 oz for every 15 g of carbohydrate = 6.3%) may be appropriate. Research has shown that solid food (Neufer et al., 1987; Lugo et al., 1993; van der Brug et al., 1995) and honey (Lancaster et al., 2001) are easily digested during exercise and are as effective as liquids in increasing blood glucose and enhancing performance. A pinch of table salt can be added to juices or low-sodium solids as necessary for events lasting longer than 3–4 hours (Gisolfi and Duchman, 1992). Having athletes count carbohydrate intake before or during exercise or plan their supplementation strategy according to the guidelines listed in Table 14.1 is often a useful tool to help them optimize their performance. Sources of carbohydrates are listed in Table 14.2 and can be used along with the carbohydrate content on the food label for these purposes.

TABLE 14.1
Summary of Macronutrient and Fluid Guidelines for Athletes

Goals	Macronutrient Recommendation	Fluid Recommendation
Daily Needs		
Optimize liver and muscle glycogen stores; ensure adequate hydration	Low intensity or skill based: 3–5 g CHO/kg BW Moderate exercise (~1 hour/day): 5–7 g CHO/kg BW Endurance program (moderate to high intensity of 1–3 hours/day): 6–10 g CHO/kg BW Extreme program (moderate to high intensity of 4–5 hours/day): 8–12 g CHO/kg BW	Drink enough fluid to achieve urine that is pale yellow in color
Pre-Event		
Maintain blood glucose and top off glycogen stores, provide fluids, and prevent both hunger and gastrointestinal distress Ensure adequate hydration before onset of exercise	1–4 g CHO/kg BW in the 1–4 hours period before exercise; smaller meals (1–2 g CHO/kg BW) should be consumed in close proximity to exercise to allow for gastric emptying; larger meals (3–4 g CHO/kg BW) maybe consumed when more time is available **Specific strategies** Consume familiar, well-tolerated, high-CHO foods that are low in fiber, simple sugars, and sodium (Rodriguez et al., 2009) Liquid meals (such as fruit smoothies) may be more tolerable when preexercise nausea/GI distress is present; experimenting with new foods and beverages should be done during practice/training and not before major competitions	5–10 mL fluid/kg BW in the 2- to 4-hour period before exercise to achieve urine that is pale yellow in color **Specific strategies** Consume fluid enough in advance to allow for urination of excess fluid before exercise Fluid replacement beverages formulated for sport provide about 6%–8% CHO by volume and may be advantageous when both fluid and CHO are desired
During Event		
Maintain blood glucose concentrations and preserve CHO oxidation Avoid fluid deficits in excess of 2% of BW	Brief exercise <45 minutes: Not needed Sustained, high-intensity exercise (45–75 minutes): Small amounts/mouth rinsing Endurance exercise and stop-and-start sports (1–2.5 hours): 30–60 g/hour Ultraendurance exercise (>2.5–3 hours): Up to 90 g/hour **Specific strategies** Intake of CHO and fluid should be initiated shortly after the start of exercise to maximize time for sugar and nutrients to reach the bloodstream High-GI foods may be more rapidly absorbed CHO choices providing multiple transportable sugars (glucose, fructose) will promote higher rates of oxidation of endogenous CHO	0.4–0.8 L fluid/hour as a general guideline; specific recommendation should be customized to the athlete's sweat rate, tolerance, exercise intensity, and duration, and the environmental conditions **Specific strategies** Fluid replacement beverages provide 6%–8% CHO by volume while simultaneously meeting fluid needs

(Continued)

TABLE 14.1 (CONTINUED)
Summary of Macronutrient and Fluid Guidelines for Athletes

Goals	Macronutrient Recommendation	Fluid Recommendation
	After Event	
Ensure rapid recovery, replace liver and muscle glycogen, and optimize muscle protein synthesis	1–1.2 g CHO/kg BW for the first 4–6 hours after exercise 0.25–0.3 g protein/kg BW as soon as possible after exercise **Specific strategies** Foods with a high GI (Burke et al., 1993; Jozsi et al., 1996; Mondazzi and Arcelli, 2009) or those containing both CHO and protein (~1 g protein to 3 g CHO) (Ivy et al., 2002) may promote a more rapid rate of muscle glycogen synthesis by stimulating greater insulin secretion	Consume 125%–150% of BM (i.e., fluid loss) during the exercise session (1 kg BM loss is approximately 1 L of fluid loss) **Specific strategies** Emphasize sodium and potassium (along with fluid) with prolonged exercise, high sweat rate, salty sweat, and extreme environmental temperatures (Maughan et al., 1996; Sawka et al., 2007)

Source: Burke LM et al., *J Sports Sci* 29 (Suppl. 1):S17–27, 2011; Phillips SM, Van Loon LJ, *J Sports Sci* 29 (Suppl. 1):S29–38, 2011; Thomas DT et al., *J Acad Nutr Diet* 116 (3):501–28, 2016.
Note: BW = body weight; CHO = carbohydrate.

14.2.2 NUTRIENT INTAKE AFTER EXERCISE

The focus of food and fluid intake after exercise is on the recovery and optimization of muscle protein synthesis. Postexercise nutrition is particularly important following prolonged or strenuous exercise when carbohydrates and possibly also protein immediately after exercise are needed to promote recovery. These efforts are particularly important during multievent competitions or when exercise training is to be resumed the following day (Burke et al., 2011; Phillips and Van Loon, 2011).

Evidence suggests that consuming protein along with carbohydrates after endurance or resistance training provides both the trigger and the amino acids necessary for the building and repair of muscle tissue (Rodriguez et al., 2007) and maximally stimulating muscle protein synthesis (Roy et al., 1997; Levenhagen et al., 2001; Tipton et al., 2001; Roy et al., 2002; Miller et al., 2003; Phillips and Van Loon, 2011). Although the exact timing of the postexercise window is not well constrained, athletes interested in skeletal muscle gain should consume protein as soon as possible after exercise (Thomas et al., 2016). Including fat during the recovery period may also be needed after periods of high-volume endurance training to replace skeletal muscle lipid stores (Larson-Meyer et al., 2002, 2008).

TABLE 14.2

Carbohydrate and Protein Content of Vegetarian and Vegan Foods

Food	Carbohydrate	Protein (g)
Egg, 1 whole	–	7
Cow's milk, all types, 1 cup	12	8
Cheese, most varieties, 1 oz	–	7
Cottage cheese, ½ cup	–	14
Hummus, ⅓ cup	15	7
Meatless burger, soy based, 1 patty (3 oz)	7	14
Meatless burger, vegetable and grain based, 1 patty (2.5 oz)	7	7
Nuts and seeds, 2 tbsp[a]	–	7
Nut spreads (peanut, almond, cashew, soy nut), 1 tbsp	–	7
Pulses (most beans, peas, lentils), ½ cup	15	7
Tempe, plain, ¼ cup (1.5 oz)	–	7
Tofu, ½ cup (4 oz)	–	7
Bread, 1 slice or 1 oz	15	3
Grains, cooked (rice, pasta, oats, grits, etc.), ⅓–½ cup	15	3
Vegetables—starchy, cooked (potato, sweet potato, winter squash, etc.), ⅓–1 cup	15	3
Vegetables—nonstarchy, raw or cooked, varies	5	2

Source: American Dietetic Association, *Choose Your Foods: Exchange Lists for Diabetes,* Alexandria, VA, American Diabetes Association Inc., 2014.

Note: Information on the food label for commercially available foods and sports products should supplement this source.

[a] serving size varies by type of tree nut.

The goal for postexercise fluid is to replace fluid loss during exercise and ensure adequate rehydration. Because not 100% of fluid ingested is retained, an amount greater than that lost is needed to optimize recovery (Burke et al., 2011; Shirreffs and Sawka, 2011). Consumption of certain fluids, including milk (Maughan et al., 2016) and sodium-containing sport beverages (Shirreffs et al., 1996), may result in greater fluid retention than plain water. Athletes participating in intense, prolonged workouts should also include sodium and potassium in the recovery snack or meal (Maughan et al., 1996; Sawka et al., 2007). While vegetarians are likely to naturally gravitate toward potassium-rich foods (e.g., fruits and vegetables), many may avoid sodium-containing foods either intentionally or unintentionally. Sodium intake is important to replace losses after heavy or prolonged training (i.e., the typical sweat loss is about 50 mEq/L or 1 g sodium/hour) (Sawka et al., 2007; Rodriguez et al., 2009). Thus, more liberal intakes of sodium are often appropriate in the athletic population. Appropriate intake can be ensured by use of iodized table salt to taste and selection of sodium-containing foods, such as pretzels and commercially available vegetarian products.

As with pre- and during-event nutrition, having athletes count carbohydrate and protein intake in their snacks or meals naturally selected postexercise, or plan their supplementation strategy according to the guidelines, is useful at least initially. This exercise can help athletes ensure that they are optimally refueling according to their training and competition goals. Athletes, for example, may only need to focus on consuming a complementary source of protein immediately after exercise when they are in a training phase designed to promote skeletal muscle growth. Select sources of carbohydrates and proteins are listed in Table 14.2 and can be used along with the information listed on the food label.

14.3 SPECIAL CONCERNS FOR THE VEGETARIAN ATHLETE DESIRING WEIGHT REDUCTION

It is not uncommon for athletes—including those following plant-based diets—to struggle to maintain a healthy body weight or desired weight or body fat losses for performance or health purposes. The desire to lose weight may be real in the slightly overweight to obese athlete and driven by genetic factors or lifestyle influences (poor eating habits, overeating, and sedentary lifestyle when not training). Vegetarian athletes are not necessarily immune from the social and metabolic factors that may predispose individuals to weight gain, including going to college, taking a new job, getting married, having children, or going through menopause. For example, freshman team athletes may gain weight during their first year because they play less during games or matches yet eat as much as their junior and senior teammates. They may also lack nutrition knowledge and cooking skills that predisposes them to weight gain. Adult athletes may have weight creep up because real-life responsibilities either decrease the time they can spend exercising or provide an environment that encourages overeating. The desire to lose weight or body fat may also be unrealistic as driven by aesthetic, weight class, or expected performance gains. Unrealistic weight expectations and the potential dangers to health and performance are defined as BM that cannot be maintained without drastic eating or exercise habits and are reviewed in the following section.

14.3.1 GUIDELINES FOR ATHLETES REQUIRING BODY MASS OR BODY FAT LOSS

When weight reduction is required, weight loss should be accomplished slowly and not using extreme techniques or fad diets or behaviors. Weight reduction plans should be undertaken in the off season or base phase of training, well out from the competitive season (Thomas et al., 2016), because the diminished energy intake can compromise nutrient intake, exercise performance, and training-induced gains. The general recommendation is to achieve a slight energy deficit on a well-balanced diet to promote a slow rate of weight loss (Thomas et al., 2016). Energy intake should be ~250–500 kcal/day less than required, with an emphasis on higher protein (that is, ~2.0 g protein/kg BM/day). In this regard, one study found that provision of higher protein (2.3 vs. 1.0 g protein/kg BM/day) on an energy-restricted diet helped athletes retain muscle mass during active weight and body fat losses (Mettler et al., 2010). Another found that fat-free mass and performance were better preserved in athletes who minimized weekly loss to less than 1% of BM (Garthe et al., 2011). Although the higher protein recommendations on an energy-restricted diet can be challenging for athletes following a plant-based diet, emphasizing the selection of high-protein foods such as pulses, pea proteins, soy foods, quinoa, eggs, or low-fat dairy at most meals and snacks may ensure higher protein intake. Carbohydrate intake, on the other hand, can be decreased to within the lower recommended range based on training level, as shown in Table 14.1, with an emphasis on whole, higher-fiber foods. Dietary fat should be included judiciously to balance protein and carbohydrate intake. Athletes by no means should attempt to follow restrictive low-carbohydrate diets (such as the Atkins or other popular diets) or restrictive low-fat diets providing less than 20% of energy as fat. As reviewed earlier, both low-carbohydrate and extremely low-fat diets are contraindicated for optimal training, performance, and health.

14.3.2 Avoiding Low Energy Availability in Vegetarian Athletes

Athletes who are pressured to succeed in sports by achieving or maintaining an unrealistically low body weight through food restriction and strenuous and/or prolonged exercise are at the potential risk for developing disorders of low energy availability (Nattiv et al., 2007). These disorders, previously termed the "female athlete triad," can occur in both female and male athletes and include low energy intake relative to energy need, disordered eating, reduced sex hormones, altered menstrual function in females, and reduced bone density. Recently termed relative energy deficiency syndrome (REDS) (Mountjoy et al., 2014), the condition is more common in athletes participating in weight class, gravitational, and aesthetic sports (Nattiv et al., 2007). Some (Huse and Lucas, 1984; O'Connor et al., 1987; Neumark-Sztainer et al., 1997; Barr, 1999) but not all (Slavin et al., 1984; Barr, 1999) sources suggest that REDS or its individual components may be more common in vegetarians. Most experts agree, however, that the apparent increase among vegetarians is because vegetarianism is seen as a socially acceptable way to restrict food intake and mask an eating disorder (Huse and Lucas 1984; O'Connor et al., 1987; Neumark-Sztainer et al., 1997; Robinson-O'Brien et al., 2009). In other cases, the apparent increased prevalence of REDS or its components among vegetarians may be explained by study design or recruitment bias (Barr, 1999). For example, some studies have defined vegetarians as those having a "low-meat" diet and not necessarily vegetarian diet and may tend to recruit a biased sample of vegetarians (i.e., those with menstrual cycle disturbances may be more likely to volunteer for a study on menstrual cycle disturbances) (Barr, 1999). It should be noted, however, that an athlete's reasoning for proclaiming to be vegetarian is important and could help to rule out an eating disorder.

The mechanism mediating the dampened circulation of sex hormones (including estrogen, progesterone, and testosterone) with REDs is not fully understood, but it is thought to be due to disruption of normal hypothalamic reproductive function due to reduced energy availability (i.e., the energy drain hypothesis), rather than stress or an overly lean body composition (Loucks, 2003). Leptin, which is synthesized by adipocytes and has receptors on the hypothalamus, is proposed as a driving signal (Ackerman et al., 2012). The earlier literature suggests, however, that other dietary factors may play a role. In nonathletic women, Goldin et al. (1982) found that lower circulating estrogen concentrations observed in vegetarians compared with nonveg-etarians were associated with higher fiber and lower fat intakes, higher fecal outputs, and a two- to threefold higher fecal concentration of estrogen. In athletes, retrospec-tive studies have found lower intakes of energy (Nelson et al., 1986; Kaiserauer et al., 1989), protein (Nelson et al., 1986; Kaiserauer et al., 1989), fat (Deuster et al., 1986; Kaiserauer et al., 1989), and zinc (Deuster et al., 1986) and higher intakes of vitamin A (Deuster et al., 1986) and fiber (Deuster et al., 1986; Lloyd et al., 1987) in amenor-rheic athletes than in their eumenorrheic counterparts. Collectively, these findings suggest that the energy and/or nutrient composition of some vegetarian diets could predispose female vegetarian athletes to amenorrhea. Lower circulating testosterone in male athletes due to higher fiber or reduced energy intake is also possible.

As available research suggests that reproductive disruption typically occurs when energy availability (dietary energy intake minus exercise energy expenditure) is less than a threshold of 30 kcal/kg lean BM (Loucks, 2003; Nattiv et al., 2007; Thomas et al., 2016), vegetarian athletes with abnormal menstrual function or reduced testos-terone should be counseled on how to meet energy needs on a vegetarian diet, as was previously discussed. For athletes in heavy training, a diet with excessive fiber may result in lower energy intake and a potentially reduced enterohepatic circulation of sex steroid hormones (Goldin et al., 1982; Raben et al., 1992). An athlete experienc-ing amenorrhea should also be encouraged to see her team or personal physician for a thorough evaluation.

14.4 ERGOGENIC AIDS OF INTEREST TO VEGETARIAN ATHLETES

Many athletes, vegetarian athletes included, will be interested in dietary supplements at one point or another for the purposes of enhancing performance or health. While some supplements have the potential to be ergogenic, the use of supplements does not compensate for poor food choices and an inadequate diet (International Olympic Committee Consensus Group, 2011; Larson-Meyer et al., 2017). Of the many ergo-genic aids available to athletes, only a few—including caffeine, creatine, and buffers such as bicarbonate and nitrate—are supported by a strong research base (Maughan and Shirreffs, 2011; Jones, 2014). Vegetarian athletes contemplating supplementa-tion should consider the efficacy, cost, and health risk of the supplement, as well as whether its ingredients are animal or plant derived, which can vary by manufacturer (see *Vegetarian Journal's Guide to Food Ingredients* [Vegetarian Resource Group, 2017]). Although extensive discussion of supplements is beyond the scope of this chapter, supplements of particular interest to vegetarian athletes—including creatine, carnitine, caffeine, nitrate, and protein—are briefly reviewed. Interested readers are referred to additional sources for information about buffering agents that may be ben-eficial in some events requiring short (1–7 minutes) burst of intense activity that are limited by acid–base disturbances (Carr et al., 2011). Although the vegetarian diet is lower in carnitine, which is an important skeletal muscle buffer, plant-based diets do not seem to negatively affect muscle buffering capacity due to the lower carnosine content (Baguet et al., 2011). As discussed in Chapter 13, a diet high in fruits and vegetables may promote higher serum alkalinity (Hobson et al., 2012).

14.4.1 CREATINE AND CARNITINE

Creatine and carnitine are supplied by the diet from meat and other animal products but can also be synthesized endogenously from amino acid precursors (Balsom et al., 1993). As discussed previously, creatine is an important component of the high-energy phosphagen system as phosphocreatine (PCr), whereas carnitine is involved in the oxidation of fatty acids as a carrier of fatty acids across the mitochondrial membrane. Although both substances are synthesized endogenously, several studies have found lower serum concentrations of creatine and carnitine (Delanghe et al., 1989; Shomrat et al., 2000) and skeletal muscle concentrations of creatine (Harris et al., 1992; Lukaszuk et al., 2002; Burke et al., 2003) in vegetarians than in omnivores. In athletes, supplementing the diet with creatine monohydrate increases muscle PCr content and improves performance and recovery during a variety of different exercise conditions (Maughan et al., 2011). These include repeated bouts of maximal and endurance sprinting that have included cycling, running, and swimming. Creatine supplementation with resistance training also has the potential to promote gains in fat-free mass, muscle force, and power output (Maughan et al., 2011). Several (Shomrat et al., 2000; Burke et al., 2003) but not all studies (Clarys et al., 1997) have observed that creatine supplementation may be more effective in vegetarians. In these studies, vegetarian athletes who took creatine supplements experienced greater increases in skeletal muscle total creatine, PCr, lean tissue mass, work performance during strength training (Burke et al., 2003), and anaerobic performance during cycling (Shomrat et al., 2000) than their nonvegetarian counterparts. Unlike creatine, however, there is no evidence suggesting that vegetarians benefit from carnitine supplementation despite its consistent mention as a potential disadvantage of following a vegetarian diet (Thomas et al., 2016).

14.4.2 CAFFEINE, COFFEE, AND TEA

Caffeine is probably the most casually and widely used sports-enhancing supplement because of its availability and social acceptance (Paluska, 2003; McLellan et al., 2016; Maughan et al., 2018). Caffeine, and its related compounds, theophylline and theobromine, occurs naturally in plant foods, including coffee, tea, and chocolate and is also added to some soda, sports bars, and gels (Applegate, 1999; Graham, 2001). Caffeine is thought to improve performance both by acting as a CNS stimulant (affecting perception of effort, warding off drowsiness, and increasing alertness) and by facilitating force production in the muscle. Well-controlled laboratory studies have found that moderate to high doses of caffeine (3–13 mg/kg BM) taken 1 hour prior to or during exercise improve endurance performance by prolonging time to exhaustion (Graham and Spriet, 1996) and improving time-trial performance (Cox et al., 2002). Such doses, however, have the potential to induce side effects, including rapid heart rate and GI disturbances.

More recent studies have demonstrated that the vast array of physical performance metrics, including time to exhaustion, time-trial performance, muscle strength and endurance, and high-intensity sprints typical of team sports, are evident with lower doses (approximately 3 mg/kg BM or less), as are the cognitive benefits of alertness, vigilance, attention, and reaction time (Spriet, 2014; McLellan et al., 2016). The effect of lower-dose caffeine on high-intensity exercise, however, has not yet been studied. Collectively, this research suggests that vegetarian athletes who enjoy coffee, tea, or other caffeinated beverages may find it beneficial to consume such beverages in the pre-event meal, weighing of course the potential for the noted side effects. Additionally, the phytochemicals, including the catechins (Jowko, 2015), found in green tea may have antioxidant properties that may dampen oxidative stress, although there is no evidence to date of direct performance-enhancing benefits (Eichenberger et al., 2010). Furthermore, habitual caffeine intake does not appear to diminish caffeine's ergogenic properties (Paluska, 2003), and caffeine does not provoke dehydration and/or electrolyte imbalance during exercise (Armstrong, 2002).

14.4.3 DIETARY NITRATES AND BEETROOT JUICE

Beetroot juice has become a popular ergogenic aid since initial studies showed that supplementation with beetroot juice can both improve performance and lower blood pressure (Webb et al., 2008; Bailey et al., 2009). Many of the performance benefits of beetroot juice appear to be due to the high concentration of nitrate in the beetroot and attributed to its capacity to increase nitric oxide (NO) (Jones, 2014). NO modulates many physiological processes, including blood flow, muscle contractility, muscle cell differentiation, and vascular tone. The most important performance-enhancing mechanism appears to be its ability to lower the energy (or oxygen) cost of submaximal exercise, which in essence improves exercise efficiency, at least in subjects who are not highly trained. The improved efficiency is thought to occur through improved contractile function in fast twitch (type II) fibers, improved muscle oxygenation, or some combination of the above.

Of importance to the vegetarian athlete, consumption of beetroot juice seems to be more effective than supplementation with nitrate in the form of sodium or potassium nitrate (Flueck et al., 2016). In fact, NO bioavailability can be enhanced by consuming more leafy green vegetables, beets, and beetroot juice (Murphy et al., 2012; Jonvik et al., 2016). Currently, however, the optimal efficacious nitrate loading regimen is not yet known but is thought to vary between individual athletes and be generally higher in the well-trained athlete to result in the same effect. Most studies have evaluated the consumption of about 2 cups of beetroot juice for several days; however, there is some evidence that longer supplementation (<15 days) may result in greater physiological benefit. Furthermore, the amount of nitrate needed for health and performance benefits, and which is found naturally in beetroots and green leafy vegetables, is orders of magnitude less than that which leads to toxicity (Bryan et al., 2012). Increasing the intake of nitrate-rich vegetables in the diet might serve as an easy strategy for optimizing performance in the vegetarian athlete (Jonvik et al., 2017).

14.4.4 PROTEIN

As discussed in Chapter 13, protein from a supplement is not needed if the athlete is consuming adequate energy and making proper food choices (Phillips and Van

Loon, 2011). For convenience, protein-containing sports beverages and bars can be used occasionally to supplement the diet. Recent research, however, has suggested that supplemental beverages that contain only soy protein are not as effective as milk but the jury is still out (Phillips et al., 2005; Hartman et al., 2007; Wilkinson et al., 2007; Tang et al., 2009). A recent study supported a possible benefit of pea protein consumption, which was found to be as effective as whey in promoting gains in muscle mass and strength during 12 weeks of resistant training (Babault et al., 2015). In this study, 25 g of protein from either pea protein isolate or whey concentrate was consumed after training and one additional time daily for the duration of the 12-week study.

14.5 CONCLUSION

In addition to following a general healthy diet, strategies that include nutrient intake relative to training or competition, maintenance of a healthy body weight, and judicious use of supplements may help the vegetarian athlete ensure optimal performance. The consumption of carbohydrates both in the pre-event meal and during exercise is shown to increase endurance performance in events lasting 60 minutes or more and in stop-and-go activities that include team sports. The consumption of carbohydrates and proteins in the snack or meal immediately after exercise promotes glycogen resynthesis and muscle protein synthesis to ensure adequate recovery. Fluid intake before, during, and after exercise also helps prevent dehydration at a level that is detrimental to performance. When weight or body fat reduction is required, weight loss should be accomplished slowly, and not during competitive season. Certain supplements, which include creatine, caffeine, and dietary nitrate, may be of interest to the vegetarian athlete. Nutritional supplements should not be used in lieu of good food choices.

REFERENCES

Ackerman KE, Slusarz K, Guereca G, Pierce L, Slattery M, Mendes N, Herzog DB, Misra M. 2012. Higher ghrelin and lower leptin secretion are associated with lower LH secretion in young amenorrheic athletes compared with eumenorrheic athletes and controls. *Am J Physiol Endocrinol Metab* 302 (7):E800–6. doi: 10.1152/ajpendo.00598.2011.

American Dietetic Association. 2014. Choose Your Foods: *Exchange Lists for Diabetes*. Alexandria, VA: American Diabetes Association Inc.

Applegate E. 1999. Effective nutritional ergogenic aids. *Int J Sport Nutr* 9 (2):229–39.

Armstrong LE. 2002. Caffeine, body fluid-electrolyte balance, and exercise performance. *Int J Sport Nutr Exerc Metab* 12 (2):189–206.

Babault N, Paizis C, Deley G, Guerin-Deremaux L, Saniez MH, Lefranc-Millot C, Allaert FA. 2015. Pea proteins oral supplementation promotes muscle thickness gains during resistance training: A double-blind, randomized, placebo-controlled clinical trial vs. whey protein. *J Int Soc Sports Nutr* 12 (1):3. doi: 10.1186/s12970-014-0064-5.

Baguet A, Everaert I, De Naeyer H, Reyngoudt H, Stegen S, Beeckman S, Achten E et al. 2011. Effects of sprint training combined with vegetarian or mixed diet on muscle carnosine content and buffering capacity. *Eur J Appl Physiol* 111 (10):2571–80. doi: 10.1007/s00421-011-1877-4.

Bailey SJ, Winyard P, Vanhatalo A, Blackwell JR, Dimenna FJ, Wilkerson DP, Tarr J, Benjamin N, Jones AM. 2009. Dietary nitrate supplementation reduces the O2 cost of low-intensity exercise and enhances tolerance to high-intensity exercise in humans. *J Appl Physiol (1985)* 107 (4):1144–55. doi: 10.1152/japplphysiol.00722.2009.

Ball TC, Headley SA, Vanderburgh PM, Smith JC. 1995. Periodic carbohydrate replacement during 50 min of high-intensity cycling improves subsequent sprint performance. *Int J Sport Nutr* 5 (2):151–8.

Balsom PD, Soderlund EB, Sjodin D, Hultman E. 1993. Creatine supplementation and dynamic high-intensity intermittent exercise. *Scand J Med Sci Sports* 3:143–9.

Barr SI. 1999. Vegetarianism and menstrual cycle disturbances: Is there an association? *Am J Clin Nutr* 70 (3 Suppl.):549S–54S.

Below PR, Mora-Rodriguez R, Gonzalez-Alonso J, Coyle EF. 1995. Fluid and carbohydrate ingestion independently improve performance during 1 h of intense exercise. *Med Sci Sports Exerc* 27 (2):200–10.

Bryan NS, Alexander DD, Coughlin JR, Milkowski AL, Boffetta P. 2012. Ingested nitrate and nitrite and stomach cancer risk: An updated review. *Food Chem Toxicol* 50 (10):3646–65. doi: 10.1016/j.fct.2012.07.062.

Burke DG, Chilibeck PD, Parise G, Candow DG, Mahoney D, Tarnopolsky M. 2003. Effect of creatine and weight training on muscle creatine and performance in vegetarians. *Med Sci Sports Exerc* 35 (11):1946–55.

Burke LM, Collier GR, Hargreaves M. 1993. Muscle glycogen storage after prolonged exercise: Effect of the glycemic index of carbohydrate feedings. *J Appl Physiol* 75 (2):1019–23.

Burke LM, Hawley JA, Wong SH, Jeukendrup AE. 2011. Carbohydrates for training and competition. *J Sports Sci* 29 (Suppl. 1):S17–27. doi: 10.1080/02640414.2011.585473.

Carr AJ, Hopkins WG, Gore CG. 2011. Effects of acute alkalosis and acidosis on performance: A meta-analysis. *Sports Med* 41 (10):801–14. doi: 10.2165/11591440-000000000-00000.

Clarys PM, Zinzen EM, Hebbelinck M. 1997. The effect of oral creatine supplementation on torque production in a vegetarian and non-vegetarian population: A double blind study. *Veg Nutr Int J* 1:100–5.

Cox GR, Desbrow B, Montgomery PG, Anderson ME, Bruce CR, Macrides, Martin DT, Moquin A, Roberts A, Hawley JA, Burke LM. 2002. Effect of different protocols of caffeine intake on metabolism and endurance performance. *J Appl Physiol* 93 (3):990–9.

Coyle EF, Coggan A, Davis JM, Sherman WM. 1992. Current thoughts and practical considerations concerning substrate utilization during exercise. *Sports Science Exchange* Spring (7):1–4.

Currell K, Conway S, Jeukendrup AE. 2009. Carbohydrate ingestion improves performance of a new reliable test of soccer performance. *Int J Sport Nutr Exerc Metab* 19 (1):34–46.

Delanghe J, De Slypere J-P, De Buyzere M, Robbrecht J, Wieme R, Vermeulen A. 1989. Normal reference values for creatine, creatinine, and carnitine are lower in vegetarians. *Clin Chem* 35:1802–3.

Deuster PA, Kyle SB, Moser PB, Vigersky RA, Singh A, Schoomaker EB. 1986. Nutritional intakes and status of highly trained amenorrheic and eumenorrheic women runners. *Fertil Steril* 46 (4):636–43.

Eichenberger P, Mettler S, Arnold M, Colombani PC. 2010. No effects of three-week consumption of a green tea extract on time trial performance in endurance-trained men. *Int J Vitam Nutr Res* 80 (1):54–64. doi: 10.1024/0300-9831/a000006.

Flueck JL, Bogdanova A, Mettler S, Perret C. 2016. Is beetroot juice more effective than sodium nitrate? The effects of equimolar nitrate dosages of nitrate-rich beetroot juice and sodium nitrate on oxygen consumption during exercise. *Appl Physiol Nutr Metab* 41 (4):421–9. doi: 10.1139/apnm-2015-0458.

Garthe I, Raastad T, Refsnes PE, Koivisto A, Sundgot-Borgen J. 2011. Effect of two different weight-loss rates on body composition and strength and power-related performance in elite athletes. *Int J Sport Nutr Exerc Metab* 21 (2):97–104.

Gisolfi CV, Duchman SM. 1992. Guidelines for optimal replacement beverages for different athletic events. *Med Sci Sports Exerc* 24 (6):679–87.

Goldin BR, Adlercreutz H, Gorbach SL, Warram JH, Dwyer JT, Swenson L, Woods MN. 1982. Estrogen excretion patterns and plasma levels in vegetarian and omnivorous women. *N Engl J Med* 307:1542–7.

Graham EE, Spriet LL. 1996. Caffeine and exercise performance. *Gatorade Sports Sci Exchange* 9 (1).

Graham TE. 2001. Caffeine and exercise: Metabolism, endurance and performance. *Sports Med* 31 (11):785–807.

Harris RC, Soderlund K, Hultman E. 1992. Elevation of creatine in resting and exercised muscle of normal subjects by creatine supplementation. *Clin Sci* 83 (367–74):367–74.

Hartman JW, Tang JE, Wilkinson SB, Tarnopolsky MA, Lawrence RL, Fullerton AV, Phillips SM. 2007. Consumption of fat-free fluid milk after resistance exercise promotes greater lean mass accretion than does consumption of soy or carbohydrate in young, novice, male weightlifters. *Am J Clin Nutr* 86 (2):373–81.

Hobson RM, Saunders B, Ball G, Harris RC, Sale C. 2012. Effects of beta-alanine supplementation on exercise performance: A meta-analysis. *Amino Acids* 43 (1):25–37. doi: 10.1007/s00726-011-1200-z.

Huse DM, Lucas AR. 1984. Dietary patterns in anorexia nervosa. *Am J Clin Nutr* 40:251–4.

International Olympic Committee Consensus Group. 2011. IOC consensus statement on sports nutrition 2010. *J Sports Sci* 29 (Suppl. 1):S3–4. doi: 10.1080/02640414.2011.619349.

Ivy JL, Goforth HW Jr., Damon BM, McCauley TR, Parsons EC, Price TB. 2002. Early postexercise muscle glycogen recovery is enhanced with a carbohydrate-protein supplement. *J Appl Physiol* 93 (4):1337–44.

Jeukendrup A. 2014. A step towards personalized sports nutrition: Carbohydrate intake during exercise. *Sports Med* 44 (Suppl. 1):S25–33. doi: 10.1007/s40279-014-0148-z.

Jeukendrup AE. 2013. Oral carbohydrate rinse: Placebo or beneficial? *Curr Sports Med Rep* 12 (4):222–7. doi: 10.1249/JSR.0b013e31829a6caa.

Jones AM. 2014. Influence of dietary nitrate on the physiological determinants of exercise performance: A critical review. *Appl Physiol Nutr Metab* 39 (9):1019–28. doi: 10.1139/apnm-2014-0036.

Jonvik KL, Nyakayiru J, Pinckaers PJ, Senden JM, van Loon LJ, Verdijk LB. 2016. Nitrate-rich vegetables increase plasma nitrate and nitrite concentrations and lower blood pressure in healthy adults. *J Nutr* 146 (5):986–93. doi: 10.3945/jn.116.229807.

Jonvik KL, Nyakayiru J, van Dijk JW, Wardenaar FC, van Loon LJ, Verdijk LB. 2017. Habitual dietary nitrate intake in highly trained athletes. *Int J Sport Nutr Exerc Metab* 27 (2):148–57. doi: 10.1123/ijsnem.2016-0239.

Jowko E. 2015. Green tea catechins and sport performance. In *Antioxidants in Sport Nutrition*, ed. M Lamprecht. Boca Raton, FL: CRC Press.

Jozsi AC, Trappe TA, Starling RD, Goodpaster B, Trappe SW, Fink WJ, Costill DL. 1996. The influence of starch structure on glycogen resynthesis and subsequent cycling performance. *Int J Sports Med* 17 (5):373–8.

Kaiserauer S, Snyder AC, Sleeper M, Zierath J. 1989. Nutritional, physiological, and menstrual status of distance runners. *Med Sci Sports Exerc* 21:120–5.

Lancaster S, Kreider RB, Rasmussen C, Kerksick C, Greenwood M, Milnor P, Almada AL, Earnest CP. 2001. Effects of honey supplementation on glucose, insulin, and endurance cycling performance. *FASEB J* 15 (Suppl.):LB315.

Larson-Meyer DE, Borkhsenious ON, Gullett JC, Russell RR, Devries MC, Smith SR, Ravussin E. 2008. Effect of dietary fat on serum and intramyocellular lipids and running performance. *Med Sci Sports Exerc* 40 (5):892–902.

Larson-Meyer DE, Hunter GR, Newcomer BR. 2002. Influence of endurance running and recovery diet on intramyocellular lipid content in women: A ^{1}H-NMR study. *Am J Physiol* 282:E95–106.

Larson-Meyer DE, Woolf K, Burke, LA. 2017 (online before print). Assessment of nutrient status in athletes and the need for supplementation. *Int J Sport Nutr Exerc Metab.*

Levenhagen DK, Gresham JD, Carlson MG, Maron DJ, Borel MJ, Flakoll PJ. 2001. Postexercise nutrient intake timing in humans is critical to recovery of leg glucose and protein homeostasis. *Am J Physiol Endocrinol Metabol* 280 (6):E982–93.

Lloyd T, Buchanen JR, Bitzer S, Waldman CJ, Myers C, Ford BG. 1987. Interrelationship of diet, athletic activity, menstrual status, and bone density in collegiate women. *Am J Clin Nutr* 46:681–4.

Loucks AB. 2003. Energy availability, not body fatness, regulates reproductive function in women. *Exerc Sport Sci Rev* 31 (3):144–8.

Lugo M, Sherman WM, Wimer GS, Garleb K. 1993. Metabolic responses when different forms of carbohydrate energy are consumed during cycling. *Int J Sport Nutr* 3 (4):398–407.

Lukaszuk JM, Robertson RJ, Arch JE, Moore GE, Yaw KM, Kelley DE, Rubin JT, Moyna NM. 2002. Effect of creatine supplementation and a lacto-ovo-vegetarian diet on muscle creatine concentration. *Int J Sport Nutr* 12 (3):336–48.

Maughan RJ, Greenhaff PL, Hespel P. 2011. Dietary supplements for athletes: Emerging trends and recurring themes. *J Sports Sci* 29 (Suppl. 1):S57–66. doi: 10.1080/02640414.2011.587446.

Maughan RJ, Leiper JB, Shirreffs SM. 1996. Restoration of fluid balance after exercise-induced dehydration: Effects of food and fluid intake. *Eur J Appl Physiol Occup Physiol* 73:317–25.

Maughan RJ, Shirreffs SM. 2011. IOC Consensus Conference on Nutrition in Sport, 25–27 October 2010, International Olympic Committee, Lausanne, Switzerland. *J Sports Sci* 29 (Suppl. 1):S1. doi: 10.1080/02640414.2011.619339.

Maughan RJ, Watson P, Cordery PA, Walsh NP, Oliver SJ, Dolci A, Rodriguez-Sanchez N, Galloway SD. 2016. A randomized trial to assess the potential of different beverages to affect hydration status: Development of a beverage hydration index. *Am J Clin Nutr* 103 (3):717–23. doi: 10.3945/ajcn.115.114769.

Maughan RJ, Burke LM, Dvorak J, Larson-Meyer DE, Peeling P, Phillips SM, Rawson EC, Walsh NP, Garth I, Meeusen R, van Loon LJC, and Shirreffs SM. IOC consensus statement: Dietary supplements and the high-performance athlete. *Br J Sports Med* 2018 doi: 10.1136/bjsports-2018-099027.

McLellan TM, Caldwell JA, Lieberman HR. 2016. A review of caffeine's effects on cognitive, physical and occupational performance. *Neurosci Biobehav Rev* 71:294–312. doi: 10.1016/j.neubiorev.2016.09.001.

Mettler S, Mitchell N, Tipton KD. 2010. Increased protein intake reduces lean body mass loss during weight loss in athletes. *Med Sci Sports Exerc* 42 (2):326–37. doi: 10.1249/MSS .0b013e3181b2ef8e.

Miller SL, Tipton KD, Chinkes DL, Wolf SE, Wolfe RR. 2003. Independent and combined effects of amino acids and glucose after resistance exercise. *Med Sci Sports Exerc* 35 (3):449–55.

Mondazzi L, Arcelli E. 2009. Glycemic index in sports nutrition. *J Am Coll Nutr* 28 (4):455S–63S.

Mountjoy M, Sundgot-Borgen J, Burke L, Carter S, Constantini N, Lebrun C, Meyer N, Sherman R, Steffen K, Budgett R, Ljungqvist A. 2014. The IOC consensus statement: Beyond the female athlete triad—Relative energy deficiency in sport (RED-S). *Br J Sports Med* 48 (7):491–7. doi: 10.1136/bjsports-2014-093502.

Murphy M, Eliot K, Heuertz RM, Weiss E. 2012. Whole beetroot consumption acutely improves running performance. *J Acad Nutr Diet* 112 (4):548–52. doi: 10.1016/j.jand.2011.12.002.

Nattiv A, Loucks AB, Manore MM, Sanborn CF, Sundgot-Borgen J, Warren MP. 2007. American College of Sports Medicine position stand. The female athlete triad. *Med Sci Sports Exerc* 39 (10):1867–82.

Nelson ME, Fisher EC, Catsos PD, Meredith CN, Turksoy RN, Evans WJ. 1986. Diet and bone status in amenorrheic runners. *Am J Clin Nutr* 43:910–6.

Neufer PD, Costill DL, Flynn MG, Kirwan JP, Mitchell JB, Houmard J. 1987. Improvements in exercise performance: Effects of carbohydrate feedings and diet. *J Appl Physiol* 62 (3):983–8.

Neumark-Sztainer D, Story M, Resnick MD, Blum RW. 1997. Adolescent vegetarians. A behavioral profile of a school-based population in Minnesota. *Arch Pediatr Adoles Med* 151:833–8.

Nicholas CW, Williams C, Phillips G, Nowitz A. 1995. Influence of ingesting a carbohydrate-electrolyte solution on endurance capacity during intermittent, high intensity shuttle running. *J Sports Sci* 13 (4):283–90.

O'Connor MA, Touyz SW, Dunn SM, Beumont JV. 1987. Vegetarianism in anorexia nervosa? A review of 116 consecutive cases. *Med J Aust* 147:540–2.

Paluska SA. 2003. Caffeine and exercise. *Curr Sports Med Rep* 2 (4):213–9.

Pfeiffer B, Stellingwerff T, Zaltas E, Jeukendrup AE. 2010a. CHO oxidation from a CHO gel compared with a drink during exercise. *Med Sci Sports Exerc* 42 (11):2038–45. doi: 10.1249/MSS.0b013e3181e0efe6.

Pfeiffer B, Stellingwerff T, Zaltas E, Jeukendrup AE. 2010b. Oxidation of solid versus liquid CHO sources during exercise. *Med Sci Sports Exerc* 42 (11):2030–7. doi: 10.1249/MSS.0b013e3181e0efc9.

Phillips SM, Hartman JW, Wilkinson SB. 2005. Dietary protein to support anabolism with resistance exercise in young men. *J Am Coll Nutr* 24 (2):134S–9S.

Phillips SM, Van Loon LJ. 2011. Dietary protein for athletes: From requirements to optimum adaptation. *J Sports Sci* 29 (Suppl. 1):S29–38. doi: 10.1080/02640414.2011.619204.

Raben A, Kiens B, Richter EA, Rasmussen LB, Svenstrup B, Micic S, Bennett P. 1992. Serum sex hormones and endurance performance after a lacto-ovo vegetarian and a mixed diet. *Med Sci Sports Exerc* 24 (11):1290–7.

Robinson-O'Brien R, Perry CL, Wall MM, Story M, Neumark-Sztainer D. 2009. Adolescent and young adult vegetarianism: Better dietary intake and weight outcomes but increased risk of disordered eating behaviors. *J Am Diet Assoc* 109 (4):648–55.

Rodriguez NR, DiMarco NM, Langley S. 2009. Position of the American Dietetic Association, Dietitians of Canada, and the American College of Sports Medicine: Nutrition and athletic performance. *J Am Diet Assoc* 109 (3):509–27.

Rodriguez NR, Vislocky LM, Gaine PC. 2007. Dietary protein, endurance exercise, and human skeletal-muscle protein turnover. *Curr Opin Clin Nutr Metab Care* 10 (1):40–5.

Roy BD, Luttmer K, Bosman MJ, Tarnopolsky MA. 2002. The influence of post-exercise macronutrient intake on energy balance and protein metabolism in active females participating in endurance training. *Int J Sport Nutr* 12 (2):172–88.

Roy BD, Tarnopolsky MA, MacDougall JD, Fowles J, Yarasheski KE. 1997. Effect of glucose supplement after resistance training on protein metabolism. *Clin J Sport Med* 8 (1):70

Sawka MN, Burke LM, Eichner ER, Maughan RJ, Montain SJ, Stachenfeld NS. 2007. American College of Sports Medicine position stand. Exercise and fluid replacement. *Med Sci Sports Exerc* 39 (2):377–90.

Sherman WM, Brodowicz G, Wright DA, Allen WK, Somonsen J, Dernbach A. 1989. Effects of 4 h preexercise carbohydrate feedings on cycling performance. *Med Sci Sports Exerc* 21 (5):598–604.

Shirreffs SM, Sawka MN. 2011. Fluid and electrolyte needs for training, competition, and recovery. *J Sports Sci* 29 (Suppl. 1):S39–46. doi: 10.1080/02640414.2011.614269.

Shirreffs SM, Taylor AJ, Leiper JB, Maughan RJ. 1996. Post-exercise rehydration in man: Effects of volume consumed and drink sodium content. *Med Sci Sports Exerc* 28 (10):1260–71.

Shomrat A, Weinstein Y, Katz A. 2000. Effect of creatine feeding on maximal exercise performance in vegetarians. *Eur J Appl Physiol Occup Physiol* 82 (4):321–5.

Slavin J, Lutter J, Cushman S. 1984. Amenorrhea in vegetarian athletes [letter]. *Lancet* 1984 (1):1474–5.

Spriet LL. 2014. Exercise and sport performance with low doses of caffeine. *Sports Med* 44 (Suppl. 2):S175–84. doi: 10.1007/s40279-014-0257-8.

Stellingwerff T, Cox GR. 2014. Systematic review: Carbohydrate supplementation on exercise performance or capacity of varying durations. *Appl Physiol Nutr Metab* 39 (9):998–1011. doi: 10.1139/apnm-2014-0027.

Tang JE, Moore DR, Kujbida GW, Tarnopolsky MA, Phillips SM. 2009. Ingestion of whey hydrolysate, casein, or soy protein isolate: Effects on mixed muscle protein synthesis at rest and following resistance exercise in young men. *J Appl Physiol* 107 (3):987–92.

Thomas DE, Brotherhood JR, Brand JC. 1991. Carbohydrate feeding before exercise: Effect of glycemic index. *Int J Sports Med* 12:180–6.

Thomas DT, Erdman KA, Burke LM. 2016. Position of the Academy of Nutrition and Dietetics, Dietitians of Canada, and the American College of Sports Medicine: Nutrition and Athletic Performance. *J Acad Nutr Diet* 116 (3):501–28. doi: 10.1016/j.jand.2015.12.006.

Tipton KD, Rasmussen BB, Miller SL, Wolf SE, Owens-Stovall SK, Petrini BE, Wolfe RR. 2001. Timing of amino acid-carbohydrate ingestion alters anabolic response of muscle to resistance exercise. *Am J Physiol Endocrinol Metab* 281 (2):E197–206.

van der Brug GE, Peters HP, Hardeman MR, Schep G, Mosterd WL. 1995. Hemorheological response to prolonged exercise—No effects of different kinds of feedings. *Int J Sports Med* 16 (4):231–7.

Vegetarian Resource Group. 2017. *Vegetarian Journal's Guide to Food Ingredients.* http://www.vrg.org/ingredients/.

Webb AJ, Patel N, Loukogeorgakis S, Okorie M, Aboud Z, Misra S, Rashid R et al. 2008. Acute blood pressure lowering, vasoprotective, and antiplatelet properties of dietary nitrate via bioconversion to nitrite. *Hypertension* 51 (3):784–90. doi: 10.1161/HYPERTENSIONAHA.107.103523.

Wilkinson SB, Tarnopolsky MA, MacDonald MJ, MacDonald JR, Armstrong D, Phillips SM. 2007. Consumption of fluid skim milk promotes greater muscle protein accretion after resistance exercise than does consumption of an isonitrogenous and isoenergetic soy-protein beverage. *Am J Clin Nutr* 85 (4):1031–40.

Wright DA, Sherman WM, Dernbach AR. 1991. Carbohydrate feedings before, during, or in combination improve cycling endurance performance. *J Appl Physiol* 71 (3):1082–8.

Wu CL, Williams C. 2006. A low glycemic index meal before exercise improves endurance running capacity in men. *Int J Sport Nutr Exerc Metab* 16 (5):510–27.

Index

Page numbers followed by f and t indicate figures and tables, respectively.

Printed in the United States
by Baker & Taylor Publisher Services